Essentials of Paediatric Urology

Edited by

David FM Thomas FRCP FRCPCH FRCS
Consultant Paediatric Urologist
Leeds Teaching Hospitals;
Reader in Paediatric Surgery
University of Leeds
Leeds, UK

AMK Rickwood MA FRCS
Formerly Consultant Paediatric Urologist
Alder Hey Children's Hospital
Liverpool, UK

Patrick G Duffy FRCS(I)
Paediatric Urologist
Great Ormond Street Hospital for Sick Children
London, UK

MARTIN DUNITZ

© 2002 Martin Dunitz Ltd, a member of the
Taylor & Francis group

Published 2002 by Martin Dunitz Ltd,
The Livery House, 7–9 Pratt Street, London NW1 0AE

Tel.: +44 (0) 20 74822202
Fax: +44 (0) 20 72670159
E-mail: info.dunitz@tandf.co.uk
Website: http://www.dunitz.co.uk

Although every effort has been made to ensure that all owners of
copyright material have been acknowledged in this publication, we
would be glad to acknowledge in subsequent reprints or editions any
omissions brought to our attention.

The Author has asserted his right under the Copyright, Designs and
Patents Act 1988 to be identified as the Author of this Work.

Although every effort has been made to ensure that drug doses and
other information are presented accurately in this publication, the
ultimate responsibility rests with the prescribing physician. Neither
the publishers nor the authors can be held responsible for errors or
for any consequences arising from the use of information contained
herein. For detailed prescribing information or instructions on the
use of any product or procedure discussed herein, please consult
the prescribing information or instructional material issued by
the manufacturer.

A CIP record for this book is available from the British Library.

ISBN 1 90186 525 8

Distributed in the USA by
Fulfilment Center
Taylor & Francis
7625 Empire Drive
Florence, KY 41042, USA
Toll Free Tel.: +1 800 634 7064
E-mail: cserve@routledge_ny.com

Distributed in Canada by
Taylor & Francis
74 Rolark Drive
Scarborough, Ontario M1R 4G2, Canada
Toll Free Tel.: +1 877 226 2237
E-mail: tal_fran@istar.ca

Distributed in the rest of the world by
ITPS Limited
Cheriton House
North Way
Andover, Hampshire SP10 5BE, UK
Tel.: +44 (0) 1264 332424
E-mail: reception@itps.co.uk

Composition by Scribe Design, Gillingham, Kent
Printed and bound in Spain by Grafos, SA

Contents

Contributors

Helen M Carty FRCR FRCPI FRCP FRCPCH FFRRCSI
Professor of Paediatric Radiology
Radiology Department
Alder Hey Children's Hospital
Liverpool, UK

H K Dhillon FRCS
Perinatal Urologist
Great Ormond Street Hospital for Sick Children
London, UK

Patrick G Duffy FRCS(I)
Paediatric Urologist
Great Ormond Street Hospital for Sick Children
London, UK

J David Frank MB FRCS
Department of Paediatric Urology
The Bristol Royal Hospital for Children
Bristol, UK

David CS Gough FRCS FRCS(E) FRACS DCS
Consultant Paediatric Urologist
Department of Paediatric Urology
Royal Manchester Children's Hospital
Manchester, UK

Henri Lottmann MD FEBU
Consultant in Paediatric Urology
Fondation Hopital Saint-Joseph;
Hopital Necker-enfants
Paris, France

Nicholas P Madden MA FRCS
Consultant Paediatric Surgeon/Urologist
Chelsea and Westminster Hospital;
St Mary's Hospital
London, UK

Padraig S Malone MB MCh FRCSI FRCS
Consultant Paediatric Urologist
Southampton University Hospitals NHS Trust
Southampton, UK

Pierre DE Mouriquand MD FRCS(Eng)
Professor of Paediatric Urology
Head of the Department of Paediatric Surgery
Claude-Bernard University - Lyon I
Debrousse Hospital
Lyon, France

AMK Rickwood MA FRCS
Formerly Consultant Paediatric Urologist
Alder Hey Children's Hospital
Liverpool, UK

David FM Thomas FRCP FRCPCH FRCS
Consultant Paediatric Urologist
Leeds Teaching Hospitals;
Reader in Paediatric Surgery
University of Leeds
Leeds, UK

Richard S Trompeter MB FRCP FRCPCH
Consultant Paediatric Nephrologist
Great Ormond Street Hospital for Sick Children
London, UK

Duncan T Wilcox MD FRCS
Consultant in Paediatric Urology
Guy's and St Thomas's Hospital;
Great Ormond Street Hospital for Sick Children
London, UK

Christopher RJ Woodhouse MB FRCS FEBU
Reader in Adolescent Urology, The Institute of Urology;
Honorary Consultant Urologist,
Great Ormond Street Hospital for Sick Children;
Clinical Director or Urology, St Peter's Hospital
(The Middlesex Hospital)
London, UK

Preface

The genitourinary system is affected by a broad spectrum of disorders in childhood. These range from complex anomalies managed by specialist paediatric urologists to common conditions such as testicular maldescent, urinary infection and incontinence, which constitute a substantial part of everyday practice for urologists, general paediatric surgeons and paediatricians.

Essentials of Paediatric Urology provides a concise and up to the minute account of the diagnosis and current management of the urological conditions of childhood, with the requirements of the non-specialist very much in mind. We have aimed to combine a didactic and accessible format with a factual content which is, as far as possible, evidence-based.

The authors include some of Europe's leading paediatric urologists. All are experts in their field and most are regular contributors to the British Association of Paediatric Urologists' postgraduate teaching course held annually in Cambridge.

Surgeons preparing to sit the Intercollegiate Examinations in Urology and Paediatric Surgery or the Fellowship of the European Board of Urology will find the syllabus amply covered by *Essentials of Paediatric Urology*.

In addition *Essentials of Paediatric Urology* is designed to serve as a source of easy reference for paediatricians, paediatric nephrologists and nurse specialists.

DFM Thomas
AMK Rickwood
PG Duffy

Dedication

To our wives: Marilyn, Valerie and Zara

Acknowledgements

Our sincere thanks to Sue Gamble, Judith Ball, Lyn Goodall and Angela Wright for their invaluable help in the preparation and editing of the manscript. We are also most grateful to the Medical Illustration Department of St James's University Hospital for their unrivalled professionalism and unfailing ability to meet the most unrealistic of deadlines.

The publication of *Essentials of Paediatric Urology* represents an opportunity to acknowledge our debt to Robert Whitaker, Emeritus Paediatric Urologist and Fellow of Selwyn College Cambridge; a great teacher, good friend and founder of the postgraduate course, which provided the impetus to produce this book.

We are also grateful to our publishing team at Martin Dunitz Ltd, especially Alan Burgess and his colleague Abigail Griffin: they ensured that the book made crucial deadlines.

DFM Thomas
AMK Rickwood
PG Duffy

Embryology

1

David FM Thomas

Topics covered
Genetic basis of genitourinary malformations
Embryogenesis

Upper urinary tract
Lower urinary tract
Genital tracts

Introduction

Paediatric urology is largely devoted to the treatment of congenital anomalies, and therefore a working knowledge of the embryology of the genitourinary tract provides the key to understanding the scientific basis of the speciality. Conventional descriptive embryology already provides us with a detailed picture of the origins of many of the structural anomalies encountered in paediatric urological practice. In addition, the science of molecular biology is now beginning to reveal how the tightly orchestrated sequence of embryological development is initiated and regulated at the cellular and molecular level. Advances in our understanding of normal embryological development are paralleled by increasing insight into the molecular basis of inherited malformations and genetic disease. The culture of embryonic stem cells and research into therapeutic cloning may ultimately pave the way to the availability of a wide range of human cells for tissue reconstruction or regenerative repair. However, research of this nature raises important ethical issues, and for this reason the use of human embryonic tissue in medical research is governed by statute under the regulation of the Human Fertilisation and Embryology Authority.

Although it concentrates predominantly on the clinical embryology of the genitourinary tract, this chapter will also touch on some of the relevant aspects of molecular biology.

Genetic basis of genitourinary tract malformations

Chromosomal abnormalities

The nuclear DNA of the normal human somatic cell is represented by 23 pairs of chromosomes: 22 pairs of autosomes and one pair of sex chromosomes, a karyotype expressed as 46XY (male) or 46XX(female)

As a result of the two meiotic divisions during gametogenesis each spermatazoon or definitive oöcyte carries only one, unpaired, copy of each autosome and one sex chromosome. Fusion of the nuclear DNA of the gametes at the time of fertilisation restores the normal diploid status to the fertilised zygote.

Major chromosomal abnormalities occur either during the formation of the gametes (gametogenesis) or during the first few cell divisions of the fertilised zygote. Examination of spontaneously aborted embryos reveals a high percentage of profound chromosomal abnormalities inconsistent with survival of the embryo. The most serious chromosomal abnormalities compatible with survival to term are trisomy 21 – Down's syndrome (47XX or 47XY) – and trisomies 13 and 18.

Trisomies result from the failure of a pair of chromosomes to separate fully during gametogenesis, with the result that an additional copy of a chromosome or fragment of chromosome becomes incorporated into the nucleus of a gamete (usually by a process termed translocation or non-disjunction).

A similar process of faulty separation affecting the sex chromosomes is encountered in, for example, Turner's syndrome (45XO karyotype) and Klinefelter's syndrome (47XXY).

Abnormalities of the sex chromosomes often occur in mosaic form, mosaicism being defined as the presence of two chromosomally distinct cell lines derived from the same zygote. In addition to translocation and non-disjunction, structural defects involving identifiable segments of chromosomes include deletion, inversion, duplication and substitution.

The genetic imbalance arising from structural chromosomal abnormalities is expressed as profound

Table 1.1 Chromosome defects associated with urinary tract anomalies

Chromosome defect or syndrome	Frequency (%)	Genitourinary anomalies
Turner's syndrome 45X0	60–80	Horseshoe kidney Duplication
Trisomy 18 (Edwards' syndrome)	70	Horseshoe kidney Renal ectopia Duplication Hydronephrosis
Trisomy 13 (Patau syndrome)	60–80	Cystic kidney Hydronephrosis Horseshoe kidney Ureteric duplication
4p (Wolf–Hirschorn syndrome)	33	Hypospadias Cystic kidney Hydronephrosis
Trisomy 21 (Down's syndrome)	3–7	Renal agenesis Horseshoe kidney

disturbances of embryological development across a number of systems, including the genitourinary tract (Table 1.1).

Gene mutations occur in structurally intact chromosomes at the level of the nucleotides comprising the individual genes. Such mutations are not visible on microscopy but are amenable to study by techniques such as PCR (polymerase chain reaction) and FISH (fluorescent in situ hybridisation). The role of individual genes can be elucidated by studying the effects of so-called 'knock out' deletion in transgenic mice.

Specific gene mutations have been identified in a number of inherited conditions affecting the genitourinary tract, e.g. autosomal dominant polycystic kidney disease, X-linked Kallmann's syndrome and renal coloboma syndrome (mutation of the *PAX2* gene encoding for a transcription factor expressed during development of the eye and urinary tract).

However, the majority of the congenital anomalies encountered in paediatric urology do not have such a clearly defined genetic basis. Most are either sporadic or inherited as autosomal dominant traits with variable expression and penetrance. Current evidence indicates that their aetiology is likely to involve the interaction of multiple genes, rather than a single gene mutation. The extent to which external factors in the fetal or the wider environment influence the expression of genes involved in regulating the development of the genitourinary tract is poorly understood.

Embryogenesis

Human gestation spans a period of 38 weeks, from fertilisation to birth. Conventionally, pregnancy is divided into three trimesters, each of 3 months' duration. The formation of organs and systems (embryogenesis) takes place principally between the third and 10th weeks of gestation. Throughout the remainder, the fetal organs undergo differentiation, branching, maturation and growth.

In each ovulatory cycle a small number of germ cells (primary oöcytes) within the ovary are stimulated to resume the long-arrested meiotic division. Of these, usually only one progresses to be extruded from the ovary into the fallopian tube at the midpoint of the menstrual cycle. At the time of fertilisation the protective zona pellucida of the oöcyte is penetrated by the fertilising spermatazoon, thereby triggering the final meiotic division to create the definitive oöcyte and second polar body (consisting of non-functional DNA). Fertilisation is defined as the fusion of the nuclear DNA of the male and female gametes (spermatazoon and definitive oöcyte). In the ensuing 5 days the fertilised zygote undergoes a series of mitotic doubling cell divisions termed cleavage (Figure 1.1).

Implantation of the sphere-like mass of cells (blastocyst) into the uterine endometrium occurs approximately 6 days after fertilisation. Proliferation of the

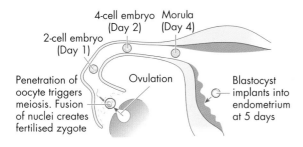

Figure 1.1 Key stages in the 5–6 days from fertilisation to implantation.

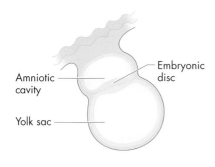

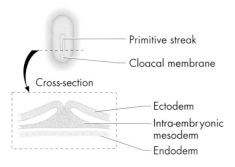

Figure 1.2 Embryonic disc at 16 days. Formation of intraembryonic mesoderm by inpouring of cells at the primitive streak.

embryonic cell mass over the ensuing 10 days is accompanied by the appearance of two cavities, the amniotic cavity and the yolk sac. The embryo is destined to develop from the cells interposed between these two cavities. The ectodermal tissues of the embryo derives from the layer of cells on the amniotic surface of the embryonic disc, whereas the endodermal derivatives have their origins in the layer of cells adjacent to the yolk sac (Figure 1.2). Inpouring of cells from the amniotic surface via the primitive streak creates a third layer of embryonic tissue, the intraembryonic mesoderm, which subdivides into paraxial, intermediate and lateral plate mesoderm. It is from the intermediate block of intraembryonic mesoderm that much of the genitourinary tract is derived. Segmentation and folding of the embryo begins during the third and fourth weeks of gestation, and towards the end of this period the precursor of the embryonic kidney begins to take shape.

Upper urinary tract (Figure 1.3)

In the cervical portions of the paired blocks of intermediate mesoderm the primitive precursor of the kidney, the pronephros, first appears in the fourth week of gestation. This structure rapidly regresses in the human embryo. The midzone mesonephros, however, continues to differentiate, giving rise to tubular structures which, although ultimately destined to contribute to the definitive gonad, function briefly in an excretory role. In the mesenchyme lying lateral to the developing mesonephros, the mesonephric ducts appear, advancing caudally to fuse with the terminal portion of the hindgut (the primitive cloaca).

Figure 1.3 Embryonic precursors of the upper urinary tract, metanephros (kidney), ureteric bud.

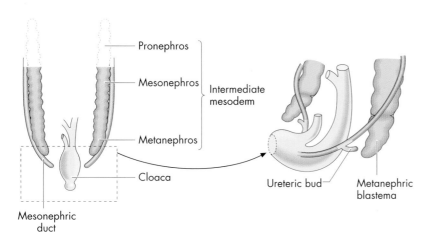

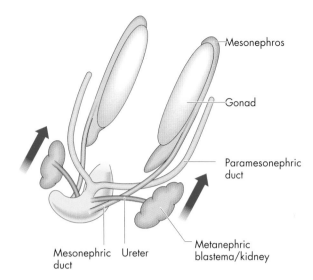

Figure 1.4 Embryonic genitourinary tract at 6–8 weeks.

Canalisation of the mesonephric ducts creates a patent excretory unit which is believed to function transiently.

At the beginning of the fifth week, however, the ureteric buds arise from the distal portion of the paired mesonephric ducts and advance towards the most caudal portion of the blocks of intraembryonic mesoderm – the metanephros. Fusion of the ureteric bud and metanephros at around 32 days initiates the process of nephrogenesis. Between the sixth and 10th weeks the lobulated embryonic kidneys ascend up the posterior abdominal wall, deriving their blood supply sequentially at different levels until the definitive lumbar position is achieved (Figure 1.4)

Nephrogenesis

The formation of nephrons within the developing kidney is an example of 'reciprocal induction'. The ureteric bud derivatives give rise to the renal pelvis, major calyces, minor calyces and collecting ducts, whereas the glomeruli, convoluted tubules and loop of Henle are derived from metanephric mesenchyme. Urine production commences at around the 10th week, when continuity is established between the distal convoluted tubules and collecting ducts. Proliferation of the ureteric bud derivatives ceases at around 15 weeks, but new generations of nephrons continue to appear within the renal cortex until 36 weeks. At that time the process of nephrogenesis ceases and the number of nephrons within each kidney remains fixed for life. There is considerable variation in the number of nephrons

within a normal kidney, with a median value of approximately 700 000. Nephrogenesis is being intensively studied to identify the molecules responsible for cell-to-cell signalling. Among the many so far identified are growth factors, transcription factors (DNA-binding proteins that regulate gene expression) and adhesion molecules. The renin–angiotensin system has recently been found to play an important role in regulating early differentiation and development of the urinary tract. Two different tissue receptors are responsible for mediating the actions of angiotensin 2. Whereas stimulation of the angiotensin type 1 receptor promotes cellular proliferation and the release of growth factors, stimulation of the angiotensin type 2 receptor, which is expressed mainly in the embryo and fetus, mediates apoptosis (programmed cell death) and diminished cell growth. Differing patterns of renal malformation are observed in transgenic 'knock out' mice, depending on whether the gene encoding for the type 1 or the type 2 receptor is deleted. The wealth of information being yielded by molecular biology is rapidly advancing our understanding of inherited renal disease and congenital malformations of the urinary tract.

Clinical considerations

The normal embryological development of the upper tract is heavily dependent on the role of the ureteric bud. Faulty or failed interaction between the ureteric bud and metanephric mesenchyme results in renal agenesis or differing patterns of renal dysplasia.

Renal agenesis

One or both kidneys may be congenitally absent, either as part of a syndrome or as an isolated anomaly. The origins of renal agenesis include:

- Intrinsic defect of embryonic mesenchyme. The association between unilateral renal agenesis and ipsilateral agenesis of the paramesonephric duct derivatives in girls provides evidence of a fundamental defect of mesenchymal tissue (see below).
- Failed induction of nephrogenesis.
- Involution of a multicystic dysplastic kidney. This common renal anomaly has been shown to involute both in utero and in postnatal life to mimic the findings of renal agenesis.

The empirical recurrence risk of bilateral renal agenesis is 3.5%. In contrast, unilateral renal agenesis is often a 'silent' condition and its inheritance is poorly documented.

Renal dysplasia

The kidney is present, although often abnormally small. The internal architecture is disordered and characterised by the presence of immature 'primitive' undifferentiated tubules and the inappropriate (metaplastic) presence of cartilage and fibromuscular tissue. Renal dysplasia results from faulty interaction between the ureteric bud and metanephric tissue, or from a major insult to the embryonic and fetal kidney, e.g. severe obstructive uropathy.

Cystic anomalies

The patterns of cystic renal disease and their aetiology are considered in Chapter 10. Evidence suggests that the faulty development of the ureteric bud is implicated in the causation of **multicystic dysplastic kidney**.

Abnormalities of renal ascent and fusion

This spectrum of renal anomalies including pelvic kidney, horseshoe kidney and crossed renal ectopia dates from the sixth to the ninth weeks of gestation, when the embryonic kidney is ascending to its definitive lumbar position. Horseshoe kidney has a reported autopsy incidence of 1:400 (Figure 1.5). Fusion of the lower poles of metanephric tissue interferes with the normal process of renal ascent, vascularisation and rotation. **Pelvic kidney** (Figure 1.6) and **crossed fused renal ectopia** (Figure 1.7) provide further examples of anomalies resulting from defects of ascent and fusion of the embryonic kidney.

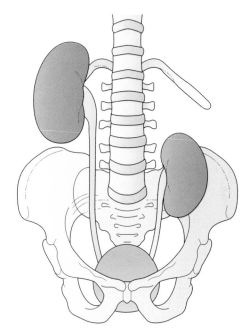

Figure 1.6 Abnormality of ascent – pelvic kidney.

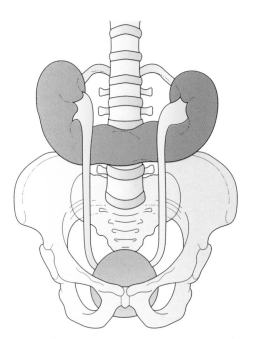

Figure 1.5 Abnormality of renal ascent and fusion – horseshoe kidney.

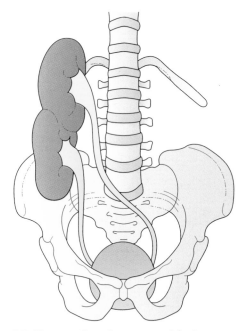

Figure 1.7 Abnormality of ascent and fusion – crossed fused renal ectopia.

Fetal renal function

The homoeostatic excretory role of the kidney after birth is fulfilled in intrauterine life by the placenta. For this reason, anephric fetuses may survive until term. The fetal kidneys, however, do serve the important role of producing increasing volumes of urine, the most important constituent of amniotic fluid. By the 36th week of gestation it is estimated that fetal urine accounts for approximately 90% of the amniotic liquor. Impairment of fetal urine excretion as a result of renal damage (agenesis or dysplasia) or obstructive uropathy causes oligohydramnios and consequent moulding deformities of the fetus and pulmonary hypoplasia (an adequate volume of amniotic fluid is an essential factor in normal fetal lung development).

Lower urinary tract (Figure 1.8)

The lower urinary tract originates from the cloaca, the section of primitive hindgut into which the mesonephric ducts and embryonic ureters drain. Between the fourth and sixth weeks of gestation the urorectal septum descends towards the perineum and the folds of Rathke ingrow laterally to subdivide the cloaca into the urogenital canal anteriorly and the anorectal canal posteriorly. While the bladder is taking shape in the upper portion of the urogenital canal, the distal ureter and mesonephric duct begin to separate. The mesonephric ducts migrate caudally to join into the developing posterior urethra, whereas the ureters remain relatively fixed at their point of entry in the developing bladder (Figure 1.9). By a process of induction the embryonic urothelium stimulates the adjacent pelvic mesenchyme to undergo differentiation into the detrusor, smooth muscle component of the bladder wall.

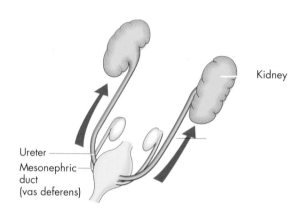

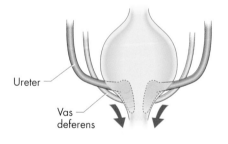

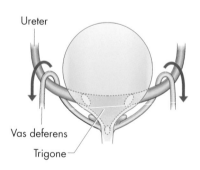

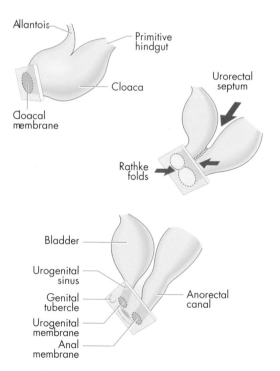

Figure 1.8 Compartmentalisation of cloaca into the urogenital compartment and anorectum by the descent of the urorectal septum – 4–6 weeks.

Figure 1.9 Changing anatomical relationships of ureters and mesonephric duct derivatives.

In the female the urethra is derived entirely from the distal portion of the urogenital canal, whereas in the male the urogenital canal gives rise to the posterior urethra and the anterior urethra is created by the closure of the urogenital groove. The allantois protrudes from the dome of the fetal bladder like an elongated diverticulum, extending into the umbilical cord. Subsequently, the obliterated allantois persists as the median umbilical ligament. Rarely, the allantois remains patent, giving rise to a congenital umblical urinary fistula (patent urachus) or an encysted remnant.

Clinical considerations

The spectrum of **cloacal anomalies** encountered in clinical practice correlates closely with varying degrees of failed or incomplete descent of the urorectal septum. The embryological origins of **bladder exstrophy** and **epispadias** are less readily apparent, but probably result from early defects of the cloacal membrane. **Incomplete ureteric duplication** results from bifurcation of the ureteric bud. **Complete ureteric duplication** is characterised by a pattern of ureteric anatomy in which the ureter draining the upper pole paradoxically enters the urinary tract more distally than the lower pole ureter (in some cases draining ectopically into the vagina). This anatomical configuration (encompassed by the **Mayer Weigert** law) occurs when the mesonephric duct separates from the embryonic lower pole ureter and descends towards the developing posterior urethra (with a tendency to take the upper pole ureter with it).

Genital tracts

In essence, the internal and external genitalia of both sexes are genetically 'programmed' to differentiate passively as female unless switched down a male pathway by the genetic information carried by the testis-determining gene (*SRY*). Until the sixth week of gestation the genitalia of both sexes share identical embryonic precursors. Differentiation of the gonads and genital tracts is initiated by the migration of primordial germ cells from the yolk sac, across the coelomic cavity to condensations of primitive mesenchyme in the lumbar region of the embryo. By a process of reciprocal interaction the germ cells and surrounding mesenchyme form the primitive sex cords within the embryonic gonad. At around this time (6 weeks) the paired paramesonephric ducts appear as cords of coelomic epithelium lying lateral to the mesonephric ducts. From this stage onwards, the pathways of male and female differentiation diverge.

Female

Internal genitalia (Figure 1.10)

Although the primitive sex cords degenerate, secondary sex cords derived from genital ridge mesoderm enfold the primordial germ cells to form primitive follicles. Differentiation of the genitalia down a female pathway may not be determined entirely by the absence of the *SRY* gene. Normal development of the ovary does appear to at least be partly dependent on the presence the two normal X chromosomes, as females with a single X chromosome (XO karyotype) typically have poorly formed streak or dysgenetic ovaries. In the female the initial phase of gametogenesis (transition from primordial germ cell to primary oöcyte) occurs within the fetal ovaries. During fetal life these primary oöcytes embark on the first phase of meiotic division before entering a long phase of arrested division, which resumes again only at puberty. In the absence of testosterone the mesonephric ducts regress (leaving only

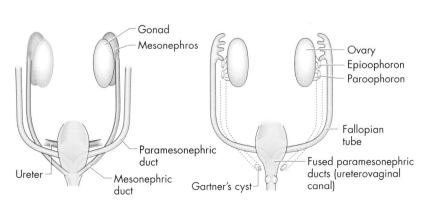

Figure 1.10 The undifferentiated genital tract is genetically programmed to proceed down the pathway of female differentiation unless switched down the male pathway by the *SRY* gene.

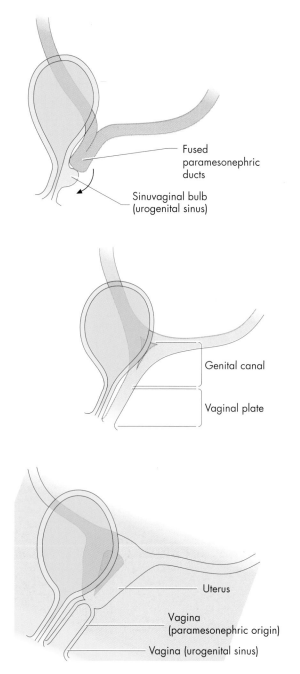

Fused paramesonephric ducts

Sinuvaginal bulb (urogenital sinus)

Genital canal

Vaginal plate

Uterus

Vagina (paramesonephric origin)

Vagina (urogenital sinus)

Figure 1.11 Development of the lower female genital tract between 10 and 20 weeks.

vestigial remnants – the epioöphoron, paroöphoron and Gartner's cysts). The paramesonephric ducts persist in the form of the fallopian tubes. Distally, the fused portions of the paramesonephric ducts give rise to the uterus and upper two-thirds of the vagina.

At the junction of the paired paramesonephric ducts with the urogenital sinus a condensation of tissue, the sinuvaginal bulb, develops. Between the 10th and 20th

weeks of gestation displacement of the sinuvaginal bulb in the direction of the fetal perineum separates the developing vagina from the urethra. During this process, canalisation of the vagina occurs. The upper two-thirds of the vagina is derived from the paramesonephric ducts, whereas the distal third has its origins in the urogenital sinus and the introitus and external genitalia are derived from ectoderm (Figure 1.11).

External genitalia

In the absence of androgens, the external genitalia of the embryo and fetus progress down a pathway of female differentiation. The genital tubicle gives rise to the clitoris, the urogenital sinus contributes the vestibule of the vagina, the urogenital folds persist as the labia minora, and the labioscrotal folds persist as the labia majora.

Male

Internal genitalia (Figure 1.12)

Current evidence indicates that differentiation of the male genitalia is initiated by a single testis-determining gene (*SRY*) located on the Y chromosome and then mediated through other Y chromosomal and autosomal 'downstream' genes. The gene product expressed by the *SRY* gene is responsible for stimulating the medullary sex cords to differentiate into secretory pre-Sertoli cells. From the seventh week onwards these pre-Sertoli cells secrete antimüllerian hormone (AMH) – otherwise termed müllerian inhibiting substance (MIS), a glycoprotein that plays a central role in subsequent differentiation of the male genital tract.

In the male the paramesonephric ducts disappear completely, with the exception of vestigial remnants (the appendix testis and utriculus). At least three important properties are ascribed to MIS:

1. MIS is responsible for regression of the paramesonephric ducts.
2. Production of testosterone by the Leydig cells of the embryonic testis is stimulated by MIS from the ninth week of gestation. During the 12th to 14th weeks of gestation the fetus is exposed to very high levels of androgenic stimulation.
3. The first stage of testicular descent is mediated by the action of MIS on the gubernaculum, which anchors the embryonic testis in the vicinity of the developing inguinal canal.

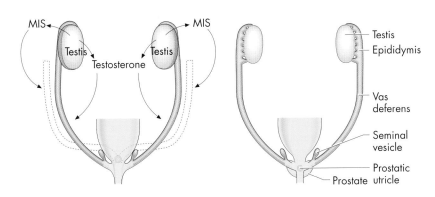

Figure 1.12 Differentiation of the male genital tract in response to müllerian inhibitory substance and testosterone.

In contrast to the germ cell differentiation initiated in the female embryo, male primordial germ cells are inhibited from further division within the embryonic gonad and only proceed to gametogenesis after puberty. In response to testosterone secreted by the fetal testis, the mesonephric duct derivatives differentiate between the eighth and 12th weeks of gestation to give rise to the epididymis, rete testis, vas deferens, ejaculatory ducts and seminal vesicles.

The development of the prostate gland is also dependent upon androgenic stimulation and provides a further example of reciprocal induction. Proliferation and branching of the endodermal lining of the urethra (which gives rise to the ducts and glanular acini of the prostate gland) induces differentiation of surrounding mesenchyme to form the capsule and smooth muscle, a process that ceases after the 15th week of gestation.

External genitalia (Figure 1.13)

The differentiation of male external genitalia is dependent upon a number of factors, including the production of testosterone by the fetal testis, the conversion of testosterone into dihydrotestosterone, and the presence of androgen receptors within the target cells. Androgenic stimulation of the genital tubercle results in the development of the male phallus. From the seventh week of gestation the male urogenital sinus advances on to the phallus as the urethral groove. Ingrowth of this urethral groove is associated with the appearance of urethral plate tissue destined to canalise and form the definitive male anterior urethra. Closure of the urethra is complete by around 15 weeks, with ingrowth of ectoderm from the tip of the glans forming the terminal portion of the urethra.

The testis

Tesicular descent is believed to occur in two distinct phases, the first initiated by MIS, the second under the stimulus of testosterone. The evidence of extensive experimental studies in rats indicates that the gubernaculum plays a key role in testicular descent (although the precise mechanism may be subject to some species variation). The gubernaculum extends from the testis down to the region of the labioscrotal swellings, anchoring the fetal testis in the proximity of the future inguinal canal. Under the influence of testosterone a second, more active phase of testicular descent occurs between 25 and 30 weeks, when the gubernaculum shrinks and contracts in length, pulling the testis down the inguinal canal into its definitive scrotal position. During the course of its descent the testis is accompanied by a sac-like protrusion of peritoneum, the processus vaginalis.

Clinical considerations
Abnormalities of female internal genitalia

Faulty development of the paramesonephric duct derivatives is responsible for a variety of congenital malformations. Unilateral agenesis of paramesonephric duct derivatives (absent fallopian tube, hemiuterus etc.) may be accompanied by unilateral renal agenesis, suggesting a fundamental underlying defect of the original ipsilateral intermediate mesoderm. Agenesis of the upper two-thirds of the vagina (Rokitansky syndrome) reflects a failure of the paramesonephric ducts to fuse distally and merge with the urogenital sinus. Other abnormalities of paramesonephric duct derivatives, e.g. uterine duplication, are commonly associated with cloacal abnormalites.

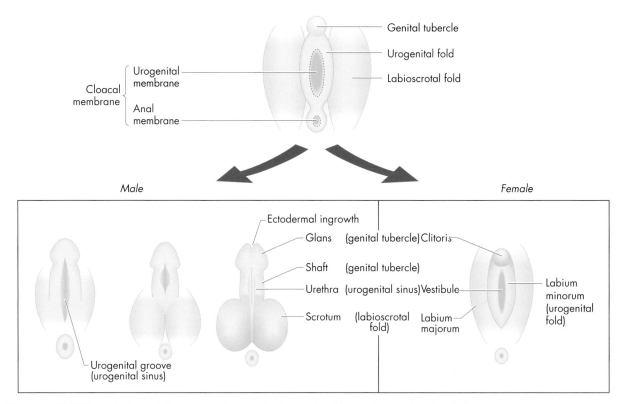

Figure 1.13 Differentiation of the external genitalia determined by androgenic stimulation.

Female external genitalia

The aetiology and classification of intersex disorders is considered in more detail in Chapter 21. The most commonly encountered intersex disorder in western Europe is virilisation of the external genitalia in a female with a 46XX genotype resulting from congenital adrenal hyperplasia. In these females the internal reproductive tract differentiates normally but the external genitalia undergo virilisation in response to high levels of circulating androgens of adrenal origin.

Male internal genitalia

The rare genetically determined syndrome of MIS deficiency is characterised by bilateral undescended testes accompanied by the presence of persistent paramesonephric duct structures, including fallopian tubes and uterus. With the exception of the undescended testes the external genitalia virilise normally, as this is not dependent on MIS.

In the syndrome of androgen insensitivity the external genitalia exhibit a receptor defect to dihydrotestosterone (the derivative of testosterone active in the peripheral tissues). As a result, the external genitalia differentiate passively down the female pathway despite a male phenotype and normal internal male internal genitalia.

Male external genitalia

Hypospadias results from varying degrees of incomplete closure of the urethral groove (although distal glanular hypospadias may simply represent failure of ectodermal ingrowth). Severe hypospadias, particularly when accompanied by cryptorchidism and a persistent müllerian utriculus, is evidently the outcome of a generalised virilisation defect. However, although isolated endocrinopathies have occasionally been identified in such cases, as yet no single endocrine defect has been implicated in the aetiology of hypospadias.

Similarly, there is no single unifying aetiology for cryptorchidism. Bilateral cryptorchidism is more likely to represent the influence of an endocrinopathy or imbalance of the pituitary-gonadal axis, whereas local mechanical factors (possibly related to the gubernaculum or the processus vaginalis) are likely to play a more important role in the unilateral cryptorchidism.

The combination of a blind-ending vas and histological findings of calcification and haemosiderin in 'nubbins' of residual testicular tissue suggests that most cases of so-called testicular 'agenesis' result from testicular torsion in utero.

Key points

- The genitourinary tract is commonly affected in children with chromosomal abnormalities.
- The ureteric bud plays a pivotal role in nephrogenesis and the embryological development of the upper tract. A number of important congenital anomalies can be ascribed to defects of the ureteric bud.
- The undifferentiated genital tract of both sexes is 'programmed' to differentiate passively down a female pathway unless positively directed down a male pathway by the presence of the *SRY* gene and associated downstream genes and their products.
- Although single gene mutations have been implicated in the aetiology of some inherited genitourinary abnormalities, most of the conditions encountered in paediatric urology occur on a sporadic basis or result from the interaction of multiple genes.

Further reading

De Mello D, Reid L M. The kidney/lung loop. In: Thomas DFM (ed) *Urological disease in the fetus and infant*. Oxford: Butterworth-Heinemann, 1997: 62–77

Haycock G B. Development of glomerular filtration and tubular sodium reabsorption in the human fetus and newborn. *Br J Urol* 1998; 81(Suppl. 2): 33–38

Hutson J M, Terada M, Baiyun Z, Williams M P L. Normal testicular descent and aetiology of cryptorchidism. *Advances in anatomy, embryology and cell biology*. Berlin: Springer Verlag, 1996: 132

Larsen W J. Development of the uro-genital system. In: Larsen W J (ed) *Human embryology*. Edinburgh: Churchill Livingstone, 1993: 276–277

McNeal J E. Anatomy and embryology. In: Fitzpatrtick J M, Kane R J (eds) *The prostate*. Edinburgh: Churchill Livingstone, 1989: 3–9

Thomson J A, Itskovitz-Eldor J, Shapiro S S et al. Embryonic stem cell lines derived from human blastocysts. *Science* 1988; 282: 1145–1147

Woolf A S. Molecular control of nephrogenesis and the pathogenesis of kidney malformations. *Br J Urol* 1998; 81(Suppl. 2): 1–7

Renal physiology and renal failure

2

Richard S Trompeter

Topics covered
Fetal and neonatal renal function
Renal impairment in infancy and childhood

Medical management
Renal replacement therapy

Renal physiology in the fetus and newborn

The adaptation of the neonate, particularly the premature, to extrauterine life depends on the ability of the immature kidney to maintain normal homeostasis. The physiology of the developing kidney and the specific metabolic demands of the newborn infant may be grossly changed by a variety of pathologic processes. As a consequence, neonatal nephrology is characterised by features distinct from the rest of paediatric nephrology.

In the later stages of pregnancy the fetus is in a physiological volume expansion. Amniotic fluid is swallowed, absorbed by the gastrointestinal tract and 'recycled' by excretion into the amniotic cavity via the kidneys. Fetal urine is the major constituent of amniotic fluid and production increases with gestational age, i.e. approximately 10 ml/hour at 23 weeks' gestation and approximately 30 ml/hour at 32 weeks' gestation until the end of pregnancy. Oligohydramnios is usually a consequence of renal dysfunction or urinary tract obstruction.

The formation of new nephrons (nephrogenesis) in humans is confined to intrauterine life and is complete by 36 weeks' gestation, but in premature infants born before 36 weeks the normal pattern of nephrogenesis continues after birth. Nephrogenesis may be affected by a number of prenatal factors, of which early urinary tract obstruction poses a particularly potent threat.

In the fetus, glomerular filtration rate (GFR) is proportional to body weight, but even when the fetal GFR has been corrected for body weight it remains considerably reduced, corresponding to 30–50% of the weight-corrected adult value. Creatinine is not a useful indicator of fetal renal function because it crosses the placenta freely and fetal plasma creatinine levels mirror those in the maternal circulation. However, amniotic fluid volume is a crude index of urine production and hence of fetal renal function. Moreover, measurement of electrolytes and osmolality in amniotic fluid and fetal urine can also provide an approximate guide to fetal renal function. Normal fetal urine is characterised by a high flow rate (>5 ml/kg/h) with low osmolality and relatively low sodium concentration. However, these data are not always a reliable reflection of fetal renal function and should be interpreted in the context of the clinical picture and ultrasound findings.

The GFR at birth correlates closely with gestational age, being approximately 5 ml/min/m^2 in premature infants born at 28 weeks' gestation and 12 ml/min/m^2 in infants born at term (40 weeks). Postnatally there is a sharp increase in GFR, which doubles by 2 weeks of age. However, it is not until 2 years of age that the corrected GFR reaches the corresponding adult-corrected value.

The low renal blood flow (RBF) and GFR in newborn infants are of considerable relevance to clinical management, for example in the interpretation of laboratory results and calculation of fluid requirements and drug dosages, especially in ill premature babies. Although the neonatal kidney can cope with most normal demands its functional reserve is limited and may be overwhelmed by common neonatal stresses. Several vasoactive systems, such as the renin–angiotensin system, intrarenal adenosine, the prostaglandins and atrial natriuretic peptide, are upregulated in the neonatal period and are probably essential for the maintenance of GFR. Overstimulation of the renin–angiotensin system (for example by hypoxia) or its inhibition by angiotensin-converting enzyme inhibitors can both predispose to renal failure.

Water metabolism

Newborn infants are born in a state of overexpansion of extracellular water, which is inversely proportional to the maturity of the neonate. Following delivery an acute isotonic volume contraction occurs, with corresponding weight loss. This phenomenon, which is part of the normal physiological adaptation to extrauterine life, is most pronounced and prolonged in premature infants.

The renal control of water balance is not fully developed at birth. In response to hypotonic fluid challenge term and preterm neonates produce urine with an osmolality of 50 and 70 mmol/kg, respectively. Despite the capacity for increasing urine flow and water clearance, renal excretion of a waterload is prolonged – presumably as a result of the reduced GFR. As a consequence, newborn infants are poorly equipped to cope with fluid overload and are at greater risk of dilutional hyponatraemia.

The capacity of the neonatal kidney to produce concentrated urine is also limited, and in the first week of life the maximum urine concentration achieved by preterm and term neonates following fluid restriction is 600 and 800 mmol/kg, respectively. This limited concentrating capacity reflects reduced responsiveness of the immature kidney to vasopressin and the inability to maintain a deep corticomedullary osmotic gradient.

Sodium balance

Newborn infants have a limited capacity to conserve sodium when challenged by sodium restriction, and a limited ability to excrete sodium in response to a sodium load. In the first week of life urinary sodium excretion is high and inversely proportional to the maturity of the neonate. Premature infants have an obligatory urinary sodium loss with consequent negative sodium balance. Plasma sodium and chloride concentrations often fall to low levels and urinary sodium excretion remains high relative to plasma sodium. This imbalance is thought to result from renal immaturity, rather than redistribution of sodium within body fluid compartments.

Disturbances in plasma sodium include:

- *Early-onset hyponatraemia* (plasma sodium <130 mmol/l) occurring in the first week of life,

which is due to water retention and sodium depletion;
- *Late-onset hyponatraemia*, usually the result of inadequate sodium intake, renal sodium wasting and free water retention;
- *Early-onset hypernatraemia* (plasma sodium >150 mmol/l). This is usually iatrogenic in aetiology, resulting from repeated administration of hypertonic sodium bicarbonate solution to correct acidosis in severely ill neonates;
- *Late-onset hypernatraemia*, owing to sodium supplementation and inadequate free water.

The clinical consequences of excessive or inadequate sodium intake are potentially serious, and careful monitoring of sodium and water balance is essential in at-risk infants.

Potassium balance

Plasma potassium levels differ postnatally in term and preterm infants. In the term infant potassium levels fall rapidly in the first week of life (although there is considerable individual variation). In contrast, a gradual rise in plasma level occurs in preterm infants, reaching a maximum at about the third to fourth weeks of life. Elevated plasma potassium levels may be a consequence of hypoxia, metabolic acidosis, catabolic stress, oliguric renal failure and inadequate excretion by the immature distal nephron. Renal tubular unresponsiveness to aldosterone and low ATPase activity in potassium-secreting epithelial cells of the distal nephron contribute to impaired potassium excretion.

Acid–base balance

Compared to adults, neonates are characterised by a degree of acidosis which is both respiratory and metabolic in aetiology and which is usually accompanied by cardiopulmonary compensation. The capacity of the newborn infant to excrete an acid load is limited, but the renal threshold for bicarbonate resorption increases with advancing maturation as the renal acidification mechanisms develop. Later-onset metabolic acidosis in premature infants is usually mild and rarely associated with clinical symptoms. However, more severe acidosis is associated with poor feeding and growth failure. Supplements may be needed to ensure that plasma bicarbonate concentration is maintained above 17 mmol/l.

Renal impairment in infancy and childhood

A major reduction in the number of functioning nephrons as a result of congenital or acquired damage gives rise to two distinct but related pathological states. First, because damaged nephrons are incapable of repair or regeneration, renal dysfunction supervenes. A series of secondary physiologic, metabolic and hormonal changes then develops as renal function progressively declines. Treatment is therefore directed at decreasing the rate of progression of chronic renal failure (CRF) and replacing diminished or absent renal function. The principal consequences of untreated CRF in children include:

- Growth retardation
- Sexual immaturity
- Psychomotor or intellectual retardation.

Treatment must be initiated very early in the course of renal dysfunction and should generally increase in intensity in parallel with disease progression. Chronic renal failure supervenes when the GFR decreases to less than 25–30% of normal (corresponding to a plasma creatinine concentration of approximately 150 mmol/l). Clinical manifestations are usually apparent when function has declined to this level.

Incidence

Data derived from the United States and European registries indicate that the incidence of chronic renal failure is approximately 10–12 per million children in the age group 0–19 years. The number of children receiving treatment is small compared to adults, and so there are fewer centres specialising in the treatment of renal failure in this age group.

The term end-stage renal disease (ESRD) is used to describe the phase when renal dysfunction has progressed to the point where native renal function has failed and the individual becomes dependent on either dialysis or renal transplantation for survival. According to data from the North American Pediatric Renal Transplant Cooperative Study, the most common renal disease diagnoses in children aged 0–17 years undergoing transplantation were hypoplastic–dysplastic kidneys, obstructive uropathy, focal segmental glomerulosclerosis, reflux nephropathy and systemic immunological disease. Congenital renal disorders accounted for 50% of renal failure in children under the age of 5 years.

Chronic renal failure

Measurement

In adults the progression of renal disease can be demonstrated by a significant decline from a predictable adult value for GFR, but in children this calculation is more difficult as both absolute and actual GFR must be adjusted for surface area during early childhood. In addition, corrected values for GFR normally increase in the first year of life. Against this background of evolving function it is more difficult to define the progression of renal impairment. Formulae based on the logarithmic value for serum creatinine concentration or reciprocal serum creatinine concentration versus time have been derived to predict the interval before dialysis or transplantation is required. However, the predictive value of these formulae is subject to the limited reliability of creatinine clearance as a measure of GFR in the later stages of deteriorating function. As a broad guide, the serum creatinine concentration at 6 months of age can be used to predict the timing of renal replacement therapy (Table 2.1).

Table 2.1 Relationship between renal function at 6 months and onset of ESRD

Serum creatinine μmol/l at 6 months of age	Prognosis (predicted age of onset of end-stage renal disease)
<150	Good
150–300	ESRD 10+ years
200–350	ESRD 5–10 years
350–600	ESRD <5 years
>600	Uncertain outcome

The point at which dialysis becomes necessary varies between individual children, but once the serum creatinine exceeds 500 μmol/l it becomes unlikely that even the most optimal medical management can avert the need for renal replacement therapy.

Growth and development

Growth failure and poor intellectual development in children with CRF are multifactorial but the principal factors are malnutrition, renal osteodystrophy, salt wasting, metabolic acidosis, anaemia and hormonal changes.

Malnutrition

Malnutrition in children with CRF is characterised by food refusal, anorexia, nausea and vomiting. Anorexia is common to all children with CRF and may be secondary to increased levels of gastric polypeptide. In addition, an increased incidence of foregut motility disorder predisposes to gastrointestinal reflux and vomiting. Growth velocity in childhood is greatest in the first year of life, and thus the impact of chronic disease and malnutrition is correspondingly more severe in this age group. Early therapeutic intervention is vital in order to prevent growth failure. Indications for intervention include:

- Failure to maintain expected weight despite adding calorie supplements to the diet;
- Recurrent vomiting, despite the use of prokinetic medications;
- Parental stress.

In a significant percentage of infants voluntary oral intake is inadequate to meet energy or volume requirements, and feeding by nasogastric, nasojejunal or gastrostomy tube is advisable to ensure adequate water and dietary intake. Supplemental feeding is given either by bolus or as a continuous overnight infusion. Infants who are tube fed at night can be fed ad libitum during the day. However, in some cases it is necessary to administer the entire diet via tube feeding. Provided oral stimulation is maintained during this period, the majority of children will learn to eat normally following successful renal transplantation.

In infancy the dietary protein intake can be easily controlled, and the most appropriate food is either human milk or a humanised milk formula with a low phosphate content. At any given level of protein intake, increasing the overall energy intake will enhance the efficient utilisation of protein. Most humanised milks have a protein to calorie ratio of 2–3 g of protein per 100 kcal (8–12% calories as protein). Human milk has a protein to calorie ratio of 1.6 per 100 kcal (approximately 6% calories as protein). Infant formulas containing 1.6–2 g of protein per 100 kcal are safe and meet the recommended dietary allowance (RDA) for protein in infancy.

When practical, the serum urea level should be kept below 20 mmol/l by maintaining adequate calorie intake and ensuring that sufficient water is available to avoid extracellular fluid volume depletion. There is a consensus that dietary intake should approximate to 100% of the recommended daily allowance of carbohydrate for the appropriate height and age. Calculated energy intake may need to be increased in children with a low weight to height ratio. Energy supplements such as polyunsaturated corn oil, complex carbohydrates or medium-chain triglycerides are widely favoured because of their high calorie density and low cost.

A typical growth pattern in infancy and childhood is illustrated in Figure 2.1. In this case growth (weight) remains below the 3rd percentile and deviates from this with the onset of puberty. Figure 2.2 illustrates the growth pattern for both height and weight in an infant in whom nasogastric tube feeding was instituted at the age of 2 years, with resulting

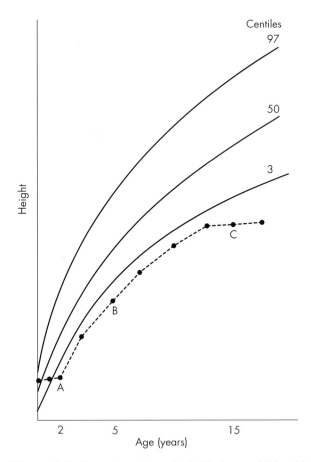

Figure 2.1 Growth pattern (height) in a child with untreated chronic renal failure. Growth maintained below the third centile with downward deviation from the centile at puberty.

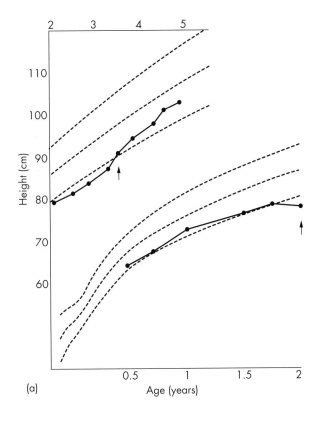

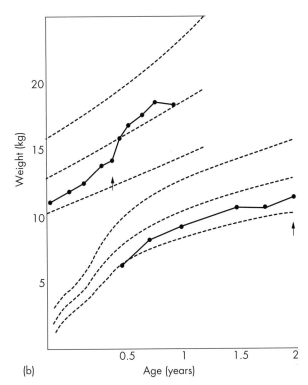

(a)

(b)

Figure 2.2 (a) Impact on growth (height) of the introduction of nasogastric enteral feeding in a 2-year-old child with CRF. (b) Improved weight gain following the introduction of nasogastric feeding in the same child.

improvement in both weight and height. At approximately 3 years of age overnight feeding was commenced, with a marked further improvement in both weight and height reflected in growth lines crossing the percentiles.

Renal osteodystrophy (Figure 2.3)

Disorders of mineral metabolism in children with CRF invariably affect skeletal growth and development, with resultant bone deformities and, in most cases, deceleration of linear growth. The crucial role played by the kidney in bone and mineral homoeostasis includes:

- Regulating calcium, phosphorus and magnesium metabolism;
- Participating in the catabolism of parathyroid hormone (PTH);
- Excreting albumin and β_2-microglobulin;
- Synthesising calcitriol or 1,25-hydroxy vitamin D_3.

The primary site of vitamin D synthesis is located in the proximal nephron, where 25-hydroxy vitamin D is converted by the action of the 1α-hydroxylase enzyme to 1,25-dihydroxy vitamin D_3 (calcitriol), its most potent and active metabolite (Figure 2.3). In renal

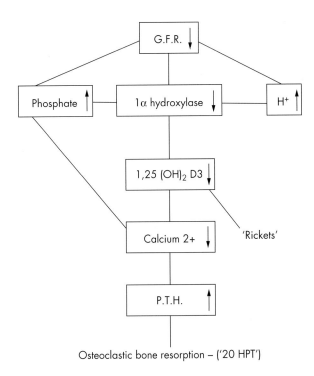

Figure 2.3 Pathogenesis of renal osteodystrophy.

failure enzymatic activity decreases, leading to reduced production of calcitriol and the development of secondary hyperparathyroidism. In addition, urinary excretion of aluminium and β_2-macroglobulin is impaired and may also contribute to certain forms of renal osteodystrophy.

Secondary hyperparathyroidism

This common feature of ESRD has a number of contributory factors:

- Phosphate retention
- Hypocalcaemia
- Impaired calcitriol synthesis
- Alterations in secretion of parathyroid hormone (PTH secretion and reduced sensitivity of the skeleton to the calcaemic actions of PTH).

Clinical manifestations

Osteodystrophy can present with non-specific signs and symptoms, or may even go unnoticed. A reduction in physical activity can be a subtle early symptom. It is important to be aware that radiographic changes are not always a reliable guide to the severity of the underlying bone disease.

Approximately 30–50% of children with CRF exhibit short stature, and in 60% of children receiving regular dialysis treatment their growth velocity is below the normal range. In early renal osteodystrophy bone pain is non-specific, but as the disease progresses may be localised to the lower back and weight-bearing joints in ambulatory patients. The onset of a limp demands thorough evaluation because of the prevalence of slipped femoral epiphysis. All epiphyses can be affected and the prevalence of fracture is high.

Skeletal deformity is a major manifestation of long-standing untreated CRF in children, with the patterns of deformity being age related. In younger children skeletal abnormalities are similar to those caused by vitamin D-deficient rickets, i.e. rachitic rosary, metaphysial widening at the wrist and ankle, craniotabes and frontal bossing, whereas deformities of the long bones, particularly the lower extremities, are more evident in older children, i.e. valgus and varus deformity of the knee.

Muscle weakness and a waddling gait are characteristic of the myopathy associated with CRF and resemble the proximal muscle weakness seen in patients with vitamin D deficiency. Although soft tissue calcification is seen more frequently in adults it can also occur in children with ESRD, the most commonly affected sites being blood vessels, lung, kidney, myocardium, central nervous system and gastric mucosa. The aetiology of soft tissue calcification is usually a high serum calcium-phosphate product resulting from poor control of secondary hyperparathyroidism.

The principal radiographic features of renal osteodystrophy relate to increased bone resorption, typically at the subperiosteal or endosteal surfaces of cortical bones. The extent of bone resorption correlates with parathyroid hormone levels and the sites involved characteristically include the distal ends of the clavicles, ischial and pubic surfaces, the sacroiliac joints, the junction of the metaphysis and diaphysis of long bones, and the phalanges. The radiological appearances are characterised by a diffuse 'ground-glass' appearance, generalised mottling, and focal lucent or sclerotic areas.

Treatment of osteodystrophy

Even in the earliest phase of chronic renal insufficiency, i.e. a GFR of 50–80 ml/min/1.73 m², some patients develop a rise in parathyroid hormone. If left untreated, the severity of secondary hyperparathyroidism worsens in parallel with the progressive decline in renal function.

1. *Dietary manipulation.* When GFR falls to less than 30 ml/min/1.73 m³ phosphate excretion decreases and it is necessary to restrict dietary phosphate intake. Phosphorus is present in nearly all foods and its highest concentration is in meat and diary products. The average dietary phosphate intake is between 900 and 1500 mg/24 h of which approximately 50% is absorbed. Restriction to less than 800 mg/24 h is desirable, but this diet may become unpalatable, with implications for long-term compliance with treatment. The use of phosphate-binding agents then plays an integral role in management.

2. *Phosphate-binding agents.* Calcium-containing salts such as calcium carbonate and calcium acetate are currently the major phosphate-binding agents used to limit intestinal phosphate absorption. Calcium carbonate is the most widely used calcium salt, as it is inexpensive, well tolerated, and contains 40% elemental calcium. The dosage is matched to dietary intake and the agent should be taken with

or immediately after food. Hypercalcaemia is the most important complication associated with long-term use.

3. *Vitamin D therapy.* Vitamin D replacement is indicated in patients with CRF. Various vitamin D sterols have been used to control secondary hyper-parathyroidism, including dihydrotachysterol, 25-hydroxy vitamin D_3, 1α-hydroxy vitamin D_3 and 1,25-dihydroxy vitamin D_3. Of these, vitamin D_3 is the most widely used vitamin D analogue and, at a dosage of 0.02–0.1 mg/kg/day, it is both safe and effective. Hypercalcaemia is the major side-effect, but calcium levels will fall in response to a temporary reduction or cessation of therapy.

Assessment of therapy

Serial measurements of total serum calcium, ionised calcium, phosphate and intact PTH levels are important when assessing the efficacy of dietary and therapeutic intervention. Calcium and phosphate levels should be maintained within normal ranges for age (total calcium 2.41–2.77 mmol/l; ionised calcium 1.16–1.45 mmol/l; phosphate 1.2–2.1 mmol/l), whereas intact PTH levels should be suppressed to below 5.4 pmol/l.

Sodium chloride and bicarbonate

Obligatory urinary salt loss is a common feature of CRF in infants with structural abnormalities of the urinary tract – notably renal dysplasia (with or without posterior urethral valves). As the sodium concentration of most infant formula feeds is low, affected infants are frequently in negative sodium balance. Salt and sodium bicarbonate supplementation is therefore required to maintain adequate extracellular fluid volume and prevent metabolic acidosis. Sodium chloride is added to the feed or diet until the serum sodium concentration rises to 135–140 mmol/l. Up to 5 mmol/kg body weight per day may be required but the level of supplementation is decreased if oedema or hypertension supervenes.

Treatment of anaemia

The availability of recombinant human erythropoietin (r-Hu EPO) has proved a major advance in the treatment of anaemia associated with CRF or ESRD in children. The benefits include:

- Correction of the anaemia of renal failure, and improvement in tissue oxygenation, exercise tolerance and haemostatic activity;
- Improved myocardial function resulting from reduction in the ventricular hyprtrophy associated with anaemia;
- Reduced risk of developing HLA antibodies by obviating the need for blood transfusion.

Subcutaneous administration is practical in predialysis patients and those on peritoneal dialysis, whereas the intravenous route is used to administer erythropoietin to those on haemodialysis. Most children require between 100 and 200 international units per kg body weight per week, and it is often necessary to prescribe iron in conjunction with r-Hu EPO to treat the functional iron deficiency. The target haemoglobin concentration should be 10 g/dl.

Therapy of growth failure

Even with assiduous control of nutrition, bone disease, anaemia, salt wasting and acidosis, the majority of children probably do not achieve their genetic growth potential. Recombinant human growth hormone is effective in improving growth velocity both before and after renal transplantation.

Renal replacement therapy

A detailed review of chronic dialysis and renal transplantation in children is beyond the scope of this chapter. As a modality of long-term treatment **peritoneal dialysis** (PD) is extremely successful in children of all ages, including very small infants. Continuous cycling peritoneal dialysis (CCPD) using an automated cycler overnight has become the system of choice, allowing relative freedom from therapy during the day (Figure 2.4). However, continuous ambulatory peritoneal dialysis (CAPD) using a portable or wearable system is also widely used, and is not dependent on access to expensive machines.

A reliable peritoneal catheter is the cornerstone of successful PD and this should be inserted by a surgeon who is well practised in the technical aspects of renal failure surgery. Exemplary PD technique and attention to detail are necessary if complications such as peritonitis are to be avoided.

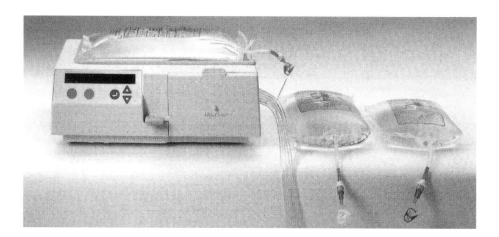

Figure 2.4 Modern compact peritoneal dialysis machine for automated overnight home treatment.

Chronic haemodialysis (HD) may be required while a patient is being assessed for peritoneal dialysis, or when it has been necessary to abandon PD following repeated infections or a loss of ultrafiltration capacity. Chronic haemodialysis is not the long-term management of choice, as it invariably relies on access to a dialysis centre and the services of highly skilled nursing and support staff. This form of dialysis is dependent on adequate vascular access, such as internal jugular catheters or an arteriovenous fistula.

Haemodialysis treatment is performed intermittently and its effectiveness is therefore transient.

Renal transplantation is the treatment of choice for any child with ESRD. Successful transplantation overcomes the problems of providing adequate nutrition, corrects renal osteodystrophy, improves growth, and avoids the frequently disfiguring operations associated with dialysis access.

Cadaveric and/or living-related renal transplantation is an accepted procedure in children of all ages and with better techniques for tissue typing and improved immunosuppression, graft survival is as good as for adult patients. Nevertheless, transplantation in this age group continues to pose challenges. In particular, the selection and availablity of donor kidneys is problematic, and it may be best to avoid using donor kidneys derived from children aged less than 2 years. Allograft rejection remains the most common cause of graft loss and the early diagnosis and treatment of rejection is still the biggest challenge for those involved in the care of the transplant recipient.

The care of infants and children with CRF/ESRD and their families is complex and depends on a multidisciplinary approach using the skills of doctors, nursing staff, dieticians, teachers, psychologists and social workers. Although it is now technically possible to treat CRF/ESRD in an infant or child of virtually any age or size, the parental expectation of such treatment must be explored before embarking upon a course of lifelong therapy. After careful consideration, some parents of small infants with very severe renal pathology may opt for non-treatment in view of the profound impact of CRF/ESRF and its treatment on the quality of life of affected children.

Key points

- The immature kidney has a limited capacity to respond to physiological stress. Careful management of fluid and electrolyte balance is particularly important in sick or compromised infants.
- Chronic renal failure in children is rare. Its management is complex and demands the expertise and resources of a skilled multidisciplinary team.
- Renal transplantation is the treatment of choice for end-stage renal failure in children.
- Chronic renal failure and its treatment carry major implications for quality of life. In some situations parents may take the ethically justifiable decision not to initiate treatment.

Further reading

Barratt TM, Avnel ED, Harmon WE (eds). *Paediatric nephrology*, 4th edn. Baltimore: Lippincott Williams & Wilkins, 1999: Chapters 1–6 pp 1–101; 71–80 pp 1151–1339

Imaging

Helen M Carty

Introduction

Nowadays, imaging departments play an important role both in diagnosis and in treatment (interventional radiology). However, the scope of interventional radiology is more limited in children than in adults, and diagnostic imaging therefore makes a greater contribution to paediatric urology.

Diagnostic imaging

Imaging of the urinary tracts is intended to seek information on anatomy, function or, frequently, both. Because none of the forms of imaging currently available fully satisfies these objectives (Table 3.1) it is often necessary to undertake some combination of examinations. In paediatric urological practice ultrasonography almost always represents the starting

Table 3.1 Relative merits of imaging studies in the assessment of urinary tract anatomy and renal function

	Anatomy	Function
Abdominal radiography	+	–
Ultrasound	+++	–
Intravenous urography	++++	++
MCUG	++++	–
Scintigraphy - DMSA	+	++++
Renography - MAG3/DTPA	++	++++
CT	++++	++
MRI	++++	+

point, but what, if anything, should follow depends on several considerations, including the clinical picture, the findings on ultrasonography, an appreciation of the limitations of ultrasonography, and a knowledge of the indications, advantages, drawbacks and pitfalls of other means of imaging.

The most commonly employed imaging studies are:

- Ultrasonography
- Micturating cystourethrography
- Indirect MAG3 cystography
- DMSA scintigraphy
- Dynamic diuresis renography

Abdominal X-ray

Although this is often a starting point in the investigation of abdominal or loin pain, the diagnostic yield is low and abnormal findings of urological relevance are generally restricted to the detection of urinary tract calculi, spinal anomalies, abdominal or pelvic mass lesions and constipation.

Films should be exposed to include the abdomen from diaphragm to pubis. The paucity of perirenal fat in children may mask renal outlines, and the abundance of gas shadows in infants tends to obscure renal and ureteric stones. In the case of spinal anomalies, those involving the sacrum are the most readily overlooked.

Ultrasonography

Ultrasonography is almost invariably the investigation of first choice for children suspected of having urinary tract pathology.

Advantages

General

- Zero burden of irradiation
- Low cost
- Painless
- Reproducible
- Portable.

Urological

- Image quality independent of renal function
- High sensitivity in the detection of renal stones and cysts, and in conditions causing dilatation of the urinary tracts.

Limitations

General

- Observer dependence.

Urological

- Low sensitivity in the detection of renal scarring (Figure 3.1) and of minor degrees of ureteric dilatation associated with the lower grades of vesico-ureteric reflux;
- Inadequate anatomical delineation of complex malformations (notably duplication anomalies);
- Imperfect demonstration of the level of obstruction (principally in respect of ureteric stones).

Technical considerations

The examination is undertaken with the child normally hydrated. The bladder should be full, because if it is not distal ureteric dilatation may not be visualised, as may intravesical lesions such as uretero-coele (Figure 3.2). Because infants are apt to void once the abdomen is exposed, the examination at this age should commence with the bladder. Any examination performed without a full bladder is incomplete, and this should be recorded in the report. Bladder wall thickness is measured, as should residual urine volume where possible. Significant residual volumes are those exceeding 10% of expected capacity, as adjusted for age (see Chapter 14). A degree of hydronephrosis may result solely from an overfull bladder, and if this is suspected the kidneys should be re-examined following voiding.

Interpretation

Renal pelvic dilatation up to 10 mm in anteroposterior diameter, without accompanying calyceal dilatation, is within the range of normality and usually represents an extrarenal pelvis. Thickening of the bladder wall, especially if associated with significant residual urine, is indicative of bladder outflow obstruction.

Renal volumes are useful in monitoring growth and can be compared with normogram tables. The normal kidney is less echogenic than the liver, and the cortex

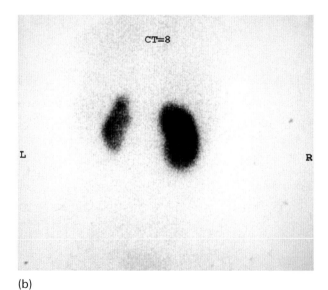

(a)   (b)

Figure 3.1 Limitations of ultrasound in respect of renal scarring. (a) Normal ultrasound appearances, but (b) DMSA scintigraphy demonstrates a small scarred kidney.

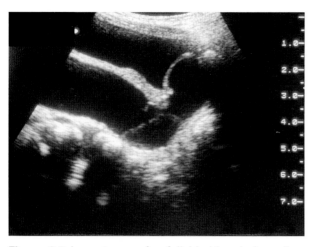

Figure 3.2 Importance of a full bladder during ultrasound examination. A duplex-system ureterocoele is seen within the bladder and the dilated upper polar ureter is visible retrovesically.

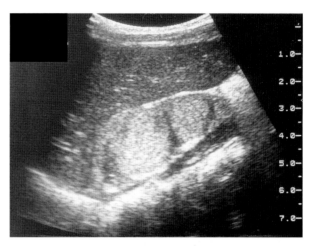

Figure 3.3 End-stage kidney. Ultrasonography shows hypoplasia with loss of the normal internal architecture.

has a higher echogenicity than the medulla. During the first 3 months of life, however, kidneys may be more echo-bright than the liver, although they should be of normal size and configuration and should retain corticomedullary differentiation. End-stage kidneys are also echo-bright but lose their normal internal architecture (Figure 3.3). The renal sinus is 'echo-bright' because of fat (Figure 3.4) and is usually single, whereas splitting of the echo is indicative of a duplication anomaly.

Abdominal pelvic masses

Ultrasound is also the investigation of first choice for children presenting with these lesions and can usually determine the organ of origin, the presence of solid or cystic components, and the presence of calcific deposits (Figure 3.5) or fat and of liver metastases. In suspected renal tumours, further relevant features are the condition of the contralateral kidney, the integrity of the capsule, and the presence or otherwise of tumour thrombus within the renal vein or inferior vena cava. Haemorrhagic necrosis within a lesion may appear as 'solid', a consideration to be borne in mind if planning biopsy under ultrasound control, as tissue must be obtained from viable and not necrotic areas.

Doppler ultrasonography

Doppler studies, of the renal artery or vein as appropriate, are helpful in some circumstances, such as:

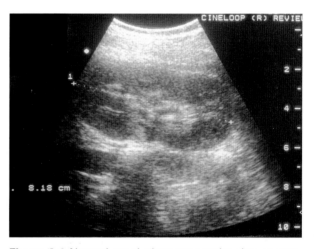

Figure 3.4 Normal renal ultrasonography demonstrating a single bright renal sinus echo.

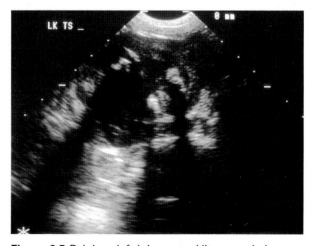

Figure 3.5 Painless left loin mass. Ultrasound shows a large left kidney with loss of normal architecture and multiple calcific densities, appearances strongly suggestive of xanthogranulomatous pyelonephritis.

- assessment of tumour extension within the renal vein or inferior vena cava
- following renal transplantation
- in cases of suspected renal vein thrombosis
- the investigation of hypertension.

Intravenous urography

Although largely supplanted by ultrasonography, intravenous urography retains a role in providing information in the following areas:

- Providing more detailed anatomy of lesions detected, but not positively diagnosed, by other means (principally duplication anomalies (Figure 3.6) and anomalies of position or fusion);
- Delineating the level of obstruction, principally ureteric obstruction due to stones;
- Investigating renal trauma when computerised tomography or DMSA scintigraphy are unavailable.

Advantages
General

- Availability
- Modest burden of irradiation.

Urological

- High anatomical definition.

Limitations
General

- Need for injection
- Risk of allergic reaction (rare in children)
- Medium burden of irradiation.

Urological

- Images dependent on renal function
- Limited functional information
- Low sensitivity in the detection of early pyelonephritic damage
- Imperfect demonstration of permanent renal scarring.

Technical considerations

A minimum series of exposures should comprise a full-length control film, a film 3 minutes post injection

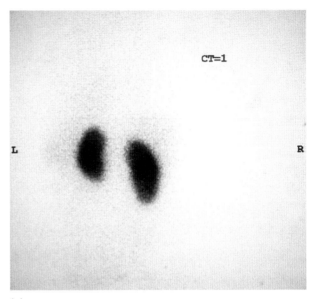

(a)

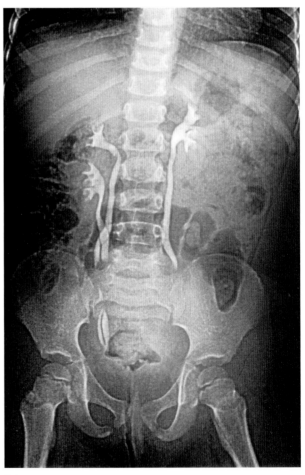

(b)

Figure 3.6 Uncomplicated renal duplication. (a) DMSA scintigraphy shows a slightly enlarged but otherwise normal right kidney. (b) Intravenous urography confirms this as being due to uncomplicated duplication.

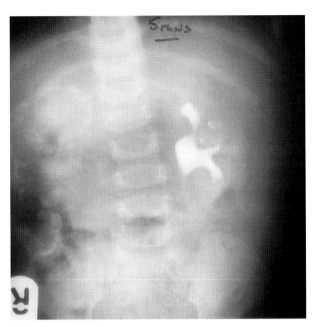

Figure 3.7 Gross hydronephrosis appearing as a 'shell nephrogram' on intravenous urography: dilated urine-filled calyces are outlined by contrast pooled within the intrarenal collecting system.

(which is limited to the renal areas and to demonstrate the nephrogram), and a third, full-length, radiograph at 15 minutes. These may be supplemented, as necessary, by oblique, prone or delayed images. In the presence of gross hydronephrosis, dilated calyces appear on early films as radiolucent against a background of contrast pooling in the collecting tubules ('shell nephrogram'; Figure 3.7). Although hydronephrosis in children is most commonly due to pelviureteric junction obstruction, delayed films (up to 2 hours post injection) may be needed to positively confirm obstruction as being at this level and not more distal, usually at the ureterovesical junction.

Micturating cystourethrography (MCUG)

Although it is not an examination to be undertaken lightly, MCUG:

- represents the only means of imaging urethral anatomy;
- is generally accepted as the most reliable means, in common use, of positively confirming or excluding vesicoureteric reflux;
- finds occasional use in the demonstration of vesical lesions (e.g. diverticula) and in the investigation of urethral trauma or bleeding.

Advantages

Excellent anatomical delineation of the bladder and urethra and good anatomical visualisation of refluxing ureters, including assessment of peristalsis.

Limitations

High burden of irradiation (including the genital area), pain and distress associated with the need for catheterisation, and the risk of introducing urinary infection.

Technical considerations

The burden of irradiation may be minimised by removal of the grid during screening and by using one of the several available radiation reduction devices. Catheterisation should be performed in the X-ray department by individuals expert in the technique; tepid cleansing solutions are used and retaining tapes, which hurt when removed, are kept to a necessary minimum. Preliminary insertion of the catheter under general anaesthetic is advisable for unusually apprehensive children, and also for girls found to have adherent labia minora. As a rule, MCUG should be delayed 4–6 weeks beyond the eradication of any infective episode. Children suspected as having vesicoureteric reflux should be maintained on antibiotic prophylaxis beforehand, and those found to have reflux should be prescribed an antibiotic in therapeutic dosage for 5 days, followed by prophylactic dosage thereafter.

The examination should document the presence and grade of reflux (Figure 3.8), plus the quality of ureteric peristalsis, and whether this occurs during filling, voiding, or both. Some children, including those with ureteric ectopia, reflux only when micturating, and failure to secure voiding views represents an incomplete examination.

Steep oblique or true lateral views are needed to demonstrate posterior urethral valves and ectopically inserted ureters adequately. In boys the entire penile urethra should be screened, so as not to miss the rare anterior urethral lesions (Figure 3.9).

Alternatives to micturating cystourethrography

Such examinations, despite reducing or eliminating the drawbacks of MCUG, are essentially limited to the exclusion or confirmation of vesicoureteric reflux, and

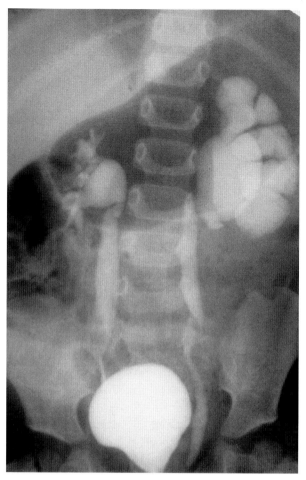

Figure 3.8 Contrast cystography showing bilateral vesicoureteric reflux. On the left side the pelvicalyceal dilatation is disproportionately greater than that of the ureter as a result of concomitant pelviureteric junction obstruction.

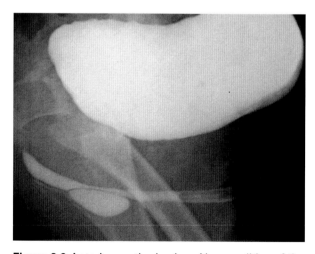

Figure 3.9 Anterior urethral valve. Abnormalities of the anterior urethra may be missed if screening is confined to the posterior urethra and the urethra is not demonstrated in its entirety.

provide little or no information as to the grade of reflux and none as to ureteric peristalsis or bladder or urethral anatomy.

Direct radionuclide cystography

The radionuclide is introduced via a catheter. During filling and voiding, with the child sitting or lying in front of the gamma camera head, the examination records both images and time–activity curves. Although reliable in excluding vesicoureteric reflux and entailing only a modest radiation dose, this investigation is best employed for children with known reflux being managed conservatively, or as a study following antireflux surgery.

Ultrasound cystography

Ultrasonic contrast medium is introduced via a catheter and vesicoureteric reflux is detectable as reflective echoes within the kidney. Although it is non-irradiating, this examination does not exclude minor grades of reflux.

Indirect MAG3 cystography

This may follow conventional MAG3 renography but is restricted to children able to micturate when required to do so. After drinking, the child voids upright in front of the gamma camera and into an appropriate receptacle. Time–activity curves are created for the renal and bladder areas (Figure 3.10) and the images are also recorded, usually using 1- and 5-second frames. No catheterisation is involved and the irradiation dose is modest. A further advantage is that information on differential renal function can be obtained if the study is combined with conventional renography. The principal limitation is low sensitivity in detecting lesser grades of vesicoureteric reflux. The examination is also unreliable in the presence of dilated upper urinary tracts with retained isotope.

Because this investigation is necessarily limited to cooperative children its use lies mainly in excluding clinically significant vesicoureteric reflux in older girls troubled by recurrent urinary tract infections and for the follow-up of known reflux.

DMSA scintigraphy

Technetium-labelled dimercaptosuccinic acid (DMSA) is a chelate extracted – but not excreted – by the renal tubules. Its uptake is limited to functioning

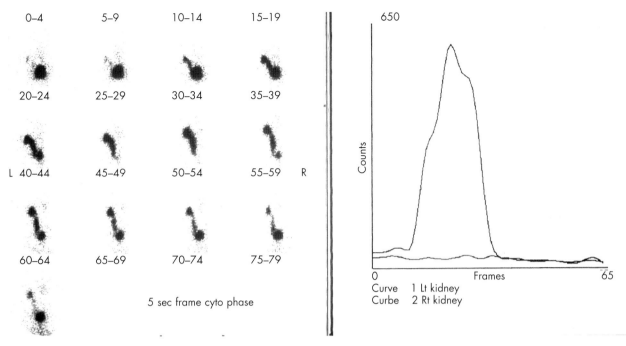

0-4   5-9   10-14   15-19

20-24   25-29   30-34   35-39

L 40-44   45-49   50-54   55-59   R

60-64   65-69   70-74   75-79

5 sec frame cyto phase

650

Counts

0   Frames   65
Curve   1 Lt kidney
Curbe   2 Rt kidney

Figure 3.10 Indirect isotope cystography. Right-sided vesicoureteric reflux is evident on both the time–activity curves and the images.

tissue and thereby reflects relative rather than absolute renal function. DMSA plays a valuable role:

- as the best (but not infallible) means of documenting the presence and progression of renal scarring;
- in identifying small (and sometimes ectopic) kidneys and 'cryptic' duplication anomalies
- in assessing kidney function following trauma or surgery, and differential function between the moieties of duplex kidneys.

Advantage

- Identification of functioning renal tissue.

Limitations

- Need for injection
- Medium burden of irradiation
- Limited anatomical information
- Indifferent image quality in neonates
- Problems of interpretation.

Technical considerations

The adult dose, 80 MBq, is scaled down according to the child's weight and images are acquired not less than 2 hours after the injection. Sedation is unnecessary, as in the event of movement, the scanning can be stopped and then restarted. A full examination comprises posterior oblique projections in addition to the standard posterior view: the former can only be obtained in cooperative children. Additional, anterior, images are obtained of ectopic or low-lying kidneys. Minimally functioning kidneys, which may lie ectopically, are best sought with the normal contralateral organ screened off.

Interpretation

DMSA scintigraphy should always be viewed in conjunction with other imaging studies. Relative uptakes of normal kidneys should be equal within a tolerance of 10%.

Photopenic areas found during or shortly after acute pyelonephrotic episodes may merely represent transient 'nephronia', and to demonstrate permanent renal scarring it is necessary that DMSA scintigraphy be delayed at least 8 weeks after the eradication of urinary infection (Figure 3.11).

In the absence of oblique images shallow peripheral scars may be missed. Chronic pyelonephritis occasionally results in smooth shrinkage of the kidney, without peripheral scarring, and if both kidneys are equally affected the scan may be misinterpreted as 'normal': intravenous urography is advisable if this possibility is suspected on clinical grounds. Conversely, a 'small'

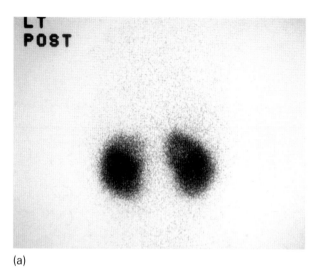

(a)

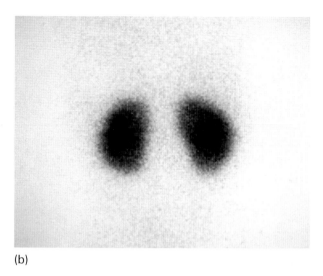

(b)

Figure 3.11 Transient nephronia. (a) Initial DMSA scintigraphy, undertaken during an episode of acute pyelonephritis, shows photopenia in the left upper pole. (b) No abnormality is visulised on a follow-up scan 8 months later.

kidney may simply reflect uncomplicated duplication of the contralateral organ, not necessarily detected by ultrasonography: if clinically relevant, the issue is determinable by intravenous urography (see Figure 3.6).

Dynamic diuresis renography

This examination is principally employed in the further investigation of suspected supravesical obstructive uropathies detected by ultrasound. The radiopharmaceutical of choice, technetium-labelled dimercaptoacetyltriglycine (MAG3), is excreted by tubular secretion, with 80% being extracted during the first pass. This agent provides a high signal-to-background ratio and hence good images. Effective renal plasma flow, a reflection of absolute renal function, can be calculated for each kidney. Although normal values have yet to be established for children they are known to change with age and are low in neonates. Time–activity curves during the excretory phase are used to distinguish between obstructive and non-obstructive hydronephrosis (Figure 3.12).

The alternative agent, diethylenetriamine penta-acetic acid (DTPA), being excreted via the glomeruli, can be used to calculate the glomerular filtration rate but, because of poorer extraction, gives flatter, less readily interpretable time–activity curves.

Advantages

- Can be performed in children of any age, including neonates;

- Small burden of irradiation;
- Assessment of differential renal function;
- Distinguishes between obstructive and non-obstructive uropathies.

Limitations

- Need for injection;
- Modest anatomical information;
- Problems of interpretation.

Technical considerations

The adult dose, 80 MBq, is reduced according to calculation of the child's surface area and is administered in a state of normal hydration. The diuretic frusemide is conventionally injected 16 minutes after the onset of the study, but in infants with tenuous venous access it is better given simultaneously with the radiopharmaceutical. Although sedation may be needed for infants and young children, current software programmes do allow some compensation for movement.

Interpretation

Images and time–activity curves should be considered together. Delayed perfusion is better appreciated from viewing the images, as is the configuration of the upper renal tracts in cases of hydronephrosis or hydroureteronephrosis. If frusemide is given simultaneously with the radiopharmaceutical the calculation

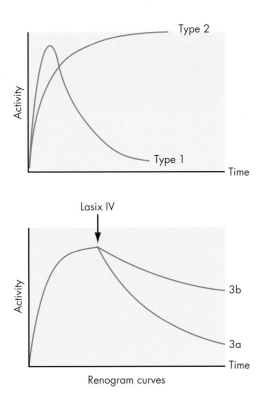

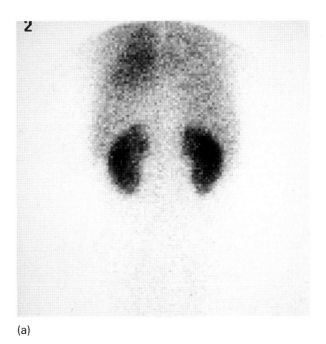

(a)

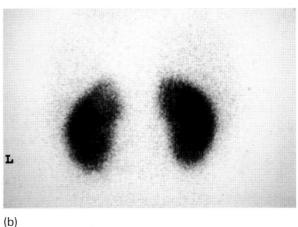

(b)

Figure 3.12 Dynamic diuresis renography. Line diagrams of time–activity curves. (a) Normal (type 1) and obstructed (type 2) patterns. (b) Equivocally non-obstructed (type 3a) and equivocally obstructed (type 3b) drainage curves.

Figure 3.13 Renal scarring on MAG3 renography and DMSA scintigraphy. (a) The first, summed, image on MAG3 renography shows a scar in the left upper renal pole. (b) This is confirmed on DMSA scintigraphy.

of divided renal function based on uptake in the first 3 minutes may be misleading in young children. In particular there is a tendency for the investigation to yield an overestimate of function in a contralateral obstructed kidney, and in these circumstances it is better to calculate differential function from isotope uptake in the first minute post injection. Estimates of differential function are also unreliable in ectopic kidneys because of distance from the camera. However, time–activity curves remain valid in respect of obstruction versus non-obstruction.

The first image during renography, representing the nephrogenic phase before excretion, may disclose renal scarring. Although such a positive finding correlates well with DMSA scintigraphy (Figure 3.13), the converse does not hold, partly because the count rate is lower and partly because oblique views are unobtainable. A rise in the count rate during the excretion phase is indicative of vesicoureteric reflux (Figure 3.14). The limitations of diuretic renography in the diagnosis of obstruction are considered in more detail in Chapter 6.

Captopril renography

This examination is sometimes employed in the investigation of hypertension. In the presence of renal artery stenosis standard renography is usually normal, but, if repeated along with the antihypertensive agent captopril, shows a decline in function owing to decreased efferent arterial constriction. Reduced blood flow may also result in prolonged cortical retention of MAG3.

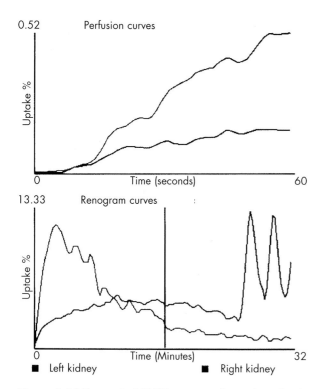

Figure 3.14 Dynamic MAG3 renography: a late rise in the time–activity curve of the poorly functioning left kidney is indicative of vesicoureteric reflux.

Table 3.2 Indications for CT

Abdominal or pelvic mass
Trauma
Renal abscess
Nephrocalcinosis (rarely)
Pyonephrosis
Biopsy

Cross-sectional imaging

In the context of paediatric urology, such imaging is largely confined to the assessment of trauma and of abdominal or pelvic mass lesions.

Computerised tomography (CT)

Indications for CT are listed in Table 3.2.

Trauma

CT has advantages over ultrasound, partly because the latter may be restricted by tenderness, ileus, or associated skeletal or head injuries, and partly because

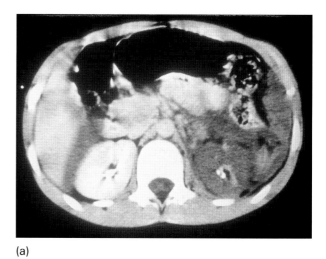

(a)

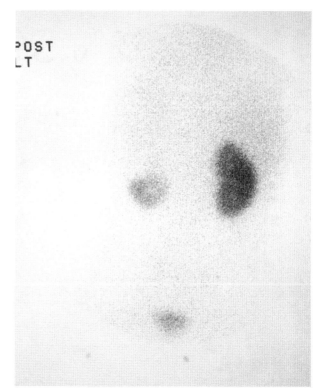

(b)

Figure 3.15 (a) CT following abdominal trauma. There is subhepatic free fluid and, in the left kidney, absence of contrast enhancement in the upper pole owing to devascularisation. (b) A subsequent DMSA scintigram demonstrated function confined to the lower renal pole.

a more complete survey of intra-abdominal injuries is obtainable. Assessment of the urinary tracts is undertaken as part of a general abdominal examination. Should bowel distension be needed, water is given via a nasogastric tube. If the bladder is catheterised the catheter is clamped at the outset. Intravenous contrast is administered, with 40% being given as a bolus prior to commencement of the examination and the remainder during the course of scanning. If renal trauma is suspected, the kidneys are examined in contiguous slices: CT is highly sensitive in detecting contusions, lacerations, perinephric fluid collections and areas of avascularity (Figure 3.15). The pelvic examination is intended to look for evidence of bladder rupture and extra- or intraperitoneal leakages of urine. As a rule, the complications of urinary tract trauma are better followed by serial ultrasonography than by further CT examinations.

Mass lesions

Because the organ of origin has usually been determined by preliminary ultrasonography, the role of cross-sectional imaging is to further characterise the lesion, including its extent (Figure 3.16), operability and, in the case of malignancy, possible metastatic spread. The choice of imaging method (CT or magnetic resonance (MRI)) depends on the suspected nature of the lesion (Table 3.3). With renal tumours both modalities are equally sensitive in respect of diagnosis and staging, although CT has an advantage in that the lungs may be scanned for metastatic spread during the same examination. Magnetic resonance imaging is indicated in the rare event of a renal tumour invading the spinal canal (Figure 3.17). Most pelvic tumours are better assessed by MRI than by CT. Pelvic pseudotumours due to an abscess (almost invariably from ruptured appendicitis) or hydro- or haematocolpos have characteristic ultrasound appearances and CT is not usually needed for diagnostic purposes. The examination may, however, be helpful when planning surgical drainage of a pelvic abscess.

Table 3.3 Preferred primary cross-sectional imaging in tumours of the paediatric genitourinary tract

CT	MR
Wilms' and other renal tumours	Neuroblastoma Pelvic rhabdomyosarcoma Sacrococcygeal teratoma Vaginal tumour Ovarian teratoma Presacral lesions Lymphoma

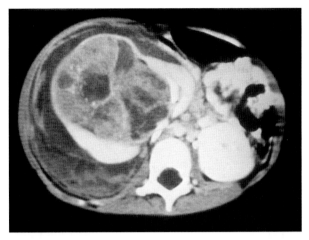

Figure 3.16 Abdominal CT in a child with Wilms' tumour showing a rim of functioning kidney tissue around the tumour, rupture of the renal capsule and a perineal fluid collection.

Renal stones and inflammatory conditions of the kidney

Although renal stones and nephrocalcinosis are usually positively identifiable by ultrasound, in case of doubt the matter can be resolved by a non-contrast enhanced CT scan. The same is true of renal abscess and pyonephrosis, and CT is sometimes helpful in planning percutaneous drainage of such lesions. Xanthogranulomatous pyelonephritis may mimic Wilms' tumour, but usually exhibits a characteristic pattern of calcific deposits and fatty densities. The role of spiral CT in the assessment of calculi in children is controversial in view of the significantly higher radiation dosage than with intravenous urography.

Magnetic resonance imaging

Over and above the absence of any irradiation, the advantages of MRI over CT are the multiplanar images and the superior delineation of bony (but not pulmonary) metastases, the interface between normal and pathological tissue and intraspinal extension of tumours. Disadvantages are the greater need for sedation, respiratory gating and the higher cost. Large calcific deposits are identifiable as a signal void, but fine and often diagnostically significant calcification may be missed.

T_1-weighted images highlight anatomy, whereas T_2 images are a better guide to pathology. Fat-suppression techniques enhance pathological diagnosis, as they differentiate between adipose and pathological

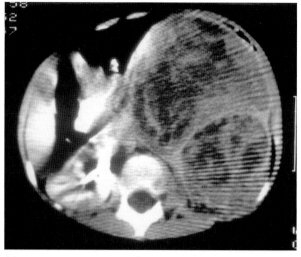

(a)

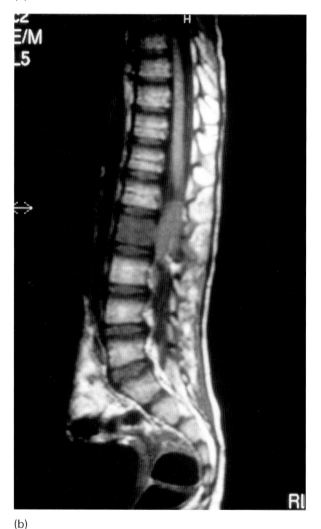

(b)

Figure 3.17 Left Wilms' tumour. (a) CT shows tumour in the region of the psoas infiltrating the vertebral body. (b) On MRI it is apparent that tumour extends into the spinal canal.

tissue, both of which may be bright, with a high signal, on T_2 sequences. Gadolinium enhancement, like contrast on CT, helps in assessing tumour vascularity, although the degree of enhancement – a measure of vascularity – is better appreciated on CT, an important consideration when planning biopsies. Necrotic tissue and pus do not enhance with gadolinium and appear as signal voids within a mass. Tumour pathology apart, the principal role of pelvic MRI lies in delineating anatomy – an advantage which is often more relevant to paediatric gynaecology than to urology.

Interventional techniques

As a rule, these should be preceded by clotting studies and any defect rectified beforehand.

Arteriography

This may be indicated in suspected renal artery stenosis (Figure 3.18) or middle aortic syndrome, and is sometimes undertaken with a view to treatment by balloon angioplasty. A further, emergency, indication exists on the rare occasion that a renal pedicle injury is suspected in time for effective surgical intervention. Some renal and bladder arteriovenous malformations are treatable by embolisation.

Venography

Selective sampling of renal veins and the inferior vena cava is sometimes indicated in children whose hypertension is thought to arise from excessive renin production. Where this is confirmed, nephrectomy may be curative.

Varicocoele embolisation represents an effective alternative to open surgery and is usually performed under local anaesthetic. Occlusion of the spermatic vein is confirmed transoperatively by Doppler examination of the scrotum, and subsequent testicular growth is monitored by ultrasound.

Antegrade pyelography and the Whitaker test

Puncture of a hydronephrotic kidney for antegrade pyelography, usually under general anaesthetic and employing a single 22 G spinal needle, is normally a straightforward undertaking and is used to delineate

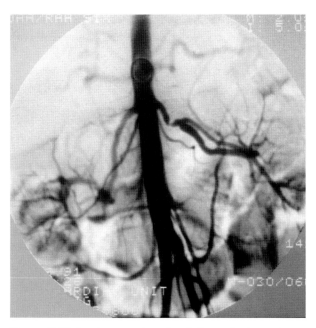

Figure 3.18 Angiogram showing left renal artery stenosis: the two right renal arteries are both normal.

complex lesions (e.g. duplication anomalies or ectopic ureters), to determine the level of obstruction, or to demonstrate ureteric polyps (which are rare lesions usually discovered incidentally during the course of investigation of unexplained hydronephrosis).

For the Whitaker test two needles are inserted, one for infusion, the other for pressure measurement. Intravesical pressure is also monitored via a urethral catheter. The investigation is indicated principally in situations where the findings of dynamic renography conflict with the clinical picture or are inherently unreliable (gross hydronephrosis, impaired renal function). Fluid is infused at 10 ml/min, and in older patients a pressure gradient between kidney and bladder rising to exceed 22 cmH_2O is taken to indicate obstruction. Whether the same values are valid in younger children has never been established.

Percutaneous nephrostomy

Performed under ultrasound control and usually under general anaesthetic, percutaneous nephrostomy is nowadays generally preferred to open surgical nephrostomy drainage. Indications include decompression and drainage of acutely obstructed or infected hydronephrosis (usually due to pelviureteric junction obstruction), and as a therapeutic trial in chronically obstructed poorly functioning kidneys. In such cases function is re-estimated after 4 weeks' drainage. Urine can be adequately drained by 5–6 FG catheters, but adequate drainage of pus requires larger catheters.

Renal biopsy

This is performed under general or local anaesthetic, depending on the child's cooperation. A biopsy needle of 16 G minimum is used, and specimens should be checked immediately to ensure that an adequate number of glomeruli has been sampled.

Tumour biopsy

Image-guided percutaneous sampling of a mass represents an alternative to open surgical biopsy, the choice being determined by the suspected nature of the lesion plus its location and vascularity. Material must be obtained from viable tumour and the specimen must be of sufficient size not only for histopathology but also for molecular genetic and cytokine studies and, ideally, when frozen, for subsequent research. For these reasons, open biopsy via a minilaparotomy has returned to favour, although even here imaging studies should be reviewed so as to select the most appropriate site for sampling.

Key points

- Careful thought is required when submitting children with urological problems to diagnostic imaging.
- It is important to have a clear understanding of the relative merits and drawbacks of each investigation.
- Do not overlook the potential radiation burden.
- Investigations should be selected according to the clinical questions to be answered and the ability of specific investigations to provide information on function or anatomy.
- Always consider the effect of the investigation on the child.

Further reading

Borthne A, Nordshus T, Reiseter T et al. MR urography: the future gold standard in paediatric urogenital imaging? *Paediatr Radiol* 1999; 29: 694–701

Krestin GP. Genitourinary MR: kidneys and adrenal glands. *Eur Radiol* 1999; 9: 1705–1714

Roebuck DJ, Howard RG, Metreweli C. How sensitive is ultrasound in the detection of renal scars? *Br J Urol* 1999; 72: 345–348

Rushton HG. The evaluation of acute pyelonephritis and renal scarring with technetium 99m-dimercaptosuccinic acid renal scintigraphy: evolving concepts and future directions. *Paediatr Nephrol* 1997; 11: 108–120

Sixt R, Stokland E. Assessment of infective urinary tract disorders. *Q J Nucl Med* 1998; 42: 119–125

Stokland E, Hellstrom M, Jakobsson B, Sixt R. Imaging of renal scarring. *Acta Paediatrica* 1999; 88 (Suppl 431): 13–21

Urinary infection

4

AMK Rickwood

Topics covered
Epidemiology of childhood urinary infection
Pathogenesis
    Infecting organisms
    Host factors

Diagnosis
    Specimen collection, urine analysis
Clinical features
Investigation
Management

Introduction

Urinary infection is the commonest mode of presentation in paediatric urological practice and there are important reasons why it should be taken seriously:

- The incidence of underlying urinary tract anomalies is far higher in children than in adults.
- Although some anomalies are of doubtful importance and represent little more than incidental findings, an appreciable proportion are of actual or potential clinical significance as causes of:
  - acute mortality, usually from urinary sepsis;
  - ongoing symptomatology and chronic ill health;
  - later morbidity, principally in the form of hypertension;
  - end-stage renal failure.

Epidemiology

Incidence

During the course of childhood some 5% of girls experience urinary infection but the proportion of boys affected throughout childhood is considerably smaller (1.5%). In the first 12 months of life, however, urinary infection is more prevalent in boys than in girls, although this risk is reduced tenfold by neonatal circumcision.

Among girls, recurrent infection is common regardless of whether or not there is any underlying urinary tract anomaly. At least 50% of girls who experience one urinary infection will suffer a second

and, of these, a similar proportion will suffer a third, those who suffer a third a fourth, and so on. However, in the absence of any underlying urinary tract anomaly there is no evidence that females who have been troubled by urinary tract infection in childhood will be any more prone to experience this complaint during adult life.

Pathogenesis of urinary tract infection

In the urinary tract, as in other systems, the occurrence of infection depends upon the balance between host resistance and the virulence of the infecting organism. *Escherichia coli* is the causative organism in some 85% of cases. Fimbriated forms of *E. coli* have the ability to adhere to receptors on the urothelial surface and are thus particularly effective at colonising the urinary tract. Other common infecting organisms, in approximately descending order of frequency, are *Proteus vulgaris*, *Klebsiella*, *Enterobacter* and *Pseudomonas*.

A number of factors impair host resistance to ascending bacterial colonisation and thus increase susceptibility to urinary infection. Of these, the most important are mechanical factors that reduce the effectiveness with which organisms are cleared from the urinary tract, namely obstruction, stasis and reflux. In this context, impaired bladder emptying due to dysfunctional voiding commonly predisposes to lower urinary tract infection, particularly in girls, whose perineum and urethra are more prone to bacterial colonisation than in boys. Other host factors of uncertain importance include reduced secretion of IgA and greater susceptibility of vaginal and urothelial cells to

Table 4.1 Incidence and pattern of urinary tract abnormalities in children presenting with urinary tract infection

			% of anomalies (n = 79)	% of series (n = 200)
VUR/renal scarring		58	(73)	(29)
*VUR only	29			
*VUR + scarring	20	} 49	(63)	(24.5)
Scarring only	9			
Total scarring		29	(37)	(14.5)
Obstructive uropathies		9	(11.5)	(4.5)
UVJ obstruction	5			
PUJ obstruction	4			
Duplication anomalies		9	(11.5)	(4.5)
Polar VUR	3			
Ureterocoele	2			
Ectopia	2			
Uncomplicated	2			
Other anomalies		3	(4)	(2)

*VUR grades I/II 30; VUR grades III/V 19.

bacterial adherence, a property that appears to be linked to blood group secretor status.

Incidence and nature of associated urinary tract anomalies (Table 4.1)

Among large series of children affected by urinary tract infection the reported incidence of anomalies varies between 30% and 50% of cases, but the proportion of these anomalies of actual or potential clinical significance is debatable. Renal scarring, which is found in 15–30% of children at initial presentation (with or without associated reflux) is certainly significant as a cause of hypertension and, occasionally, of renal failure. Obstructive uropathies, particularly urethral valves, pose a potential threat of long-term morbidity even when renal function is unimpaired, and similar considerations apply to urinary tract calculi and most examples of complete duplication anomalies. At the opposite end of the spectrum, incomplete duplications and anomalies of position and fusion are of little consequence (in the absence of other complicating features) and almost always represent incidental findings, which are unlikely to be implicated in the causation of urinary infection.

Much the most common anomaly identified in children who present with urinary infection is vesicoureteric reflux, with or without associated scarring. In the absence of scarring the significance of reflux can be difficult to gauge, as this depends both upon the grade of reflux and upon the age of the child at presentation. Grade III reflux, for example, carries a far greater risk of potential scarring, whereas grades I and II are not commonly associated with scarring at any age.

When anatomical findings of doubtful significance are excluded, urological disorders predisposing to further infection or posing a threat of significant morbidity, occur with an overall incidence of approximately 25% of children presenting with urinary infection. Within this overall figure, however, there is some variation, depending on factors such as age, gender, and the severity of infection. Thus the likelihood of finding a significant urinary tract anomaly is far greater in a 6-month-old boy presenting with a febrile illness than, for example, a 6-year-old girl with a clinical picture confined to lower urinary tract symptoms.

Diagnosis

Because the significance of childhood urinary infection is well recognised there is a risk of overdiagnosis and, in turn, overinvestigation and overtreatment. In as many as a third of suspected cases the diagnosis is not subsequently confirmed by urine culture. Spurious diagnosis of urinary infections is common among referrals from general practice and may result from imperfect collection or processing of specimens, from misinterpretation of urine culture reports or from both. It should be routine practice, when accepting such referrals, including referrals describing 'proven infection', to insist upon a sight of the urine culture report(s) and then, during the consultation, to check with the parents the mode of specimen collection and subsequent disposal. These simple measures commonly spare children the discomfort and risks of unnecessary investigation.

Specimen collection

Children who are toilet trained can usually cooperate in the collection of a conventional midstream urine (MSU) sample, but problems arise in infants and in toddlers who are still in nappies. Here the options comprise:

- **Clean catch** Such specimens, although ideal, can only be collected cleanly from boys and the process calls for a degree of parental patience which is not always forthcoming.
- **Collection bags** This represents the routine method of collection and, if properly undertaken, produces few false positive or equivocal results.
- **Catheterisation or suprapubic aspiration** These methods have no place in general practice or routine urological practice, but find occasional use in a hospital setting in certain specific situations. Catheterisation may be justifiable to obtain an urgent specimen, and suprapubic aspiration may be required when the results of bag specimens have been equivocal or unexpectedly positive or negative.

Once obtained, specimens must be properly processed, which is to say they should reach the laboratory within 2 hours of collection. When this is not feasible the sample should be refrigerated immediately (although not for longer than 24 hours) before it is forwarded to the laboratory.

Urine analysis
Urine culture and microscopy

The accepted criteria required for an unequivocal dagnosis of urinary tract infection are a pure growth of a conventional urinary pathogen with a colony count $>10^5$ organisms/ml and an associated significant pyuria (white cell count $> 5 \times 10^6$/l in boys, $> 40 \times 10^6$/l in girls). Although most positive growths satisfy all these criteria, an appreciable number fall short in one or more respects:

- **Insignificant or absent pyuria** A significant colony count which is not accompanied by pyuria represents the commonest diagnostic dilemma. The clinical relevance of this finding remains controversial, especially in respect of whether renal scarring occurs in the absence of pyuria. Conventionally, however, an acellular or hypocellular but otherwise positive MSU result is regarded as a clinically significant finding meriting both treatment and subsequent investigation.
- **Unconventional urinary pathogens** *Staphylococcus aureus* occurs as an occasional but genuine urinary pathogen in neonates and young infants. Other unconventional urinary pathogens – the most common being *Staph. albus* – are less 'significant, even if associated with pyuria. When present in collecting bag specimens this organism usually represents a skin contaminant.
- **Insignificant colony count** This finding, with or without pyuria, is of doubtful significance except, possibly, in specimens obtained by suprapubic puncture.
- **Mixed bacterial growth** With few exceptions, such growths represent contaminated specimens.

Alternatives to urine culture

In an emergency, a diagnosis of urinary infection is confirmed if microscopy of a fresh specimen, by ground glass illumination, demonstrates the presence of numerous motile organisms.

Combined dipsticks for urinary nitrites and leukocyte esterase represent a more readily available means of emergency diagnosis. However, it is important to note that although false negative tests are few (<2% of examinations), false positive reactions occur more frequently (5–10% of examinations).

Clinical features of urinary infection
Neonates and infants

With only occasional exceptions the clinical features are wholly non-specific, and consequently the great majority of cases come under the care of paediatricians rather than urologists. A sizeable proportion of urinary infections in this age group present as emergencies. Fever is an almost universal feature and is typically accompanied by vomiting. Diarrhoea is not uncommon. This clinical picture has many causes and a diagnosis of urinary infection can only be confirmed or excluded on the basis of urine culture. Presentation with outright Gram-negative septicaemia is increasingly rare nowadays. Other non-specific features include failure to thrive or frank weight loss and, in neonates, prolonged jaundice.

Haematuria is an occasional localising symptom although this is usually apparent as a bloodstained nappy. Urine microscopy and culture are needed to confirm a urinary tract origin and the presence of urinary infection.

Urinary infection in male infants occasionally presents with epididymo-orchitis. Some mothers suspect that something is amiss because the urine is malodourous: they are often right.

Children aged 2 years and older

Even at 2 years of age most children are able to give some account of their symptoms, although this is least reliable with respect to abdominal pain. By 4 years of age, and often earlier, an accurate history can nearly always be obtained. Symptoms associated with urinary infection fall into two categories, those relating to the kidneys (pyelonephritis) and those relating to the bladder and urethra (cystourethritis) (Table 4.2), and any one patient may complain of either or both.

Upper urinary tract symptomatology

It is doubtful whether upper urinary tract infection ever occurs without a fever. Although the fever resulting from pyelonephritis is typically high, any temperature exceeding 38°C should be regarded as suspicious

Table 4.2 Symptoms of urinary tract infection

Lower urinary tract	Upper urinary tract
Frequency/nocturia	Fever
Dysuria	Vomiting
Hesitancy	General malaise
Secondary enuresis	Loin pain
Suprapubic pain	Upper/central abdominal pain

of renal involvement. Although the occurrence of fever is usually documented reliably in children admitted as emergencies, it is more difficult to ascertain in children referred as outpatients, either because the temperature was never measured during the acute episode or because the temperature reading is not recorded in the referring letter. Consequently, in most outpatient referrals, the occurrence or otherwise of fever must be inferred from other features of the illness. Rigors represent a sure sign of an elevated temperature, and a history of vomiting is, likewise, strongly suggestive of upper urinary tract infection in the absence of any alternative explanation. Other, less reliable, features include general malaise, listlessness, anorexia and nausea. Parents' judgement in this respect tends to be unreliable, with their presumed diagnosis of fever often being based on nothing stronger than an observation that the child felt hot or, as is typically described, 'burning up'. Negative evidence is frequently more trustworthy. If a child with predominantly lower urinary tract symptoms is reported as having been entirely well except when voiding, it is highly unlikely that the episode represented a febrile upper tract infection.

Upper abdominal pain is an occasional symptom of renal infection but may be difficult to distinguish from the non-specific pattern of central abdominal pain, a very common complaint in children. True loin pain is rare and, if prolonged, with or without vomiting, is more likely to signify urinary obstruction than infection.

Lower urinary tract symptomatology

As in adults, symptoms of lower urinary tract infection typically consist of dysuria, frequency and urgency, but in practice only a minority of children experience a 'full house' of symptoms and dysuria is the commonest complaint. If abdominal pain is present it is invariably located in the suprapubic region. In girls, vulval soreness is a frequent complaint but one to be viewed with suspicion. If other symptoms, particularly dysuria, precede the vulval soreness the diagnosis of urinary infection is likely to be correct, but, if the sequence is reversed (vulval irritation preceding the symptom of 'stinging' on voiding) a diagnosis of vulvovaginitis is more probable. As previously indicated, children with lower urinary infections are usually otherwise well, and many continue to attend school during the course of their illness.

The occurrence of haematuria in association with documented urinary infection is not in itself an indicator of the severity of infection. Haemorrhagic cystitis is the most likely explanation but when *Proteus* is isolated from the urine this should always arouse suspicion of calculi; stones can be present in the upper urinary tract even in the absence of constitutional symptoms. In boys referred with a diagnosis of haematuria (with or without documented infection) it is important to take a careful history, as this may have been postmicturition bleeding rather than true haematuria. This symptom is usually due to urethritis.

Another, uncommon, presenting feature of urinary infection in boys is epididymo-orchitis. If urinary infection is confirmed, investigation is indicated to identify any predisposing urological abnormality, such as urethral obstruction distal to the ejaculatory ducts, or ureteric duplication with an upper pole ureter draining ectopically into the ejaculatory duct. In other instances, mainly older boys, the urine is found to be entirely clear of infection and the aetiology is presumed to be viral.

Asymptomatic bacteriuria

Studies undertaken during the 1970s found that the prevalence of 'asymptomatic bacteriuria' in 5-year-old girls was 1–2%. Closer attention, however, revealed that a number of these children did have trivial urinary symptoms, such as urgency and urinary malodour. In addition, investigation disclosed that approximately 20% had urinary tract anomalies which, although mostly minor in nature, did include some instances of renal scarring. Because subsequent trials found no difference in prognosis between those treated and those untreated, it was concluded that asymptomatic bacteriuria is benign. However, these children were all identified and studied at an age when fresh renal scarring is rare, and it remains possible that asymptomatic bacteriuria among children of preschool age is not necessarily 'benign'.

Differential diagnosis

As previously indicated, vulvovaginitis represents the principal differential diagnosis in girls. This condition, most prevalent at 3–6 years of age, is the more likely diagnosis if the vulval soreness precedes other symptoms, if it is accompanied by vaginal discharge; or if dysuria occurs as an isolated symptom not accompanied by bladder symptoms, such as frequency, suprapubic pain or secondary enuresis.

Urine analysis in girls with vulvovaginitis is typically equivocal, with insignificant or unconventional growths (usually of *Staph. albus*), acellular growths or sterile pyuria. Balanoposthitis is the only common confusing diagnosis in boys, but there is always a history of simultaneous (and often preceding) preputial inflammation, sometimes accompanied by purulent discharge. As with vulvovaginitis, urine specimens taken during an acute episode tend to yield equivocal results.

Clinical indicators of urinary anomalies

In general the clinical features of a childhood urinary infection give little clue to the presence or otherwise of an underlying urinary tract anomaly. However, the likelihood is increased in the presence of the following:

- **A positive family history** Vesicoureteric reflux has a strong genetic basis. Duplication anomalies and upper tract obstructive uropathies may also run in families, although genetic factors play a smaller role in these conditions.
- **Febrile urinary infections** Almost all published series have found that children suffering from febrile urinary infections have an increased incidence of urinary tract anomalies compared to children with afebrile infections. In one large prospective series the presence of renal scarring (as opposed to uncomplicated reflux) was almost exclusively confined to children who had suffered febrile infections. However, these findings have yet to be confirmed by comparable studies.

There are three further clinical features that have historically been thought to carry an increased incidence of urinary anomalies, but which have lately been called into question:

- **Recurrent infection** In contrast to previous work, several recent studies have failed to demonstrate an increased incidence of anomalies despite a history of repeated infections. The newer findings probably reflect changing referral practice and the tendency to refer children after their initial infection.
- **Age** Although historical studies found an inverse correlation between the incidence of anomalies and age, this no longer appears to be the case, at least for urinary tract anomalies as a whole. However,

with respect to renal scarring the risk is clearly age related, being maximal in infancy, declining progressively in the first 4 years of life, and being low thereafter.

- **Gender** Contrary to common belief, most studies find no significant difference in the incidence of anomalies between boys and girls.

Investigation

All children, regardless of gender, merit investigation after their first urinary tract infection. Unfortunately, there is no such consensus as to what constitutes an appropriate investigative protocol.

Ultrasound

In any scheme of things, ultrasonography represents the investigation of first choice. This examination reliably detects obstructive and pseudo-obstructive dilatation, most urinary calculi, and clinically significant duplication anomalies. Other, more subtle, indicators of pathology include disparity in renal size (>1 cm difference in length measurement), abnormalities of renal echotexture, and distal ureteric dilatation suggestive of vesicoureteric reflux. False positive results are uncommon, and therefore all children with positive findings on ultrasound should undergo further investigation along the lines shown in Figure 4.1. Ultrasound investigation of the urinary tract should always include an examination of the bladder, which in a child who is old enough to void on volition should include views before and after voiding.

By contrast, normal ultrasound findings are frequently unreliable in respect of both vesicoureteric reflux (false negative rate ≈ 25–50%) and renal scarring (false negative rate ≈ 15–45 %). Although there is no consensus as to what further investigations, if any, should be undertaken in the event of a normal ultrasound scan, there is general agreement that three groups of children always merit further investigation in addition to ultrasound:

- Those under 2 years of age, partly because of the enhanced risk of scarring in this age group and partly because the majority have experienced febrile infection(s);
- Those aged 2 years of age and older who present with febrile infections;
- Those with a positive family history of vesico-ureteric reflux.

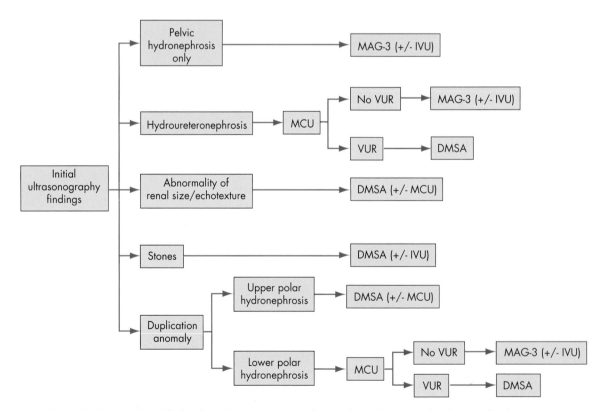

Figure 4.1 Investigative protocol following ultrasonography for the investigation of urinary infection.

DMSA scintigraphy

When further investigations are pursued following normal ultrasonography, DMSA scintigraphy is the examination of first choice. In addition to the categories listed above, some authorities also advocate this investigation for:

- children in the age range 2–4 years suffering *afebrile* urinary infection(s);
- children over 4 years of age who have suffered *recurrent* afebrile urinary infection(s).

Micturating cystography

Cystography, in one form or another, should be advised as a matter of routine if an abnormality (scarring, dysplasia, small kidney) is demonstrated on DMSA scintigraphy. However, an exception may be made for older children presenting with a single infection, as the risk of further renal damage is low and if reflux were identified it is unlikely that active treatment would be undertaken.

Even if the findings on DMSA scintigraphy are normal, cystography should nevertheless be routinely advised for the following groups:

- Children under 2 years of age
- Children aged 2–4 years of age with *febrile* urinary infection(s)
- Children aged 2–4 years of age with a positive family history of vesicoureteric reflux
- Children aged 4 years or over suffering *recurrent febrile* infections.

Although some authorities advocate cystography for all children aged 2–4 years regardless of symptomatology, and for those aged over 4 years with recurrent afebrile infections or a positive family history of reflux, the balance of current evidence supports a more selective approach.

Once the decision has been taken to proceed to cystography the options comprise **contrast cystography**, with the requirement for urethral catheterisation, or **indirect MAG3 cystography**. This latter has the disadvantages that the necessary cooperation from the child is seldom forthcoming before 3½ years of age, and it is relatively insensitive for detecting lesser grades of reflux.

Regardless of other considerations a **conventional contrast MCU** should be advised for the following:

- Children who are too young to cooperate with indirect isotope cystography. Although this is not contentious in children under 2 years of age, difficulties arise in those aged 2–3½ years and for whom it may be reasonable to defer the investigation until the child is old enough for indirect cystography, while administering antibiotic prophylaxis in the interim;
- Boys in whom there is any suspicion of bladder outflow obstruction;
- Any child who, if found to have reflux, is likely to require surgical treatment;
- Any child with a duplication anomaly and/or urethral ureteric ectopia.

In other circumstances indirect MAG3 cystography is usually sufficient, with the proviso that, in the event of a normal examination, contrast cystography should be performed subsequently if the child experiences further febrile urinary infections.

Abdominal X-ray

Because urinary calculi are not always detected on ultrasonography, this examination is worthwhile in children presenting with *Proteus* infections and/or infective haematuria.

Intravenous urography

The few remaining indications for this examination, in the context of urinary infection, are discussed in Chapter 3.

Management

Antibiotic treatment should be commenced promptly on suspicion of the diagnosis of urinary infection, once a specimen has been obtained. The choice of antibiotic and route of administration are determined principally by the severity of the infection and the age of the child. The intravenous route is preferred for infants (who are at greatest risk of renal scarring) and older children with marked systemic symptoms and a clinical picture suggesting pyelonephritis. Gentamicin remains a very effective agent for intravenous use, although it is necessary to monitor blood levels to minimise the risks of ototoxicity and nephrotoxicity. Alternatives include ampicillin, injectable cephalosporins or ciprofloxacin (which, although not fully licensed for paediatric use in the United

Kingdom, may be justified in view of its efficacy against *Pseudomonas* infection). Oral agents commonly used for the treatment of urinary infection include trimethoprim in therapeutic dosage, ampicillin and oral cephalosporins. Failure to respond may indicate infection with an antibiotic-resistant organism, but it is also worth bearing in mind that another common cause is vomiting of the antibiotic. Treatment with oral antibiotics should be continued for 5–7 days and the MSU checked subsequently to ensure that the infection has been eradicated. It may be prudent to maintain prophylaxis pending the results of investigations, for example in infants, in children whose symptomatology suggests pyelonephritis, or where preliminary investigation with ultrasound has already revealed a possible urological abnormality.

Even potent intravenous antibiotics may be inadequate when severe infection or pyonephrosis occurs within an abnormal urinary tract, and unless there is a prompt response to treatment some form of intervention should be considered to drain the infected urine and thus reduce the risk of progressive renal damage. For bladder outflow obstruction or vesicoureteric reflux this can usually be achieved by inserting a urethral or suprapubic catheter, but in the case of supravesical obstruction at the pelvi-ureteric or vesicoureteric junction percutaneous nephrostomy drainage under general anaesthesia may be required.

The following clinical situations also merit particular consideration:

- **Children under 4 years of age** As this is the age group at greatest risk of fresh or progressive renal scarring, antibiotic prophylaxis is advisable at least until investigation is completed. The referring GP should be formally advised to this effect.
- **Girls with no identifiable urinary tract anomaly** In most instances the episodes are well spread out and can be treated on an *ad hoc* basis. A minority of girls, however, are troubled more frequently and a few experience almost continuous symptomatic urinary infection. Although their symptoms relate only to the lower urinary tract, inevitably, over a period of time, they tend to be submitted to the full gamut of investigations, including contrast cystography, intravenous urography and even cystoscopy. These investigations invariably yield either negative results or, at worst, low-grade

vesicoureteric reflux. Dysfunctional voiding can be incriminated as an important contributory factor in a substantial proportion of these girls, particularly when accompanied by other features such as daytime wetting. Pre- and postvoid ultrasound imaging of the bladder is often informative by demonstrating significant postvoid residual urine, which predisposes to ascending bacterial colonisation and infection. Active treatment of bladder dysfunction is an important aspect of overall management, and this is considered in more detail in Chapter 13.

Other girls have a normal pattern of micturition and where conservative measures such as high fluid intake, attention to hygiene and drinking cranberry juice fail, a prolonged period (6–12 months) of antibiotic prophylaxis may be curative. A small percentage of older children are resistant to all measures and continue to experience recurrent or near-continuous asymptomatic or low-grade lower urinary tract infection. The parents of these girls can be reassured that there is no risk of renal damage (which is a worry for many parents) and that the complaint is almost always self-limiting, typically through the course of puberty.

Key points
- Approximately 40% of children of both genders suffering urinary infection have some underlying urinary tract abnormality, most commonly vesicoureteric reflux with or without associated renal scarring.
- All children who have experienced a urinary infection should be investigated. Wherever possible, however, it is important to establish a definite diagnosis of urinary infection before submitting a child to any investigation more invasive than ultrasonography.
- Ultrasonography is always the investigation of first choice. False positive findings are rare but ultrasound frequently gives false negative results, particularly in respect of vesicoureteric reflux and renal scarring. Consequently these conditions cannot be excluded on the basis of a normal ultrasound scan.
- Although clinical features are not a reliable guide to the presence of a urinary tract anomaly the incidence of underlying anomalies is far higher in

children suffering febrile urinary infections than those with purely lower tract symptoms.

- Although there is still some controversy as to which children with normal ultrasonography require further investigation, there is general agreement that DMSA scintigraphy and contrast cystography are advisable for all infants. DMSA scintigraphy plus contrast cystography in selected cases is indicated for all older children experiencing one or more symptomatic urinary infections.

Further reading

Aggerwal VK, Verrier-Jones K, Asscher AW, Evans C, Williams LA. Covert bacteriuria: long-term follow-up. *Arch Dis Child* 1991; 66: 1284–1286

Kunin C M. Urinary tract infections in children. In: O'Donnell B, Koff SA (eds). *Pediatric urology*. 3rd edn. Oxford: Butterworth-Heinemann, 1997; 171–196

Management of urinary tract infection in children. *Drugs Thera Bull* 1997; 35: 65–69

Rickwood AMK, Carty HC, McKendrick T. Current imaging of childhood urinary infections: prospective survey. *Br Med J* 1992; 304: 663–665

Vesicoureteric reflux

5

David FM Thomas

Topics covered
Incidence and aetiology of reflux
Reflux nephropathy
Clinical features

Diagnostic imaging
Management – medical, surgical, reflux trials
Surgical options

Introduction

Vesicoureteric reflux (VUR) is one of the most important conditions in paediatric urology. In childhood its clinical significance lies in its role in symptomatic urinary infection, which may progress to chronic ill health and failure to thrive. In the longer term renal scarring (reflux nephropathy) acquired in childhood poses a threat of morbidity in later life, which may include hypertension, complications of pregnancy and end-stage renal failure.

Ureteric reimplantation was widely accepted as the standard form of treatment until the late 1970s, when the arguments underpinning the routine surgical correction of VUR were challenged by the findings of experimental and clinical studies. Advances in our understanding of the pathogenesis of reflux nephropathy and the natural history of VUR have led to a more conservative approach to the management of VUR and the adoption more selective indications for surgery.

This chapter summarises current thinking on the aetiology, diagnosis and management of VUR and highlights some of the more topical or controversial aspects of the subject, including the role of genetic factors, prenatal diagnosis, the feasibility of screening, and the surgical alternatives to conventional ureteric reimplantation.

Incidence

Our knowledge of the prevalence of VUR dates largely from the 1950s and 1960s, when micturating cystogram studies in series of healthy children demonstrated VUR in 1–2% of the general paediatric population. It is now recognised, however, that VUR may behave as an intermittent phenomenon which can be provoked in a previously non-refluxing system, for example by elevated voiding pressures (detrusor instability, bladder dysfunction) or by oedema and distortion of the ureterovesical junction during an episode of acute cystitis.

Sex ratio

Important differences in the aetiology, natural history and presentation of VUR are summarised in Table 5.1. When VUR presents clinically with urinary infection it is predominantly a disorder of females, who outnumber boys by a ratio of approximately 5:1 in

Table 5.1 Summary of gender-related differences in vesicoureteric reflux between males and females

Female
Presents clinically – usually with urinary infection
Peak incidence in early to mid-childhood – age 2–7 years
VUR generally low grade, i.e. grades I–III
Functional factors important in aetiology: dysfunctional voiding, detrusor instability, constipation

Male
Presents clinically or detected prenatally
Clinical presentation usually in infancy or early childhood – 0–2 years
Often moderate to high-grade VUR, i.e. grades III–V
Anatomical factors important in aetiology (+ intrauterine bladder dysfunction???)

most large published clinical series. However, this ratio is reversed in the first year of life, when both urinary infection and VUR are more commonly diagnosed in boys. A preponderance of males is a feature common to all published series of infants with prenatally detected VUR.

Aetiology of vesicoureteric reflux

Primary VUR has been traditionally considered to be anatomical in aetiology. This pattern is characteristically associated with a ureteric orifice sited laterally on the base of the bladder, rather than in the normal anatomical position on the trigone. The length of intramural and submucosal ureter is correspondingly shorter, resulting in deficiency of the normal 'flap valve' mechanism which predisposes to reflux. Ureteric duplication provides the clearest example of the role of the ureteric bud as a crucial determinant of the position of the ureteric orifice, the occurrence of reflux and the presence of renal dysplasia. Stephen's ureteric bud hypothesis can also be invoked to explain many of the features of primary VUR.

The tendency for the relative length of the submucosal tunnel to increase with age accounts for the spontaneous resolution of VUR.

The role of **genetic factors** in the aetiology of VUR is now well documented. In a 10-year prospective study Noe found VUR in 34% of 354 siblings of 275 children with clinically presenting reflux (see section on Screening, below). VUR has also been demonstrated in more than 50% of the offspring of women with a history of VUR. In general, where VUR does exhibit a familial pattern it behaves as an autosomal dominant trait with variable penetrance and expression, and almost certainly results from the interaction of multiple genes rather than an isolated single gene mutation.

The term **secondary VUR** describes the occurrence of reflux in response to patterns of abnormal bladder function resulting in elevated intravesical pressure. Examples include **neuropathic bladder** (Figure 5.1) and obstructed voiding associated with **posterior urethral valves**. Secondary VUR often resolves following the restoration of more physiological bladder pressures after treatment of the underlying condition.

Evidence is accumulating to indicate that the traditional distinction between primary and secondary VUR is oversimplistic. It is now clear that **non-neuro-**

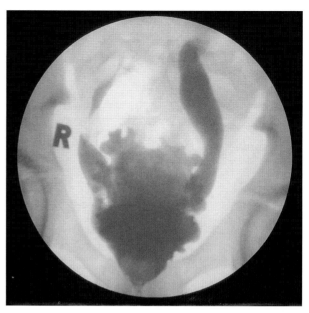

Figure 5.1 Secondary reflux. Characteristic appearances of reflux associated with trabeculated neuropathic bladder in a child with spina bifida.

pathic bladder dysfunction plays a more significant role in the aetiology of so called primary VUR than was previously recognised (Figure 5.2). This is particularly true of girls with low-grade VUR in whom voiding dysfunction, characterised by detrusor instability or detrusor–sphincter dyssynergia, is coupled with

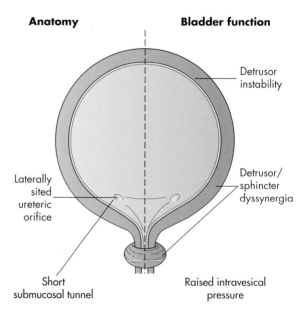

Figure 5.2 The balance between functional and anatomical factors in the aetiology of VUR.

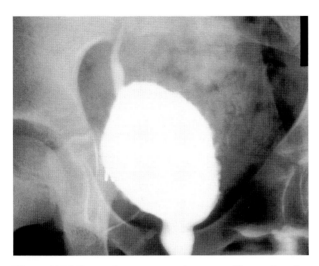

Figure 5.3 Micturating cystourethrogram illustrating the importance of bladder dysfunction in the aetiology of 'primary' VUR. Five-year-old girl presenting with wetting and recurrent UTIs. No neurological abnormality. MCU demonstrates low-grade right VUR, fine trabeculation and probable sphincter–detrusor dyssynergia. Good response to antibiotic prophylaxis, anticholinergic and voiding regimen.

'borderline' competence of the ureterovesical junction. Typically these girls present with wetting and urinary infection (Figure 5.3). Constipation is also a common and contributory feature.

The aetiology of high-grade primary VUR in infant boys has recently been called into question by the reported findings of urodynamic studies which have revealed high intravesical pressures in these infants. Increased bladder wall thickness on ultrasound and subtle radiological abnormalities of the male urethra have also been invoked as possible evidence of transient infravesical obstruction leading to elevated voiding pressures in utero and high-grade reflux – a hypothetical mechanism reminiscent of secondary VUR in boys with posterior urethral valves.

Reflux nephropathy

In children with clinically presenting VUR, DMSA imaging reveals evidence of scarring in 25–40% of refluxing units at the time of presentation. The reported incidence of hypertension in later life associated with unilateral renal scarring is of the order of 10%, rising to 20% for bilateral scarring. However, these figures, based on IVU assessment of scarring,

probably overstate the risks associated with the more subtle scars now being detected by the more sensitive modality of DMSA. For an individual with reflux nephropathy the risk of progressing to renal failure is difficult to quantify, but is now likely to be substantially less than the figure of 0.1% historically quoted in the literature.

Aetiology

Congenital

In infants with prenatally detected VUR (predominantly males with higher grades of VUR) imaging with DMSA before exposure to infection in postnatal life reveals evidence of renal damage in 15–30% of kidneys. Congenital renal damage usually takes the form of varying degrees of 'global' reduction in functioning renal parenchyma (a small smooth kidney), rather than the pattern of focal damage commonly associated with postinfective scarring. Severe damage (renal dysplasia) is predominantly a feature of grade V reflux (Figure 5.4).

Infective renal scarring

The experimental work of Hodson, and subsequently of Ransley and Risdon, highlighted the role of **intrarenal reflux** in the aetiology of renal scarring. In the human kidney (and the pig experimental model) the conical profile of the normal renal papilla provides

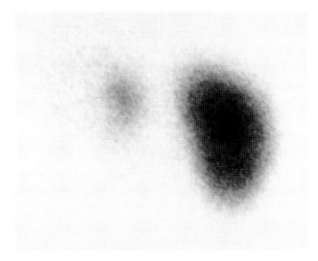

Figure 5.4 DMSA scan at around 1 month of age in an infant with unilateral grade V reflux detected prenatally; 9% differential function in the affected kidney. No urinary infection prior to DMSA imaging.

a second valve-like antireflux mechanism to protect the renal parenchyma against the reflux of potentially infected urine from the collecting system. Morphologically abnormal flat or 'compound' papillae, which may permit intrarenal reflux, are sited mainly at the poles of kidney – the areas particularly prone to pyelonephritic scarring.

The weight of experimental and clinical evidence indicates that the reflux of sterile urine at normal physiological voiding pressures does not result in scar formation. Urinary infection and intrarenal reflux are the critical elements of the scarring process.

Bacterial virulence is an important factor in the pathogenesis of both lower and upper urinary tract infection. Fimbriated strains of *Escherichia coli* are particularly successful uropathogens because of their capacity to adhere to urothelial surface receptors. Ascending bacterial colonisation of the lower urinary tract is the initial step in a process which, if unchecked, ultimately progresses to pyelonephritis. It is therefore inaccurate to describe VUR as 'causing' urinary infection, but like obstruction and urinary stasis, VUR impairs the mechanical efficiency with which organisms are cleared from the urine and thus promotes bacterial proliferation, which progresses to infection. Moreover, vesicoureteric reflux transports infected urine from the bladder to the upper tracts, where bacterial adherence and endotoxin production trigger the sequence of events which, if untreated, leads to parenchymal scarring.

The key observations and conclusions contributing to our current understanding of the nature and aetiology of renal scarring can be summarised as follows:

- Reflux of sterile urine at physiological voiding pressures does not result in renal scarring.
- Focal renal scarring requires the combination of urinary infection and intrarenal reflux.
- Renal scarring occurs maximally after the first episode of pyelonephritis (Ransley's 'big bang' hypothesis).
- The risk of renal scarring is greatest in infancy and early childhood. Conversely, the risk of infective scarring decreases significantly beyond the age of 4 years.
- To pose a risk of renal scarring, urinary infection must be sufficiently severe to give rise to symptomatic pyelonephritis. Asymptomatic bacteriuria, a relatively common finding in older girls, does not result in renal scarring.

- The bulk of any reflux-related renal damage is generally present at the time of initial presentation. Although fresh scars can develop, the risk is low if surveillance is maintained and further infections do not go unrecognised or untreated.

Presentation

Clinical

Symptomatic urinary infection represents by far the commonest mode of clinical presentation. The overall incidence of VUR in children undergoing investigation for urinary tract infection is approximately 30% (although this varies considerably according to age and gender).

In adolescents or young adults extensive reflux nephropathy occasionally comes to light following presentation with **renal failure** and **hypertension**. Urinary infection is not usually a prominent feature of recent symptomatology, and in these cases reflux nephropathy is retrospectively ascribed to unrecognised urinary infection in infancy (possibly superimposed on pre-existing renal dysplasia).

VUR may be also be identified during the course of investigations for **urinary incontinence** in girls with underlying dysfunctional voiding. **Pain** is not generally accepted as a symptom of VUR, except in the form of loin pain associated with pyelonephritis, secondary pelviureteric junction (PUJ) obstruction or some other complication.

Asymptomatic

The term **prenatally diagnosed VUR** describes a diagnostic sequence in which prenatally detected dilatation of the fetal urinary tract prompts postnatal investigation by micturating cystourethrography (MCU), which in turn reveals the presence of VUR. Primary VUR (usually moderate to high-grade in male infants) accounts for 15–20% of significant prenatally detected uropathies. Asymptomatic VUR may be detected during the course of screening the siblings and offspring of individuals with known reflux.

The investigation of UTI is described in more detail in Chapters 3 and 4.

The following considerations apply specifically to the diagnosis and evaluation of VUR:

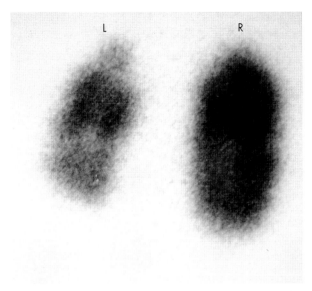

Figure 5.5 DMSA scan demonstrating renal scarring with patchy cortical damage to the left kidney on initial investigation of a child presenting with urinary infection.

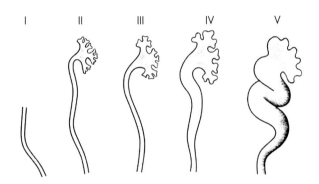

Figure 5.6 Grades of reflux (International Reflux Study Committee classification). Grade I: into ureter only; grade II: to upper tract (pelvic calyces), no dilatation; grade III: mild to moderate dilatation but minimal blunting of calyces; grade IV: moderate dilatation, loss of angles of fornices, papillary impressions in calyces still present; grade V: gross dilatation and tortuosity, and the impressions of papillae no longer visible.

- **Ultrasound** Although it is non-invasive, ultrasound has a high false negative rate when used as the front-line investigation to screen children with urinary infection. Comparing ultrasound and MCU in 272 refluxing units, one large American study found normal ultrasound appearances in 201 (74%). Of the refluxing units missed by ultrasound, 28% had grade III VUR or higher.

- **DMSA** is the most sensitive modality for visualising scarring and quantifying differential renal function (Figure 5.5). Yet when used as a screening test to identify children with VUR it has a sensitivity of less than 50%.
- **Indirect isotope cystography MAG3 or DTPA** involves an intravenous injection but is less invasive than an MCU, which requires urethral catheterisation. The radiation dose is also less. Unfortunately, this modality provides very little anatomical information and its role lies largely in follow-up.
- **Micturating cystourethrography** Although invasive, the conventional radiological contrast study remains the 'gold standard' investigation for the initial diagnosis and evaluation of VUR:
  - It permits accurate grading of the severity of VUR – information which is important when assessing prognosis and the potential for spontaneous cessation.
  - Unlike isotope cystography, MCU permits anatomical visualisation of urethral obstruction, bladder trabeculation, paraureteric diverticula etc.

  VUR is graded according to the scheme devised by the International Reflux Study Committee (Figure 5.6).
- **Intravenous urography (IVU)** is of little value, having been superseded by DMSA for the visualisation of renal scarring.
- **Urodynamic investigations** have been used for research purposes but are of limited clinical value in children with VUR associated with non-neuropathic voiding dysfunction. A careful voiding history and input/output and wetting chart are usually more instructive.

Management

The rationale for medical or 'conservative' management centres on the following observations:

- In the absence of urinary infection, VUR does not give rise to renal scarring.
- Uncomplicated primary reflux has the potential to resolve spontaneously.

Resolution rates for the five grades of VUR documented in one large study are illustrated in Table 5.2.

Table 5.2 Distribution of grades of reflux and spontaneous resolution for each grade in 844 refluxing ureters. Data from the Children's Hospital National Medical Centre, Washington. Skoog SJ, Bellman AB, Majd M, 1987

Grade of reflux	Distribution of different grades of reflux (%)	Spontaneous resolution rate for each grade (%)
I	7	83
II	53	60
III	32	46
IV	6	9
V	2	0

Medical management comprises:

- **Continuous antibiotic prophylaxis:**
  - Trimethoprim 1–2 mg/kg/day, usually as a single night-time dose.
- **Urine surveillance** Recently introduced reagent strip tests for nitrites and leukocytes now enable parents or general practitioners to make a more accurate provisional diagnosis, but where possible a freshly collected midstream specimen (MSU) should always be examined by microscopy and culture.
- **Treatment of any underlying bladder dysfunction.** A regular voiding regimen, with double voiding where there is evidence of incomplete voiding on ultrasound. Oxybutinin should be considered if the symptomatic picture suggests detrusor instability.
- **Treatment of constipation** Treatment is as for other forms of habitual constipation: a regimen comprising a faecal softener and a laxative, with the dose titrated against the child's response.
- **Commitment** Medical management should not be mistaken for benign neglect. Parental commitment is essential to ensure compliance with the medical regimen. Older children must be motivated to modify their voiding behaviour to correct voiding dysfunction. Effective arrangements are required to ensure that urine samples are collected and examined promptly to facilitate diagnosis and treatment of any breakthrough infections. **If the elements of successful medical management are absent, or where the necessary level of primary healthcare support is not available, surgery may be a safer, more reliable alternative.**

Medical or surgical management?

Randomised controlled clinical trials of medical versus surgical management have failed to demonstrate any convincing advantage of one over the other. For example, in the Birmingham Reflux Study 161 children with moderate to severe reflux were stratified by age and allocated randomly to surgery or medical treatment. After 2 years 161 children were assessed, and 104 after 5 years. No significant differences emerged between the two groups with respect to the incidence of breakthrough urinary infection, renal function, renal growth, progression of existing renal scars or incidence of new scar formation. The International Reflux Study reported broadly similar findings. Urinary infection was seen more frequently in the medically treated group (22% vs 8%), whereas new renal scarring was documented more frequently (on IVU) in those managed surgically, but in neither group was any change in glomerular filtration rate observed during the duration of the trial.

However, in everyday clinical practice medical and surgical treatment do not prove equally effective in the management of individual children with VUR. Whereas some children thrive and remain infection free on antibiotic prophylaxis, others experience symptomatic breakthrough infections which are only controlled by ureteric reimplantation. This paradox probably reflects the difficulty of designing trial methodologies that encompass the many different subpopulations of children with reflux – defined by variables such as age, gender, grade of reflux, patterns of bladder dysfunction, constipation, patient and parental compliance with voiding regimens and antibiotic prophylaxis, etc.

Practical approach to the management of VUR

Three practical conclusions can be drawn from the literature:

- Medical management can be safely adopted as the first line of treatment for the majority of children with VUR, with surgical intervention being reserved for specific indications.
- Children with underlying bladder dysfunction remain at risk of further urinary tract infections (UTIs) despite successful surgical correction of VUR.
- Medical and surgical management are both associated with a low (and comparable) risk of new scar formation.

A simplified clinical algorithm summarising the management of clinically presenting VUR is illustrated in Figure 5.7.

Clinical practice varies with respect to certain aspects of medical management, for example:

- **Duration of antibiotic prophylaxis** As a rule, the author aims to discontinue prophylaxis in girls by the age of 4 or 5 and in boys by the age of 3 or 4, provided a reliable pattern of regular and complete voiding has been established. For those whose VUR presents for the first time in later childhood, antibiotic prophylaxis is maintained until a full 12 months have elapsed since the last documented UTI and until bladder dysfunction has been successfully treated.

- **How often should the MCU be repeated in the course of medical management?** If a child is thriving and infection free on medical management there is little justification for submitting her/him to the discomfort and radiation dosage entailed in repeated MCUs. Only when the findings are likely to make a practical contribution to management should the MCU be repeated. It is not the author's practice to obtain an MCU either prior to stopping antibiotic prophylaxis or after ureteric reimplantation (an operation with a low failure rate). However, the occurrence of a symptomatic UTI after cessation of prophylaxis does merit a further MCU. Similarly, a postoperative MCU is required if UTI recurs despite antireflux surgery – although this is usually in girls who remain predisposed to cystitis because of incomplete voiding.

Indications for surgery

These are relative rather than absolute. There are two broad categories:

- **Functional** Symptomatic breakthrough infection represents the most common indication to abandon medical management and proceed to surgical intervention.
- **Anatomical** VUR associated with certain urological abnormalities, such as paraureteric diverticulum or ureteric duplication, is less likely to cease spontaneously than is uncomplicated primary reflux. The presence of coexistent abnormalities may tip the balance in favour of surgery.

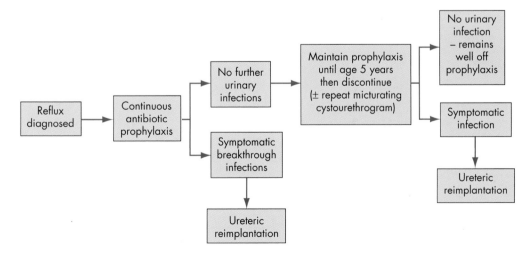

Figure 5.7 Simplified algorithm for management of reflux presenting clinically under the age of 5 years.

Neither severe renal scarring nor high-grade VUR is an automatic indication to intervene surgically. Ureteric reimplantation will not reverse any pre-existing renal damage. High-grade VUR, particularly in young boys, whether detected prenatally or presenting in infancy, has a significant tendency to cease spontaneously in the first 2 years of life. Similarly, correction of persisting high-grade VUR in older boys is of little benefit to those who remain well and infection free when off antibiotic prophylaxis. Conversely, clinical situations undoubtedly exist in which the presence of severe renal damage or high-grade VUR strongly influences the decision to adopt a surgical approach.

Management of secondary VUR

Although it may occasionally prove necessary to resort to open antireflux surgery for secondary VUR, reimplanting dilated ureters into thick-walled neuropathic or 'valve' bladder can be technically difficult and is best avoided unless there is a compelling indication. The failure rate (persisting reflux) and incidence of complications are both higher than for primary VUR. Moreover, secondary VUR associated with posterior urethral valves has a resolution rate of more than 50% following treatment of the underlying outflow obstruction, and VUR secondary to neuropathic bladder often resolves in response to bladder augmentation. Even when VUR persists it often merits no treatment other than antibiotic prophylaxis. Favourable results have been reported for endoscopic treatment Submucosal Teflon Injection (STING) and this is a technically attractive alternative to open surgery in a thick-walled bladder.

Surgical considerations

Ureteric reimplantation

The cross-trigonal advancement procedure devised by **Cohen** remains the operation favoured by the majority of paediatric urologists (Figure 5.8). The appeal of the procedure lies in its relative simplicity, its high success rate in correcting VUR (97% in one reported series of 100 consecutive Cohen reimplantations) and its low incidence of postoperative obstruction.

Postoperative stenting of the reimplanted ureter is not routinely necessary, but the bladder is drained postoperatively with either a suprapubic or a urethral catheter.

a)
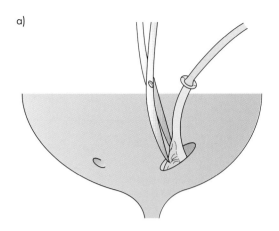

b)
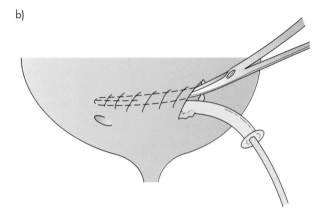

c)
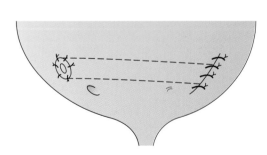

Figure 5.8 Ureteric reimplantation: Cohen technique. (a) Intravesical mobilisation of ureter. (b) Creation of submucosal tunnel. (c) Ureter reimplanted across the width of the trigone. The Cohen cross-trigonal reimplantation can be performed bilaterally and, if necessary, combined with ureteric plication of a mild to moderately dilated ureter.

An effective antireflux flap valve requires the creation of a submucosal tunnel whose length is four or five times greater than the diameter of the reimplanted ureter. Achieving this ratio when reimplanting a dilated

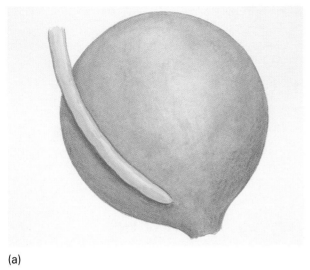

(a)

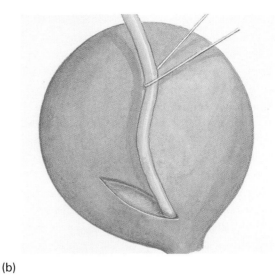

(b)

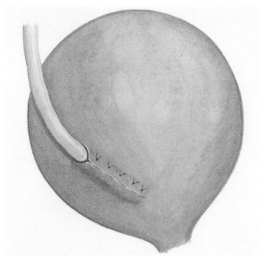

(c)

Figure 5.9 Ureteric reimplantation: Lich–Gregoir technique. Extravesical mobilisation and reimplantation in detrusor tunnel. Unsuitable for dilated ureters. (a) Refluxing ureter exposed and mobilized extravesically. (b) Detrusor muscle incised in the line of the water. Bladder mucosa exposed but not opened. (c) Detrusor closed around distal ureter to enclose it within detrusor tunnel.

ureter into a small bladder is not always technically possible, and in this situation the diameter of the distal ureter can be reduced by plication using the Starr technique. The **Politano–Leadbetter** technique, combined with a psoas hitch, may be preferable to the Cohen type of reimplantation following plication or remodelling of a grossly dilated megaureter.

Extravesical antireflux operations of the type originally described by Lich and Gregoir (Figure 5.9) are favoured by some paediatric urologists. The benefits centre on the reduced incidence of postoperative haematuria and discomfort compared with intravesical operations. However, extravesical techniques are unsuited to dilated ureters. Anecdotal concerns have also been expressed about the occurrence of postoperative voiding dysfunction, particularly following bilateral extravesical ureteric mobilisation.

Surgical alternatives to ureteric reimplantation

- **Circumcision** The role of the prepuce in predisposing to infection in boys with VUR was demonstrated by the findings of the International Reflux Study. Circumcision may be indicated on an individual basis, but without the evidence of controlled trials there is insufficient justification for routinely performing 'prophylactic' circumcision in all boys with prenatally detected or early-presenting VUR.
- **Vesicostomy** A temporary stoma between the bladder and the lower abdominal wall is an effective way of decompressing refluxing upper tracts and facilitating drainage. Vesicostomy is well tolerated and the incidence of complications is low. Cutaneous vesicostomy has largely replaced

ureterostomy in young infants whose VUR is complicated by sepsis or reduced renal function. Closure can be undertaken as an isolated procedure or in combination with definitive correction of VUR during the second or third year of life.

- **Nephroureterectomy** The role of nephrectomy is being reappraised in the light of concerns regarding the possible long-term risk of hyperfiltration damage sustained by solitary kidneys. Removal of a poorly functioning refluxing unit may be justifiable when the pathology is unilateral, function in the affected kidney is greatly reduced (less than 10% on DMSA) and the child is experiencing urinary infections. The kidney and refluxing ureter are excised in their entirety to prevent the risk of infection associated with a residual 'refluxing stump'.

- **Transureteroureterostomy (TUU)** In this procedure one ureter is reimplanted, usually by the Politano–Leadbetter technique with psoas hitch, and the contralateral ureter anastomosed to it above the level of the bladder. TUU is particularly useful for overcoming the problems arising from a previous failed ureteric reimplantation.

- **Endoscopic treatment (STING)** Developed and popularised in the mid-1980s, this innovative technique entails the endoscopic injection of a small volume of polytetrafluorethylene (PTFE 'Teflon') paste under the bladder mucosa in the region of the refluxing ureteric orifice. A European multicentre study of endoscopic treatment of 12 251 refluxing ureters in 8332 children reported successful correction of VUR with a single injection in 75% of cases. Unlike open antireflux sugery, the STING can be performed as a day case and repeated if necessary. Despite these apparent advantages, opinion remains divided on the role of the STING in the overall management of VUR.

Critics voice the following concerns about endoscopic correction:

- **Doubts about the long-term safety of implanted PTFE particles** Migration of injected particles to distant sites (including the lung and brain) has been described in experimental animals. Other authors have disputed these findings. A number of alternative materials have been studied, including silicone, cultured chondrocytes and dextran polymer. As yet none has proved as effective as PTFE for correcting reflux.

- **Inappropriate patient selection** Despite claims that the STING is being used selectively to treat clinically significant grades of reflux, the European 'trial' data suggest otherwise. In some centres the STING has clearly been employed extensively (and perhaps inappropriately) to treat children with low-grade VUR which had a high probability of resolving without any form of surgical intervention. Furthermore, the success rate for the correction of high-grade VUR is lower than for conventional reimplantation.

Long-term follow-up of VUR

The long-term risk of hypertension associated with unilateral renal scarring is considered above. The risks resulting from the subtle degrees of scarring now being detected by the more sensitive modality of DMSA renography may prove to be considerably less than those derived from historical data. Nevertheless, it is advisable for all individuals with evidence of renal scarring (regardless of whether their VUR has been managed medically or surgically) to undergo an annual check of blood pressure for life.

Prenatal diagnosis has recently highlighted the existence of a subgroup of children (boys with high-grade bilateral primary reflux) characterised by the combination of congenital renal damage and bladder dysfunction. Evidence is emerging to suggest that a small proportion of these boys may be at risk of progressing to renal failure even in the absence of infection – in a manner similar to the long-term natural history of boys with posterior urethral valves. Follow-up should be continued into adolescence, with monitoring of renal function and testing for proteinuria.

Screening for vesicoureteric reflux

Reducing the morbidity of reflux nephropathy by identifying VUR before infection has supervened is an attractive concept, but an effective screening programme for detecting asymptomatic VUR in the general low-risk paediatric population demands the availability of a non-invasive, inexpensive test of sufficient sensitivity and specificity.

DMSA and MCU are too invasive and costly to fulfil this role, and ultrasound is not sufficiently sensitive for the detection of VUR. Routine ultrasound imaging of the fetal urinary tract in pregnancy already constitutes a form of screening programme, but it identifies a subpopulation of boys with higher grades of reflux, rather than the numerically more important population at risk, namely girls with low-grade reflux. Urinary biochemical markers, including N-acetyl glucosaminidase, α_1-microglobulin and retinal binding protein, have been investigated as the possible basis of non-invasive screening tests for VUR. Unfortunately, the presence of these substances in the urine is more indicative of renal damage than of VUR itself. Furthermore, there is considerable overlap between urinary concentrations in refluxing patients and non-refluxing controls.

In current practice screening is therefore largely limited to the siblings and offspring of known patients with VUR. Opinion is divided on whether all siblings should be screened in the first instance by ultrasound, or by contrast or indirect isotope cystography. Using direct radionuclide cystography, one study found a 36.5% overall incidence of VUR in siblings. However, in siblings screened over 6 years of age the incidence fell to only 7%. Sibling screening is therefore likely to be of the greatest value in young infants, but probably serves little useful purpose in asymptomatic older siblings.

Further reading

Noe HN. The long-term results of prospective sibling reflux screening. *J Urol* 1993; 148: 1739–1742

Quinn MJ, Puri P. Vesicoureteral reflux: endoscopic treatment. In: Stringer MD, Oldham KT, Mouriquand PDE, Howard ER (eds) *Paediatric surgery and urology: long-term outcomes*. London: WB Saunders, 1998: 519–530

Ransley PG, Risdon RA, Goldy ML. High pressure sterile vesicoureteral reflux and renal scarring: an experimental study in the pig and minipig. *Contrib Nephrol* 1984; 39: 320–343

Rushton HG. Vesicoureteral reflux new concepts and techniques. *J Urol* 1997; 57: 1414–1415

Thomas DFM. Vesicoureteric reflux. In: Thomas DFM (ed) *Urological disease of the fetus and infant*. Oxford: Butterworth-Heinemann, 1997: 213–214

Verrier Jones K. Prognosis for vesico ureteric reflux. *Arch Dis Child* 1999; 81: 287–289

Yeung CK, Godley ML, Dhillon HK, Gordon I, Duffy PG, Ransley PG. The characteristics of primary VUR in male and female infants with prenatal hydronephrosis. *Br J Urol* 1997; 80: 319–327

Key points

- Voiding dysfunction plays an important role in the aetiology of 'primary' VUR, particularly in girls. Active treatment of voiding dysfunction is an important aspect of medical management.
- VUR is not a single entity. Treatment should be individualised to encompass the individual contributory factors.
- Nevertheless, medical management can be safely employed as the initial line of treatment for most children with VUR, with surgical intervention being reserved for specific indications.

Upper tract obstruction: pathophysiology and diagnosis

6

David CS Gough

Topics covered
Terminology – definition of 'obstruction'
Pathophysiology of acute and chronic upper tract obstruction

Diagnosis
    Ultrasound
    Isotope renography
    Pressure/flow study (Whitaker test)
    Urography, pyelography

Introduction

There is no universally accepted scientific definition of obstruction, despite the fact that a substantial part of paediatric and adult urological practice is devoted to diagnosing and treating this condition. However, one widely used working definition characterises obstruction as 'some impedance to flow of urine which causes gradual and progressive damage to the kidney'. The terminology used by urologists and radiologists has not been helpful in advancing our understanding of obstruction, particularly when pathological and descriptive terms such 'pelviureteric junction (PUJ) obstruction', 'idiopathic hydronephrosis', or 'vesico-ureteric junction obstruction' and 'primary mega-ureter' have been used synonymously. It is still not uncommon for these terms to be used interchangeably and they may even be applied to the same patient by different clinicians, depending on their interpretation of the investigations.

The introduction of isotope renography has proved a major advance in the diagnosis of obstruction, but even this is potentially unreliable in a number of important clinical situations.

Researchers investigating the role of different diagnostic tests have tended to assume that there is some objective definition of obstruction against which new investigations can be judged. Unfortunately this is not the case, and the proverbial 'gold standard' for the diagnosis of obstruction continues to elude us. In the absence of a definitive scientific definition of obstruction, clinical decision making will continue to be dependent on information from a number of different investigations, each with its own limitations.

Hydronephrosis

Although the term 'hydronephrosis' is often used synonymously with pelviureteric junction obstruction, this is not correct. Hydronephrosis is not a diagnosis in itself, but a descriptive term denoting pathological dilatation of the renal pelvis and calyces. When the ureter is also dilated, the corresponding term hydroureteronephrosis is used. Hydronephrosis (dilatation) may be a feature of a number of acquired or developmental urological disorders, most commonly:

- Obstruction to urinary drainage
- Vesicoureteric reflux
- Dysplasia and developmental abnormalities of the upper urinary tract
- Abnormally high urinary output ('flow uropathy').

More than one of these causes may be present in the same individual. For example, in a child with a duplex kidney there might be acquired hydronephrosis secondary to bladder outlet obstruction caused by a prolapsing ureterocoele in addition to congenital dilatation of the upper pole ureter associated with the ureterocoele. Dilatation of the lower pole of the duplex kidney might also result from reflux into the lower pole ureter, particularly in the presence of elevated voiding pressures resulting from the bladder outflow obstruction.

High urinary output is a rare cause of hydronephrosis and, when it occurs, is usually the result of nephrogenic diabetes insipidus. 'Flow uropathy' is usually bilateral and the dilatation is mild.

Pathophysiology of obstruction

Acute obstruction can be reproduced experimentally and the sequence of physiological events within the kidney is well documented. Acute obstruction is relatively uncommon in children and generally results from acute pelviureteric junction obstruction or, occasionally, impaction of a urinary calculus at the pelvi-ureteric or vesicoureteric junction. The initial sequence of pathological events in the obstructed kidney consists of reabsorption of urine from the collecting system into the interstitium, increased intrarenal pressure and decreased renal blood flow. Progressive nephron damage supervenes, with the loss of approximately 50% of functioning nephrons after 6 days and the irreversible loss of all renal function within 6 weeks. The timescale of renal damage is rapidly accelerated by the presence of urinary infection (pyonephrosis).

Chronic or partial obstruction is more difficult to diagnose and the risk of functional deterioration more difficult to predict. In the past the majority of children presented clinically with symptoms, and the decision to intervene surgically was easier to justify. With the advent of routine antenatal ultrasound, however, it is clear that mild to moderate hydronephrosis is more prevalent in healthy, asymptomatic infants than was previously recognised. In many such cases there is no evidence of active obstruction or renal impairment, and the natural history is one of progressive improvement. Even when obstruction is positively diagnosed by appropriate investigation there is nevertheless a well-documented potential for spontaneous resolution over time. Conversely, some obstructed kidneys are at risk of progressive functional deterioration which may prove irreversible. The practical dilemma, therefore, is how best to identify those infants who are likely to benefit from surgical intervention.

Investigation

Although the presence of dilatation does not necessarily denote active obstruction, it is generally true that obstruction does not occur without evidence of dilatation: the early stages of acute obstruction, e.g. by an impacted calculus, being a rare exception to this rule.

Ultrasound

The diagnostic pathway almost invariably commences with the ultrasound finding of dilatation. It is important

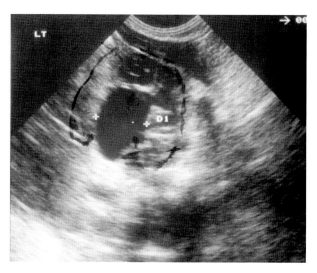

Figure 6.1 Ultrasound image demonstrating dilatation of the renal pelvis. Formal measurement of the renal pelvic anteroposterior diameter is preferable to the use of subjective descriptions such as 'mild', 'moderate' or 'gross' dilatation, or 'hydronephrosis'.

to note, however, that ultrasound cannot distinguish reliably between the different causes of dilatation, and cannot be used to establish the diagnosis of obstruction.

Although certain parameters of the ultrasound study can provide clues to the presence of obstruction, these are not always of prognostic value. For example, measurements of cortical thickness and overall renal length do not correlate closely with other parameters of obstruction. The measurement shown to be of most value is the anterior–posterior (AP) diameter of the renal pelvis measured at the renal hilum (Figure 6.1). Although in the neonate this does not normally exceed 6 mm, an AP diameter of less than 15 mm is most unlikely to denote significant obstruction posing a threat to renal function. Conversely, an AP diameter exceeding 50 mm is usually associated with diminished function, either at the time of initial assessment or during the course of follow-up.

Ureteric dilatation must always be regarded as an abnormal finding, as a ureter of normal calibre cannot be visualised on ultrasound. Because ultrasound does not reliably distinguish between the various causes of ureteric dilatation additional investigation is always merited.

Resistive index is measured by use of a Doppler ultrasound probe directed at a branch of the renal artery. Changes in arterial flow during systole and diastole result in changes in the Doppler signal, which are expressed graphically in a waveform from which

$$RI = \frac{\text{systolic} - \text{diastolic}}{\text{systolic}}$$

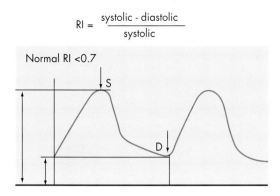

Figure 6.2 Diagrammatic representation of renal artery Doppler ultrasound pattern illustrating parameters used for the calculation of resistive index.

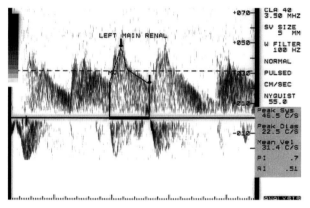

Figure 6.3 Normal Doppler ultrasound trace, normal resistive index, normal kidney.

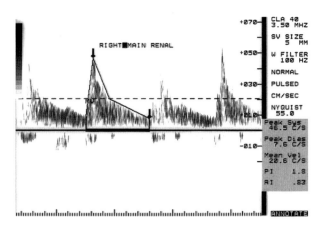

Figure 6.4 Abnormal Doppler ultrasound trace with an elevated resistive index in a normal kidney. Measurement of resistive index is not a reliable guide to the presence of obstruction in children.

the resistive index can be calculated (Figures 6.2, 6.3). An elevated resistive index has been shown to correlate with obstruction in adults, but it is far more difficult to obtain reproducible data in infants, in whom the resistive index fluctuates in response to factors such as movement and respiration. Furthermore, the few reported studies in this age group have failed to demonstrate a valid relationship between resistive index and other parameters of obstruction (Figure 6.4). For these reasons, measurement of resistive index has not found a role in routine clinical evaluation.

Isotope renography is the principal investigation used to diagnose upper tract obstruction. The first radiopharmaceutical to be used for this purpose was ^{131}I hippuran, but it was only with the availability of ^{99m}Tc DTPA (diethylenetriamine penta-acetic acid) that isotope renography became widely adopted in urological practice. The drawbacks of DTPA include

slow clearance rate, high background activity, and the requirement for the child to lie still for 30 minutes after the injection. However, DTPA has the advantage that imaging can be combined with a clearance study to permit estimation of GFR (glomerular filtration rate).

[99m]Tc MAG3 (mercaptoacetyl triglycine) is cleared largely by tubular secretion and has been widely adopted as the radiopharmaceutical of choice. Gamma camera images are superior to those of DTPA, studies can be performed more rapidly and background subtraction calculations are easier. The following components of the dynamic renogram are routinely analysed in the investigation of possible obstruction:

● **Differential renal function** This is derived by comparing isotope uptake in the two kidneys, which in turn is a measure of renal blood flow. Although different centres vary in the part of the uptake phase they use for this calculation, very similar results are achieved. Isotope uptake by the liver or spleen can interfere with the computerised analysis of differential uptake and renal handling of DTPA or MAG3, and may be significantly compromised by the presence of obstruction, resulting in considerable disparity between the figures for differential function yielded by dynamic renography compared with static scintigraphy with DMSA.

Since DMSA provides a more reproducible value for differential function when function is severely impaired, this is the preferred investigation to determine whether a poorly functioning obstructed kidney should be removed or undergo pyeloplasty. Regardless of whether differential function is assessed by DTPA, MAG3 or DMSA, it is important to note that the functional components of all these studies provides a comparative rather than absolute measure of renal function.

- **Renogram curves** Diuresis renography was pioneered by O'Reilly and associates as a means of distinguishing between obstructive and non-obstructive dilatation. The characteristics of the uptake and drainage curves fall into four patterns (Figure 6.5):

Type 1: normal uptake with prompt washout;

Type 2: rising uptake curve, no response to diuretic (obstruction);

Type 3a: an initially rising curve which falls rapidly in response to injection of lasix (non-obstructive dilatation);

Type 3b: an initially rising curve which neither falls promptly following the injection of lasix nor continues to rise. This renogram pattern was defined by O'Reilly and colleagues as equivocal, and much of their subsequent work has been aimed at eliminating the type 3b curve by modifying the technique and timing of lasix administration.

Although there is general agreement that the type 1 and type 3a curves are normal and non-obstructive, there is still disagreement regarding the clinical significance of type 2 and 3b curves. The interpretation of drainage curves is particularly problematic in the first few months of life (the period of so-called 'transitional nephrology'), when immaturity of renal tubular function may result in an impaired diuretic response to lasix. To circumvent this difficulty many paediatric urologists now base the decision on whether or not to proceed to pyeloplasty in infants with asymptomatic prenatally detected PUJ obstruction principally on differential function in the affected kidney, rather than an drainage curve data.

A cut-off figure for differential function of 40% has been widely used, but at best this represents only a very pragmatic guide to clinical management. Histological studies on parenchymal tissue obtained at the time of pyeloplasty have demonstrated pathological damage in 20% of obstructed kidneys retaining more than 40% differential function, whereas, conversely, a third of kidneys with less than 40% function showed only minor histological changes.

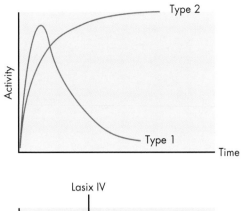

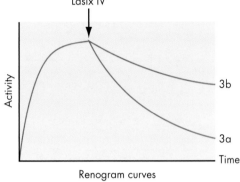

Figure 6.5 Patterns of uptake and drainage curves on isotope renography, as classified by O'Reilly and associates.

Pressure/flow studies

Developed and popularised by Whitaker in the 1970s, this investigation was designed to quantify obstruction by measuring the hydrostatic pressure within the kidney when the collecting system is directly filled with fluid at different rates of flow (Figure 6.6). Renal puncture under general anaesthesia is required and the investigation is time-consuming. For these reasons it has been largely superseded by isotope renography. Nevertheless, the Whitaker test made a significant contribution to our understanding of upper tract obstruction and still retains a role in the investigation of kidneys with poor function (which are inadequately imaged by MAG3 renography or intravenous urography) and in the diagnosis of recurrent PUJ obstruction or of vesicoureteric junction obstruction.

Urinary markers of obstructive uropathy

A number of substances such as N-acetyl-β-D-glucosaminidase (NAG) and transforming growth factor β (TGFβ) which are predominantly markers of

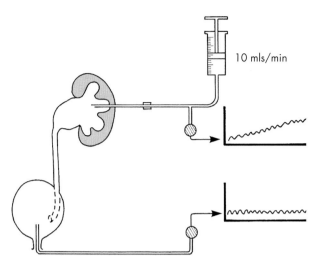

Figure 6.6 Principle of the pressure/flow ('Whitaker') test. Intrarenal and intravesical pressures are measured simultaneously at different rates of perfusion of the renal pelvis (typically 10 ml/min in adults). Obstruction is associated with an elevated pressure differential.

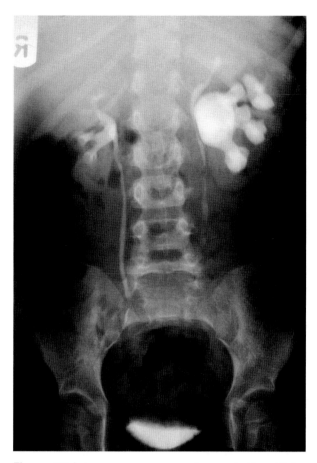

Figure 6.7 Intravenous urogram demonstrating dilatation confined to the lower pole of a duplex kidney (PUJ obstruction in an incomplete duplication – 'bifid system'). The IVU retains a useful role in delineating ureteric or caliceal anatomy in unusual variants of upper tract obstruction.

tubular damage, have been studied with the aim of identifying those obstructed kidneys at greatest risk of functional deterioration (on the rationale that glomerular damage is often preceded by tubular concentrating defects). Although this is an attractive concept the specificity has proved to be unacceptably low, with considerable overlap between 'obstructed' values and the normal range, particularly where the renal pathology is unilateral.

Intravenous urography

Although the IVU has been superseded by dynamic renography there are situations when it can provide valuable anatomical information which is not forthcoming from other imaging modalities. Examples include midureteric obstruction and retrocaval ureter (although this is also well demonstrated on CT), PUJ obstruction in the lower pole of a duplex kidney (Figure 6.7), and isolated calyceal obstruction due to infundibular stenosis. Intravenous urography is relatively easy to perform in an emergency and can sometimes provide valuable information on suspected obstruction when isotope imaging is not available. Finally, some surgeons still insist on an IVU before embarking on pyeloplasty, to demonstrate the surgical anatomy and confirm the affected side with absolute certainty.

Retrograde pyelography

Reliance on retrograde pyelography to confirm the anatomical level of obstruction immediately prior to surgery has declined following the introduction of other imaging modalities, notably ultrasound, which will provide this information by less invasive means. However, there are still rare situations in which retrograde pyelography may prove valuable if the level of obstruction is in doubt, and if this information is relevant to the choice of incision and surgical procedure.

Antegrade pyelography

Renal puncture under ultrasound guidance and the injection of contrast into the collecting system can be performed in conjunction with a pressure perfusion

(Whitaker) test, or solely as an imaging study. Antegrade pyelography is preferable to retrograde pyelography in most situations, and can be particularly helpful in visualising obstruction distal to the pelvi-ureteric junction and in the investigation of suspected cases of recurrent PUJ obstruction following previous pyeloplasty.

Diagnostic pathway

In summary, the clinical investigation of hydronephrosis is designed to answer the following questions:

- **Is the dilatation due to active obstruction?** Isotope renography is the firstline investigation but other modalities may be needed to exclude reflux and non-obstructive dilatation.
- **At what anatomical level is the obstruction (and what is the most likely pathology)?** Ultrasound generally provides this information, but intravenous urography and/or antegrade or retrograde pyelography may also be required.
- **Is the function in the obstructed kidney sufficient to justify a conservative procedure or would nephrectomy be more appropriate?** Isotope renography with ^{99m}Tc MAG3 study will generally suffice, but when renal function is grossly impaired ^{99m}Tc DMSA is a more accurate measure of function and a more reliable predictor of functional recovery.

Key points

- There is no agreed scientific diagnosis of obstruction and no 'gold standard' diagnostic test.
- Clinical management often depends on information derived from a number of different investigations, each of which is subject to technical limitations.
- Although ^{99m}Tc MAG3 is the isotope of choice for most aspects of the investigation of obstruction, ^{99m}Tc DMSA provides a more reliable assessment of differential function in the presence of renal impairment, and is a more reliable predictor of functional outcome following pyeloplasty.
- The pressure/flow (Whitaker) test has a very limited role in children, but in some circumstances intravenous urography or antegrade pyelography may provide valuable additional information.

Further reading

O'Reilly PH, Testa HJ, Lawson RS et al. Diuresis renography in equivocal urinary tract obstruction. *Br J Urol* 1978; 64: 124–129

Palmer LS, Maizels M, Kaplan WE et al. Urine levels of transforming growth factor-beta in children with ureteropelvic obstruction. *Urol* 1997; 50: 769–773

Platt JF, Robin JM, Ellis JA. Distinction between obstructive and non obstructive peylocalyecstasis with duplex doppler sonography. *Am J Radiol* 1989; 153: 997–1000

Whittaker RH. Methods of assessing obstruction in dilated ureters. *Br J Urol* 1973; 45: 15–22

Upper tract obstruction: clinical management

7

David CS Gough and David FM Thomas

Topics covered
Pelviureteric junction obstruction
  Clinical presentation
  Prenatal diagnosis
  Surgical and non-surgical management

Vesicoureteric junction obstruction
  Presentation
  Management

Pelviureteric junction obstruction

Pelviureteric junction (PUJ) obstruction is a heterogeneous disorder with a number of different anatomical causes which exhibits considerable variation in severity and natural history.

The true incidence in the paediatric population is difficult to establish, as PUJ obstruction is frequently asymptomatic. Estimates derived from antenatal screening put the incidence in the range 1:750–1:1000, but this figure is derived largely from second-trimester scanning when a substantial proportion of cases are still undetectable on ultrasound. Postnatally the calculation is complicated on the one hand by the fact that prenatally detected PUJ obstruction can resolve spontaneously, and on the other by the well documented potential for PUJ obstruction to arise de novo in previously normal kidneys. As an approximate guide, 1:1000–1:1500 individuals undergo pyeloplasty for PUJ obstruction at some stage in their childhood.

The male to female ratio is approximately equal and the left kidney is more commonly affected than the right, by a ratio of approximately 2:1. Although PUJ obstruction generally occurs as a sporadic anomaly familial inheritance has been reported, with a pattern suggesting autosomal dominant inheritance with incomplete penetrance. The incidence of PUJ obstruction is increased in the presence of other urinary tract anomalies, such as multicystic dysplastic kidney, and in children with multiple anomalies, particularly the VACTERL spectrum of anorectal and vertebral malformations.

Pathology and aetiology of PUJ obstruction

Although the appearances on intravenous urography can sometimes give a clue to the precise anatomical cause of the obstruction it is not usually until the time of surgery that this can be established with certainty.

Intrinsic obstruction (Figure 7.1a)

Typically the obstruction is caused by a short stenotic segment of ureter at the pelviureteric junction, but the narrowing may sometimes extend distally from the PUJ to involve a longer segment of upper ureter.

Ureteric folds (Figure 7.1b)

Although the PUJ is of normal calibre the proximal ureter is tortuous and kinked. This anatomical pattern is often associated with self-limiting obstruction, which gives rise to characteristic appearances on intravenous urography in later childhood, the upper ureter looking like a curly pig's tail!

'High insertion' of the pelviureteric junction

The PUJ is sited high on the dilated renal pelvis rather than at its most dependent part. Although this may contribute to poor drainage, it is generally ascribed to upwards displacement of the junction by the dilated pelvis, and as such is an effect rather than a cause of the obstruction.

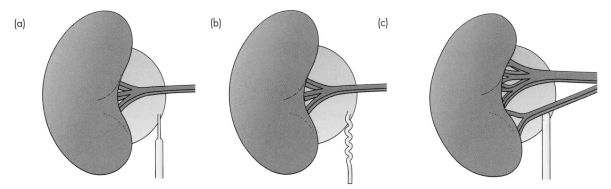

Figure 7.1 Aetiology of pelviureteric junction obstruction. (a) Intrinsic stenosis. Obstruction due to narrowing of a segment of ureter which is usually localised to the region of the pelviureteric junction but may extend over a length of several centimetres. (b) Ureteric folds. Tortuous segment of proximal ureter giving rise to varying degrees of obstruction. Straightening of this segment with growth may explain the spontaneous resolution of obstruction observed in a proportion of prenatally detected cases. (c) Extrinsic obstruction by crossing lower pole vessels.

Extrinsic obstruction: lower pole or 'crossing' vessels (Figure 7.1c)

Aberrant or 'crossing' vessels are found in approximately 30% of older children and adults presenting with PUJ obstruction, but their clinical significance is often difficult to ascertain. In some cases the lower pole vessels are simply incidental to an intrinsic PUJ obstruction, but in other instances (particularly older children presenting with intermittent loin pain), 'crossing vessels' do appear to be implicated as a genuine cause of obstruction, as evidenced by the relief of symptoms following pyeloplasty in which the pelviureteric junction is relocated anterior to the vessels. In contrast, lower pole vessels are rarely encountered in infants, being present in fewer than 5% of cases of prenatally detected PUJ obstruction coming to pyeloplasty.

Variants of PUJ obstruction

Horseshoe kidney (Figures 7.2, 7.3)

Obstructed drainage occurs either because of distortion of the proximal ureter as it loops over the renal isthmus, or because of compression of the pelviureteric junction and proximal ureter by the aberrant vessels commonly found at the renal hilum of horseshoe kidneys.

Retrocaval ureter

This rare anomaly, which more commonly affects the right ureter, is a consequence of abnormal development

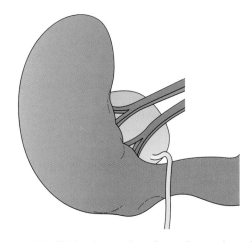

Figure 7.2 PUJ obstruction in a horseshoe kidney caused by distortion of the proximal ureter looping over the renal isthmus (or compression by aberrant vasculature).

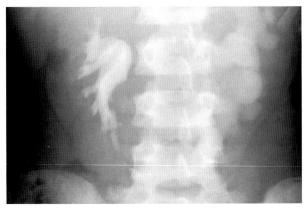

Figure 7.3 Intravenous urogram demonstrating dilatation associated with obstruction in the left limb of a horseshoe kidney.

of the posterior cardinal veins, the precursors of the inferior vena cava. A number of anatomical patterns have been described resulting in varying degrees of compression of the ureter between the vertebrae and inferior vena cava.

Intraluminal obstruction

Cases of ureteric obstruction by intraluminal fibroepithelial polyps have been reported, more often in the midureter rather than the pelviureteric junction. Ureteric folds are considered above.

Idiopathic 'functional' obstruction

Urine is normally expelled from the renal pelvis by a peristaltic contraction initiated by pacemaker sites located in each of the minor calices. Failure of peristaltic activity or discoordination of pacemaker activity is thought to account for those cases of 'obstruction' in which the pelviureteric junction is patent and there is no evidence of extrinsic compression. The phenomenon of 'functional' obstruction is more commonly encountered in adults, whereas in paediatric practice one of the anatomical factors listed above is almost invariably present.

Secondary PUJ obstruction

Gross vesicoureteric reflux, e.g. grades IV or V, can result in marked tortuosity and kinking of the proximal ureter, which in turn results in secondary obstruction of the pelviureteric junction. This phenomenon is most apparent on the MCU after voiding, with retention of urine within the obstructed pelvis, but in time this may progress to a more permanent PUJ obstruction (Figure 7.4).

Natural history of PUJ obstruction

The natural history of PUJ obstruction varies considerably. Whereas in some kidneys the obstruction resolves spontaneously, in others it becomes increasingly severe, giving rise to progressive functional deterioration. In a substantial proportion, however, the obstruction remains stable with no impact on renal function over many years. In a series of children with prenatally detected PUJ obstruction who were initially managed conservatively at Great Ormond Street Hospital, 17% came to pyeloplasty because of deteriorating function; 27% showed evidence of resolving obstruction and 56% remained stable, with persisting obstruction but no functional deterioration. To

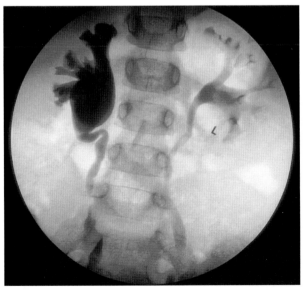

(a)

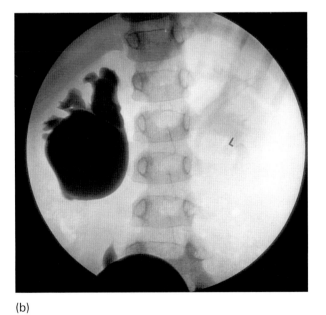

(b)

Figure 7.4 'Secondary' PUJ obstruction associated with vesicoureteric reflux. (a) Dilatation of the right renal collecting system seen on the early phase of a micturating cystogram. (b) Progressive dilatation throughout the course of the MCU study. The degree of dilatation is grossly disproportionate to the severity of the reflux. PUJ obstruction subsequently confirmed by isotope renography (performed with a bladder catheter in situ to eliminate confusion due to reflux of isotope).

confuse the picture further, it is well documented that progressive obstruction and dilatation can occur in a previously normal or mildly dilated kidney. At present broad predictions of outcome can be made on the basis of ultrasound and other parameters, but it is not possible to make a precise prediction of the outcome in an individual case.

Presentation

Prenatal ultrasound (Figure 7.5) Pelviureteric junction obstruction is the most common form of prenatally detected hydronephrosis and accounts for 30–50% of all significant uropathies detected by prenatal ultrasound. Mild to moderate obstruction does not usually give rise to detectable dilatation at the time when fetal anomaly scans are routinely performed in the second trimester, and more commonly comes to light on scans performed in later pregnancy.

The severity of the dilatation is a more accurate predictor of functional outcome than the gestational age at which the dilatation was first detected, and where the anteroposterior diameter of the renal pelvis exceeds 3.0 cm the probability of functional impairment in the obstructed kidney is between 60 and 100%, depending on the severity of dilatation.

Before the introduction of antenatal ultrasound **urinary tract infection** was the most frequent form of presentation in infants and young children and it is still relatively common for PUJ obstruction to be diagnosed during the investigation of urinary infection. Pyonephrosis may supervene, with a high fever, systemic ill health and ultrasound findings of pus and infective debris in the collecting system.

Pain is not a prominent feature of prenatally detected hydronephrosis, although some parents do sometimes comment that their child is less fractious and generally happier following pyeloplasty. Typically, pain occurs in children 4 years and upwards and is often severe and accompanied by vomiting. Unlike non-specific abdominal pain it usually extends over a period varying from several hours to several days, and examination during the acute phase often reveals both loin and abdominal tenderness. Episodes of pain are generally self-limiting, although occasionally a child presents with intractable pain which is only relieved by percutaneous nephrostomy. Older children presenting within episodic pain are more likely to have PUJ obstruction associated with crossing vessels.

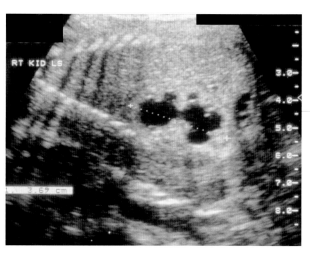

Figure 7.5 Prenatal ultrasound. Marked dilatation of a fetal kidney – PUJ obstruction confirmed by postnatal investigations.

Haematuria may occur spontaneously, but is more commonly the consequence of minor trauma – to which hydronephrotic kidneys are more susceptible.

Grossly hydronephrotic kidneys are now usually detected on prenatal ultrasound and only rarely does the condition present unexpectedly as an **abdominal mass** in the neonatal period. However, it can sometimes present as an abdominal mass in later childhood, when it can be readily distinguished from a Wilms' tumour by ultrasound and CT (Figure 7.6). A dilated kidney sometimes comes to light as an **incidental ultrasound finding** on an abdominal scan performed for unrelated symptoms such as

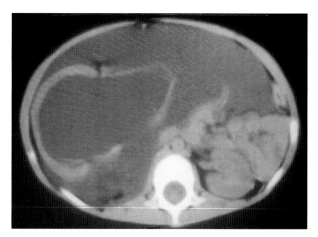

Figure 7.6 CT scan demonstrating a grossly dilated right kidney with a thin rim of renal cortex. This kidney has ruptured after trauma, leading to extensive extravasation.

nocturnal enuresis or abdominal pain. It is important to take a careful history to distinguish between pain which may genuinely be due to PUJ obstruction (see above) and non-specific abdominal pain, which is usually more transient and typically central abdominal.

Investigation

The diagnostic pathway in most cases of PUJ obstruction adopts the following sequence:

- **Ultrasound** – to demonstrate dilatation, provide information on the severity of hydronephrosis and thickness of the renal cortex and indicate the probable level of obstruction;
- **Isotope renography MAG3^{Tc99}** – to distinguish between obstructive and non-obstructive dilatation and quantify differential function; in some cases additional information is provided by:
- **DMSA scintigraphy** – to assess severely impaired renal function and inform the decision as to whether to proceed to pyeloplasty or nephrectomy;
- **Intravenous urography** – to demonstrate anatomy before surgery, particularly in variants such as retrocaval ureter or horseshoe kidney;
- **Micturating cystourethrography** – to investigate possible coexisting vesicoureteric reflux, especially when ureteric dilatation has been visualised on ultrasound.

Management

This was more straightforward in the days before prenatal diagnosis, when children with PUJ obstruction presented with symptoms and the decision to proceed to surgery could be justified on this basis. By contrast, the majority of infants with prenatally detected PUJ obstruction are healthy and entirely asymptomatic, and although there was initially a phase when pyeloplasty was performed routinely it is now undertaken more selectively.

Opinion remains divided on the precise criteria for surgical intervention, but conservative management is generally adopted for obstructed kidneys retaining normal levels of differential function (defined as greater than 40% in the affected kidney). However, functional assessment with isotopes does not correlate closely with the histological events within the obstructed kidney. In one study 21% of kidneys with greater than 40% differential function nevertheless showed evidence of significant histological damage on renal biopsies obtained at the time of pyeloplasty whereas almost a third of kidneys with less than 40% function showed only minor histological changes.

With the introduction of prenatal diagnosis and the consequent increase in the number of infants undergoing pyeloplasty, we might justifiably ask: 'Are we overdiagnosing and overtreating pelviureteric junction obstruction in children?' The findings of a recent American study, however, suggest that although there had been a trend towards much earlier surgery during the 20-year period 1970–1990, the overall pyeloplasty rate in children is unchanged.

Conservative management is initiated when differential function in the obstructed kidney exceeds 40% and the renal pelvic AP diameter is less than 20–30 mm (surgical opinion differs as to the precise figure chosen as the upper limit for conservative management).

In 15–20% of infants with prenatally detected PUJ obstruction the condition occurs bilaterally. In these cases less reliance can be placed on the renographic assessment of differential function and greater weight must be attached to the severity of the hydronephrosis. Bilateral pyeloplasty may be indicated when the dilatation is of equal severity and both drainage curves appear symmetrically obstructed. However, it is not uncommon to find a difference in the severity of hydronephrosis in the two kidneys, and it may be appropriate to operate on the more severely dilated one and monitor its less dilated counterpart.

The **indications for pyeloplasty** can be broadly summarised as:

- Symptomatic PUJ obstruction, e.g. pain, infection, palpable renal mass;
- Asymptomatic obstruction with reduced function (<40%) at the time of initial evaluation, particularly if the AP diameter of the renal pelvis exceeds 30 mm;
- Failure of conservative management, i.e. deteriorating function or increasing dilatation (which often precedes functional deterioration);
- Persisting asymptomatic obstruction where there is good preservation of function but no evidence of resolving obstruction despite prolonged follow-up. The point at which conservative management should be abandoned in such cases is the subject of debate.

Surgical options

In the debate surrounding minimal access surgery its possible role in the treatment of PUJ obstruction has not been overlooked. However, the results published to date are distinctly inferior to those obtained with conventional open surgery, and for the foreseeable future it is likely that the Anderson–Hynes dismembered pyeloplasty will remain the procedure of choice. The key points are summarised below, but for a detailed account the reader should consult a textbook of operative paediatric urology or paediatric surgery.

Surgical approach to the kidney

The anterior extraperitoneal approach is ideally suited to infants and younger children (Figure 7.7a), but access is more limited in older children with a narrower subcostal angle. Although the posterior lumbotomy (Figure 7.7b) is favoured by some surgeons because of ease of access to the kidney and reduced postoperative discomfort, it provides less flexibility to deal with lower pole vessels or unexpected operative findings. The 'supra-12 loin' approach, conserving the 12th rib (Figure 7.7c), can be employed for all age groups but gives rise to greater postoperative discomfort and carries a risk of subcostal nerve neuropraxia in infants.

Pyeloplasty – technical considerations

Once the anatomy of the pelviuretric junction has been displayed the ureter is divided and incised for a short length ('spatulated') just distal to the pelviureteric junction and a portion of the redundant dilated renal pelvis excised. For the initial stages of the anastomosis most paediatric urologists favour interrupted sutures, and even in unstented pyeloplasty it may be advisable to minimise the risk of stenosis by performing the anastomosis over a feeding tube, which is then withdrawn prior to closure of the renal pelvis.

The pyeloplasty techniques described by Culp-De Weerd (Figure 7.8) and Foley give inferior long-term results to the Anderson–Hynes operation (Figure 7.9) and are rarely used in paediatric practice.

Much has been written about the different forms of postoperative drainage, but published studies have mostly failed to demonstrate any statistically significant advantage of one method over the other. In

children the most widely used techniques include nephrostomy drainage with transanastomotic splintage, extrarenal drainage alone and, increasingly, the use of an indwelling JJ stent. Nephrostomy drainage alone is inadvisable as the diversion of urine above an unsplinted anastomosis may encourage adherence of

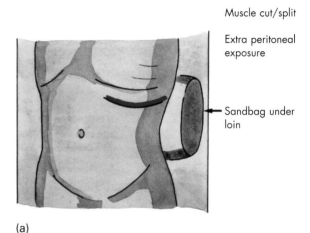

(a)

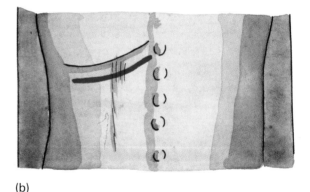

(b)

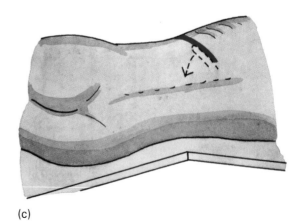

(c)

Figure 7.7 Surgical approach to the kidney. (a) Anterior subcostal incision, extraperitoneal exposure of the kidney. (b) Posterior lumbotomy. (c) 'Supra-12' loin incision.

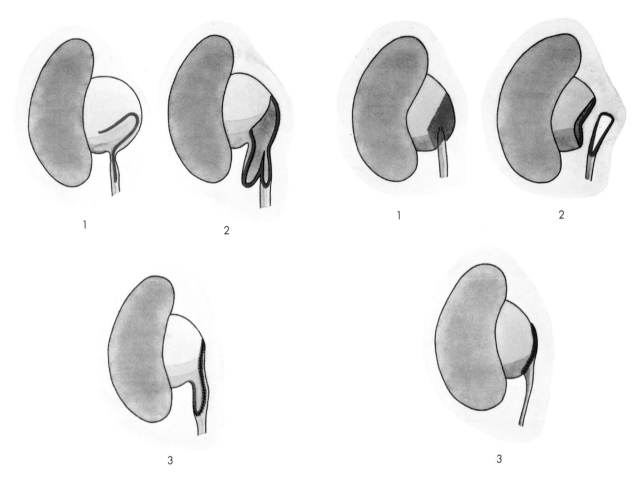

Figure 7.8 Culp-De Weerd pyeloplasty. Flap of renal pelvis rotated across the pelviureteric junction.

Figure 7.9 Anderson–Hynes dismembered pyeloplasty. The procedure of choice in children.

the edges of the anastomosis and lead to a greater risk of recurrent obstruction.

Postoperative follow-up typically comprises ultrasound and isotope renography (although it may be reasonable to omit the latter if ultrasonography at 6–12 months clearly demonstrates resolution of the dilatation, indicating that obstruction has been successfully relieved. Assessing the postoperative ultrasound appearances in a grossly dilated system can prove problematic, as considerable dilatation commonly persists for a long time despite a technically successful pyeloplasty. Similarly, it may be a matter of years rather than months before a normal drainage curve can be demonstrated on isotope renography.

Results

The Anderson–Hynes pyeloplasty gives consistently satisfactory results in children with several large

published series reporting reoperation rates in the region of only 3–5%. In infants with gross prenatally detected hydronephrosis, however, the long-term success rate may prove slightly less satisfactory.

Other surgical options

Percutaneous nephrostomy

The insertion of a pigtail catheter into the kidney to provide temporary drainage is a particularly valuable manoeuvre in children presenting with pyonephrosis, as it facilitates treatment of the infection and permits antegrade studies and assessment of recoverable function with DMSA prior to definitive surgery. Although a period of percutaneous drainage was once favoured to assess the potential recovery of function in infants with severe prenatally detected hydronephrosis, this has largely been abandoned because it rarely resulted in any useful improvement in function.

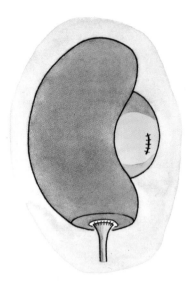

Figure 7.10 Ureterocalicostomy. The ureter is disconnected from the renal pelvis and the pelviureteric junction closed. The ureter is then anastomosed directly to the lower pole calyx. A useful procedure to facilitate dependent drainage in a grossly dilated system or horseshoe kidney and in cases of recurrent PUJ obstruction.

Ureterocalicostomy (Figure 7.10)

In this procedure the ureter is detached from the renal pelvis and anastomosed directly to the most dependent lower pole calix. Although rarely appropriate for the primary management of PUJ obstruction, ureterocalicostomy may prove more effective than pyeloplasty as a means of securing reliable drainage in recurrent PUJ obstruction or PUJ obstruction complicating horseshoe kidney.

Percutaneous endopyelotomy

To date, the published results of percutaneous endopyelotomy and laparoscopic pyeloplasty in children have been markedly inferior to those for conventional open dismembered pyeloplasty, as exemplified by a 23% failure rate with percutaneous endopyelotomy in one published series. At present these must be considered experimental procedures that should be confined to a few specialist centres. Balloon dilatation, however, does have a limited role in the treatment of mild to moderate recurrent PUJ obstruction, particularly in older children.

Nephrectomy

When deciding whether to advise pyeloplasty or nephrectomy, most paediatric urologists apply a nominal 'cut-off' for differential function in the range

10–15%. The decision to proceed to nephrectomy should be based on information derived from DMSA, as the figure yielded by MAG3 and DTPA is less reliable in the presence of renal impairment. The normality or otherwise of the contralateral kidney is clearly another important consideration. A period of temporary percutaneous drainage may indicate the potential for recovery, as considered above.

Vesicoureteric junction obstruction

The terminology used to describe and classify the different causes of ureteric dilatation (megaureter) has been a source of considerable confusion. Three broad categories are now accepted:

- **Obstructed megaureter:** the obstruction is usually intrinsic, e.g. primary stenosis of the distal ureter or vesicoureteric junction, but may occasionally be extrinsic, e.g. tumour, or secondary to scarring and fibrosis. Most cases are due to primary obstruction at the vesicoureteric junction, hence the synonym 'VUJ obstruction'.
- **Non-refluxing, non-obstructed megaureter:** the ureter is dilated but no evidence of active obstruction or reflux can be demonstrated. The aetiology of non-refluxing, non-obstructed megaureter is often unclear, but it is believed that in many cases it represents the legacy of 'burnt-out' vesicoureteric junction obstruction.
- **Refluxing megaureter.**

Obstructed megaureter
Aetiology

Obstructed megaureter is characterised by a marked discrepancy between the calibre of the distal ureteric segment and the ureter proximal to it, which is dilated and often tortuous. In most instances the obstruction is associated with the presence of a stenotic segment of variable length, extending proximally from the vesicoureteric junction (Figure 7.11). Occasionally the absolute dimensions of the distal ureter are normal and it is only narrow in relation to the dilatation affecting the remaining ureter. In the absence of any demonstrable stenosis the obstruction is presumed to be due to an adynamic distal ureteric segment, which acts as a functional obstruction by failing to propagate bolus transmission of urine into the bladder.

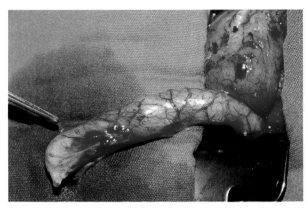

Figure 7.11 Obstructed megaureter. The ureter has been mobilised and divided at the level of the bladder. Dilatation of the ureter proximal to a short stenotic segment at the vesicoureteric junction.

The true prevalence of megaureter (both obstructive and non-obstructive) is difficult to quantify, as before the days of prenatal diagnosis many cases almost certainly failed to come to light. On the basis of information from routine prenatal ultrasound screening the incidence appears to be in the approximate range 1:1500–1:2000. Megaureter occurs more frequently in males and, as with pelviureteric junction obstruction, the left side is more commonly affected than the right. Although it generally arises on a sporadic basis it sometimes features as one of the urinary tract anomalies encountered in families with an inherited tendency to renal malformations.

Presentation

Prenatal detection

Obstructed megaureter accounts for approximately 10% of clinically significant prenatally detected uropathies. Although dilatation of the ureter may be visualised on prenatal ultrasonography it is often the dilatation of the renal collecting system that is detected initially, and indeed the presence of ureteric dilatation may not always be apparent until a postnatal scan. The distinction between obstructed and refluxing megaureters can never be made on ultrasound alone, and postnatal micturating cystourethrography is always indicated to exclude the VUR or, in boys, outflow obstruction due to posterior urethral valves.

Symptomatic presentation

Urinary infection used to be the most common form of presentation and although the condition can now be detected prenatally it continues to present in this way. Infection associated with obstructed megaureter may vary in severity from mild, predominantly lower-tract symptoms to a severe systemic febrile illness accompanied by pus and infected debris within the obstructed collecting system (pyoureteronephrosis). Other modes of presentation include **pain, abdominal swelling** (rare), or symptoms arising from the presence of calculi within the obstructed system. Calculi are more common if the patient has a single system – orthotopic ureterocoele – as a cause of the obstruction.

Investigations

Ultrasound

Ultrasound is a valuable investigation for demonstrating ureteric dilatation, particularly where renal function is poor and the excretion of radiological contrast or isotope tracer is impaired. In addition to assessing calyceal and pelvic dilatation, ultrasound should also visualise the dilated ureter throughout its course and measure the diameter of the mid and distal ureter. Where the ureteric diameter is less than 1 cm, obstruction is rarely severe and renal function is usually preserved, but even when the ureteric diameter exceeds 1 cm differential renal function is often normal, particularly when the calyceal dilatation is only mild or moderate in severity.

Micturating cystourethrogram

As already stated, this investigation should always be undertaken to distinguish between obstruction and vesicoureteric reflux as the possible cause of ureteric dilatation.

Isotope renography

Although isotope renography will reliably assess differential function, drainage curves can be very difficult to interpret and potentially misleading. In particular, the clearance of isotope from the kidney may create the appearance of a non-obstructed system with a relatively normal drainage curve, but inspection of the 'hard-copy' gamma camera image reveals that the tracer has simply emptied from the kidney into the capacious, dilated ureter (Figure 7.12). Attempts to improve the sensitivity of isotope renography by drawing regions of interest over the kidney and different portions of ureter to estimate ureteric emptying

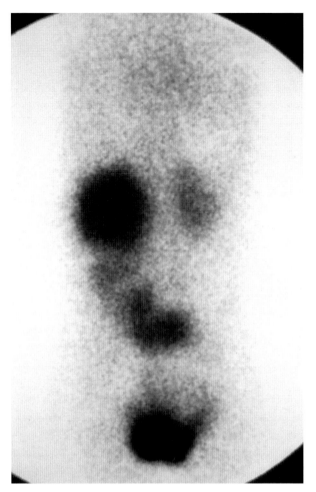

Figure 7.12 MAG3 renogram demonstrating retention of isotope within a grossly dilated right megaureter. Despite detailed analysis of renogram drainage curve data it may be extremely difficult to distinguish between obstructive and non-obstructive megaureter.

have proved unrewarding in children. Considering the controversy surrounding the interpretation of drainage curve appearances in obstructed kidneys, it is hardly surprising that there is little consensus on the interpretation of drainage curve data in diagnosing vesicoureteric junction obstruction.

Management
Prenatally detected obstructed megaureter

As with PUJ obstruction, the majority of affected infants are healthy and asymptomatic at birth and their management follows broadly similar lines. Conservative management is initiated where differential renal function is normal (defined as greater than 40%), with surgery being undertaken on a selective basis for the

indications set out below. In one published series of 17 children with prenatally detected primary VUJ obstruction managed conservatively, no instances of functional deterioration were observed during follow-up averaging 7.3 years. However, in another series of 67 children followed for a mean of 3.1 years, 17% required surgical intervention. Conservative management consists of serial ultrasound and, where indicated, further isotope scans. The optimum duration of follow-up is not known, but in practice children can probably be safely discharged after 3–5 years if there is decreasing dilatation and good preservation of differential function. However, some paediatric urologists prefer to follow these patients through childhood, with further appointments for ultrasound at 10 and 15 years of age.

Indications for surgery
Prenatally detected obstructed megaureter

Surgical intervention should be considered if differential renal function is impaired on initial assessment, but ideally the study should be repeated at 3–6 months of age before proceeding to operation. Deteriorating renal function on follow-up is a further indication for surgery, as is massive dilatation, particularly when accompanied by a palpable kidney or ureter.

Symptomatic complications
Urinary infection

A presenting infection of mild to moderate severity is not an automatic indication for surgery if the other parameters (differential function, ureteric diameter 1 cm or less) are favourable. In such cases it is reasonable to consider antibiotic prophylaxis and a trial of conservative management, but when obstructed megaureter is complicated by recurrent or severe infection (including pyonephrosis and calculi) it should be managed surgically. Other indications include **pain** or an **abdominal mass** or, occasionally, failure to thrive.

Surgical treatment

Definitive treatment consists of excising the obstructing distal segment and reimplanting the ureter into the bladder in a way that facilitates good upper tract drainage without permitting vesicoureteric reflux. However, this goal may be difficult to achieve, particularly in infants with gross ureteric dilatation, in whom the diameter of the ureter may equal the diameter of the bladder.

Wherever possible, reimplantation of a megaureter should be avoided in the first year of life, because of these technical difficulties. In addition, there is good anecdotal evidence that dissection in the perivesical tissues and region of the bladder neck in infancy can result in a degree of neurological damage, with possible impairment of continence in later childhood.

Surgical options in the first year of life

Successful medium-term drainage with a paediatric **indwelling ureteric JJ stent** has been described by a number of authors. Endoscopic insertion is not feasible in this situation, but open cystostomy, dilatation of the ureteric orifice and insertion of a JJ stent is usually well tolerated. The stent can be left in situ for up to 6 months, after which time it may be feasible to proceed to definitive treatment. It is also possible that in some infants the combination of dilatation and stent drainage may be sufficient treatment in its own right.

Although supravesical diversion by terminal or ring ureterostomy was once widely practised in infants with obstructed megaureter, the indications are now very limited. **Ureteric reimplantation** is best deferred until 12 months of age where possible, but may be considered from 6 months upwards depending on the circumstances of the case and the experience of the surgeon.

Surgical treatment from 1 year of age upwards

Mild ureteric dilatation (ureteric diameter approximately 1 cm or less)

The ureter is initially mobilised intravesically (as for a conventional ureteric reimplantation for vesicoureteric reflux; Chapter 5), the stenotic distal segment is excised and the ureter reimplanted in a conventional Cohen cross-trigonal tunnel.

Moderate to severe dilatation

The dilated ureter is identified and mobilised extravesically and the stenosed segment excised. In older children it may be feasible to reimplant the ureter using the original hiatus but because of the difficulty in creating a cross-trigonal antireflux tunnel of adequate length, a Leadbetter–Politano reimplantation is generally preferable, ideally in combination with a psoas hitch (the psoas hitch anchors the entry

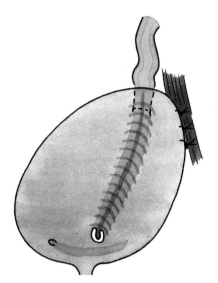

Figure 7.13 The Politano–Leadbetter reimplantation procedure combined with psoas hitch, which is often better suited to megaureters than the Cohen cross-trigonal reimplantation technique.

point of the ureter on the posterior wall of the bladder to a fixed point on the pelvic wall, thus preventing kinking of the ureteroneocystostomy during various phases of bladder filling; Figure 7.13).

To achieve the requisite ratio of ureteric length to width within the submucosal tunnel to avoid reflux, it is often necessary to resort to plication or remodelling of the distal ureter prior to reimplantation. Although tapering ('remodelling') has also been claimed to restore ureteric peristalsis this benefit is probably imaginary. Tapering carries a greater risk of devascularisation and subsequent fibrosis, but gives good long-term results if careful attention is paid to technique. Plication by the Starr or Kalicinski techniques is more straightforward but leads to a bulkier ureter and a greater risk of postoperative reflux (Figure 7.14).

Ureteric peristalsis is greatly impaired in megaureters, and therefore some form of postoperative stenting is necessary, which nowadays commonly consists of a JJ stent left in situ at the time of surgery and removed endoscopically after 6–8 weeks. Alternatively, the reimplanted ureter can be drained externally via a feeding tube for 10–14 days.

Bilateral obstructed megaureters

Because the psoas hitch procedure cannot be performed bilaterally, the technique of choice in this

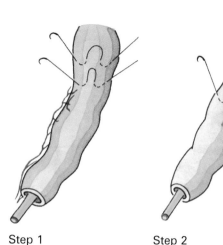

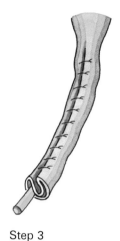

Figure 7.14 Method of ureteric plication using the Starr technique.

Step 1   Step 2   Step 3

unusual situation is a unilateral Leadbetter–Politano reimplantation with psoas hitch (after remodelling or plication if necessary), combined with transureteroureterostomy.

Follow-up

Antibiotic prophylaxis is maintained for 3–6 months and follow-up imaging by ultrasound and isotope renography is undertaken after 6–12 months. Where gross dilatation has been present preoperatively this often persists for a considerable time despite successful correction of the original obstruction, and parents should be warned that there may be very little change on the initial ultrasound appearances.

Follow-up isotope renography is best deferred for at least 6–12 months, as a demonstrable improvement in drainage curve appearances is most unlikely before this time. Even if the drainage curve is still abnormal after 12 months no action need be taken provided the child is well and differential function is maintained. However, further ultrasound and isotope renography is advisable. If no improvement is evident on ultrasound or isotope renography an IVU may be helpful, and where concern persists an antegrade contrast study may be indicated. Any postoperative vesicoureteric reflux is usually mild and self-limiting, but a more prolonged period of postoperative antibiotic prophylaxis is nevertheless advisable.

Key points

- PUJ obstruction is a heterogeneous condition with a number of different causes and a variable natural history.
- Hydronephrosis due to PUJ obstruction accounts for 35–50% of clinically significant prenatally detected uropathies. A renal pelvic diameter exceeding 30 mm is associated with a significant likelihood of functional impairment.
- Conservative management of prenatally detected PUJ obstruction is appropriate when differential function is well preserved and dilatation is mild to moderate in severity.
- When surgery is indicated the Anderson–Hynes dismembered pyeloplasty is the operation of choice.
- Reimplantation of an obstructed megaureter should be avoided in the first year of life, when it has a higher failure rate and carries a greater risk of morbidity.

Further reading

Gough DCS. The dilated urinary system. Clinical Paediatric Nephrology 2nd ed. RJ Postlethwaite (ed) Oxford: Butterworths 1994

O'Flynn K, Gough DCS, Gupta SJ et al. Prediction of recovery in antenatally diagnosed hydonephrosis *Br J Urol* 1993; 71: 478–480

Ransley PG, Dhillon HK, Gordon I, Duffy PG. The postnatal management of hydrohephrosis diagnosed by prenatal ultrasound. *J Urol* 1990; 144: 584–587

Shokeir AA, Nijman RJM. Primary megaureter: current trends in diagnosis and treatment. *BJU Int* 2000; 86: 861–868

Duplication anomalies, ureterocoeles and ectopic ureters

8

J David Frank and AMK Rickwood

Topics covered
Embryology and classification
Pathology
Clinical presentation
Investigations

Management
    Duplex-system ureterocoele
    Suprasphincteric ectopic ureter
    Infrasphincteric ectopic ureter
    Duplex-system vesicoureteric reflux
Single-system ureterocoele and ectopic ureter

Introduction

Some degree of upper urinary tract duplication is found in 0.8% of postmortem examinations, and in a rather higher proportion (2–3%) of patients undergoing intravenous urography. In approximately 40% of cases the condition is bilateral. The anomaly is transmitted as an autosomal dominant trait with incomplete penetrance, so that among members of affected families the incidence is of the order of 8%.

The great majority of duplications are incomplete, with confluence of the ureters at some point above the ureteric orifice, and as such are only exceptionally of any clinical consequence. In contrast, complete duplication anomalies are often of clinical significance in terms of symptoms, renal function or both. However, complete duplication anomalies are far rarer, affecting appreciably less than 0.1% of individuals, the majority being females. Most present clinically during childhood, and nowadays around 50% are detected by prenatal ultrasonography. In approximately 25% of cases complete duplication exists bilaterally and occasionally nonconcordantly, for example with ureteric ectopia on one side and a ureterocoele on the other.

Because duplication anomalies often take the form of ureterocoele and ureteric ectopia, this chapter also deals with their single-system counterparts.

Duplication anomalies (Table 8.1)

Embryology

Normal ureteric and renal embryogenesis is described in Chapter 1. A single ureteric bud which arises normally from the mesonephric duct but which bifurcates early, leads to some degree of incomplete duplication of the upper renal tract. Complete duplication occurs when two ureteric buds arise separately from the mesonephric duct.

An accessory ureteric bud arising caudally and subserving the lower renal pole is absorbed into the urogenital sinus, so that the ureteric orifice comes to lie superolaterally on the trigone (Figure 8.1a,b), an anatomical configuration commonly associated with vesicoureteric reflux to the lower pole of the kidney.

An accessory bud arising cephalad to the normal site on the mesonephric duct and subserving the upper

Table 8.1 Classification of complete duplication anomalies

Lower polar Vesicoureteric reflux

Upper polar
Duplex-system ureterocoele
Suprasphincteric ureteric ectopia
    Boys – vas, seminal vesicle, ejaculatory duct
    Girls – bladder neck, proximal urethra
Infrasphincteric ureteric ectopia
    Girls *only* - introitus, distal vagina

(a)

(b)

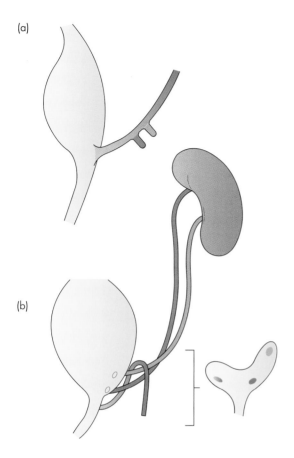

(a)

(b)

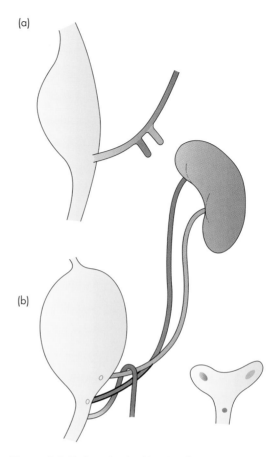

Figure 8.1 Embryological basis of complete duplication with lower pole reflux. (a) Accessory ureteric bud (red) arising caudally on the mesonephric duct (green) at around 6 weeks subsequently becomes incorporated into the superolateral portion of the trigone (b), with a short submucosal tunnel predisposing to reflux. Relative positions of ureteric orifices on trigone also illustrated.

Figure 8.2 Embryological basis of complete duplication with upper pole ureteric ectopia. (a) Accessory ureteric bud (blue) with an abnormally cephalad site of origin on the mesonephric duct (green). (b) By 12 weeks the upper pole ureter has been carried with the mesonephric duct to an abnormally distal ectopic location (Meyer–Weigart law). Relative positions of ureteric orifices on trigone/bladder neck also illustrated.

renal pole will come to enter the urinary tract in a distally ectopic location (Meyer–Weigart's law), in either the bladder, the urethra or the urogenital sinus (Figure 8.2a,b). In females, such ectopic ureters may be sited above the sphincter mechanism (suprasphincteric), close to or at the level of the striated sphincter (although usually below the bladder neck), or distal to the sphincter (infrasphincteric), either at the introitus or in the distal vagina. In males the termination is always suprasphincteric, in the vas, the seminal vesicle or, most often, the ejaculatory duct.

Pathology

As a rule, the more extreme the degree of ureteric ectopia the greater the likelihood that the developing

ureteric bud will penetrate an abnormal zone of metanephric tissue, with resultant dysplasia (Figure 8.3). Even in the absence of dysplasia the affected pole typically exhibits some degree of dilatation, the only common exception being in some girls with infrasphincteric ectopia. Ureteric dilatation may result from reflux or, if non-refluxing, may represent obstruction or dysmorphism.

Duplex-system ureterocoeles (defined as cystic dilatation of the terminal portion of the ureter draining the upper pole; Figure 8.4a,b) may lie entirely intravesically (orthotopic ureterocoele; Figure 8.4c) or, more commonly, may extend to or beyond the bladder neck (ectopic ureterocoele; Figure 8.4d). In the rare and most extreme form, caecoureterocoele, which is confined to girls, the lesion prolapses deeply

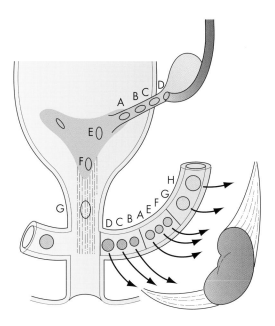

Figure 8.3 Stephen's hypothesis (see 'Further reading'). A ureteric bud arising from the normal region of origin on the mesonephric duct (AEF) makes contact with the central zone of metanephric blastema, initiating normal nephrogenesis, the formation of a healthy kidney and a ureteric orifice located on the trigone. By contrast, a ureteric bud arising from an abnormal site on the ureteric bud is more likely to make contact with a peripheral zone of metanephric blastema, with consequent renal dysplasia and an ectopic ureteric orifice.

Figure 8.4 Ureterocoeles: embryology and classification. (a) Delay in canalisation of the upper ureteric bud at around the time it makes contact with the upper pole metanephric blastema results in cystic dilatation subsequently resulting (b) in the formation of a duplex ureterocoele. (c) Single-system orthotopic ureterocoele. (d) Duplex ectopic ureterocoele. (e) Caecoureterocoele. Large ureterocoele extending distally downward from the deficient trigone towards the perineum in a plane between the urethra anteriorly and the vagina posteriorly.

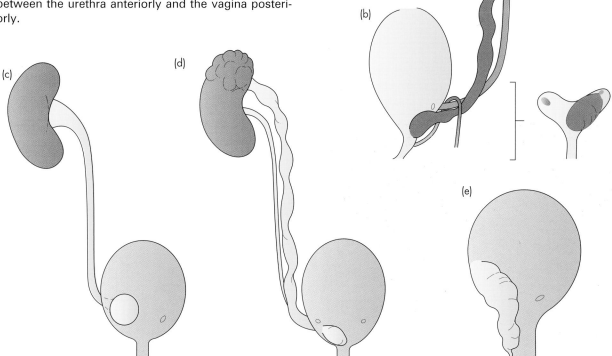

posterior to the urethra (Figure 8.4e). As would be expected, upper polar dysplasia is the rule with duplex-system ureterocoeles, so that with few exceptions useful or even normal levels of function are usually associated with orthotopic ureterocoeles, particularly single-system ureterocoeles.

In addition to the primary anomaly, duplex-system ureterocoeles may be complicated by one or more further associated or secondary phenomena:

● Vesicoureteric reflux to the ipsilateral lower pole. This is present in 50% of cases and usually moderate in degree (grades I–III). More severe degrees of lower pole reflux are generally associated with significantly impaired function of that pole.
● Obstruction of the ipsilateral upper pole polar ureter owing to the obstructing nature of the ureterocoele itself. In this situation lower polar function is usually well preserved, although lower pole drainage can sometimes be impaired by a massively dilated upper pole system.
● Bladder outflow obstruction caused by the ureterocoele (almost always an ectopic lesion).
● Compromise of the contralateral upper renal tract as a result of bladder outflow obstruction.
● Incidental contralateral vesicoureteric reflux, present in 25% of cases but seldom exceeding grade III in severity.
● Perurethral prolapse of the ureterocoele, a rare complication confined to girls.

Incidence

Duplex-system ureterocoeles occur in approximately 0.02% of individuals, 80% of them female. A slight

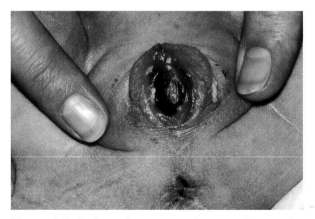

Figure 8.5 Prolapsed ureterocoele emerging at the introitus of a newborn infant.

majority are left-sided, and in 10% of cases the lesion is bilateral.

Ectopic ureter is still rarer, affecting some 0.01% of individuals, mostly females. Some degree of contralateral duplication, usually incomplete, is found in 80% of cases, and in 10% of cases of infrasphincteric ectopia the anomaly is bilateral.

The incidence of complete duplication with lower polar reflux is difficult to determine, as not all cases are detectable by prenatal ultrasonography, nor do all affected individuals present clinically. At a best estimate no more than 0.04% of the population are affected.

Clinical presentation

Duplex-system ureterocoele

Approximately 60% of children with these anomalies are currently identified by prenatal ultrasonography. Clinical presentation, usually during infancy, is most commonly with urinary infection, typically with marked constitutional upset and occasionally with Gram-negative septicaemia. Other, rarer, modes of presentation include acute or chronic urinary retention and, in females, perurethral prolapse of the ureterocoele (Figure 8.5).

Suprasphincteric ectopic ureter

These anomalies are frequently detected prenatally by virtue of dilatation of the upper pole ureter or collecting system. Clinical presentation is almost invariably with urinary infection which, in males, may be manifest as epididymo-orchitis.

Infrasphincteric ectopia (Figure 8.6)

If not picked up prenatally, the clinical presentation is classically characterised by constant dribbling of urine superimposed upon an otherwise normal pattern of micturition. The constant dribbling distinguishes this cause of incontinence from incontinence due to dysfunctional voiding, while the presence of a normal voiding pattern serves to distinguish ectopic ureter from other organic causes of incontinence, such as neuropathic bladder, epispadias and urogenital sinus anomalies. However, the history is not always so straightforward. Some girls remain dry overnight, whereas others, with intravaginal ectopia, are able to remain dry for brief periods during the day. Occasionally the clinical picture is further confused by secondary changes in the pattern of normal micturi-

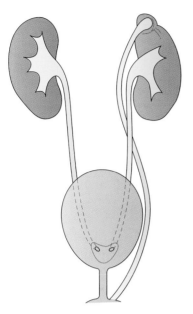

Figure 8.6 Diagrammatic representation of duplex-system infrasphincteric ureter.

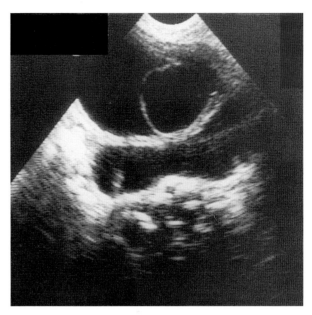

Figure 8.7 Bladder ultrasonography demonstrating a large ureterocoele within the bladder and the dilated upper pole ureter behind the bladder.

tion, for example marked urinary frequency prompted by the parents' increasingly desperate efforts get their daughter dry. Lastly, where the affected upper renal pole is severely dysplastic, the minimal quantity of urine produced pools in the vagina, becomes infected and presents as vaginal discharge.

Physical examination is usually unrewarding, although occasionally constant, slight, urinary leakage may be observed at the introitus.

Investigations

Ultrasound

Because it detects dilatation of one or other renal pole, ultrasound is the investigation of first choice. Dilatation of the *lower* pole may be due to:

- **Vesicoureteric reflux.** In this situation it is usually also possible to visualise a dilated ureter behind the bladder.
- **Pelviureteric junction obstruction** which, when it occurs in a duplication anomaly, almost always involves the lower pole (see Chapter 7).

Dilatation affecting the *upper* renal pole may be due to:

- **Duplex-system ureterocoele**, in which event the ureterocoele itself is always readily imaged within

the bladder (Figure 8.7), provided the bladder is full.
- **Ureteric ectopia**, either suprasphincteric in boys or supra- or infrasphincteric in girls. As a rule, the dilated distal ureter can be visualised behind the bladder. In some girls with infrasphincteric ectopia the upper renal pole is not hydronephrotic but is small and dysplastic, and consequently difficult or impossible to detect by ultrasonography ('cryptic duplication').

Dilatation affecting *both* renal poles is almost always due to **duplex-system ureterocoele**.

DMSA scintigraphy

This examination should be undertaken routinely to assess the distribution of function in the duplex kidney (Figure 8.8). Areas of interest drawn around the upper and lower poles enable the differential function of each moiety to be calculated. The examination also finds occasional use in detecting 'cryptic duplication' (Figure 8.9).

Cystography

Cystography is essential for patients suspected of having lower polar vesicoureteric reflux. In the presence of a *complete* duplication anomaly, reflux is

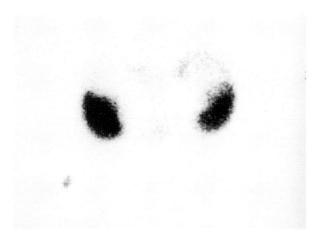

Figure 8.8 DMSA scintigrapy in a child with bilateral duplex-system ureterocoeles. Left upper renal pole is non-functioning and there is only minimal function in the thin rim of renal parenchyma overlying the grossly dilated right upper pole. Both lower poles exhibit normal function.

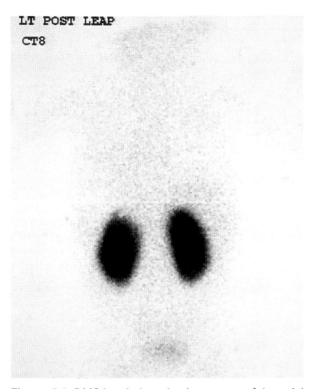

Figure 8.9 DMSA scintigraphy in a case of 'cryptic' duplication. The subtle defect at the left upper pole represents a non-functioning, non-dilated moiety.

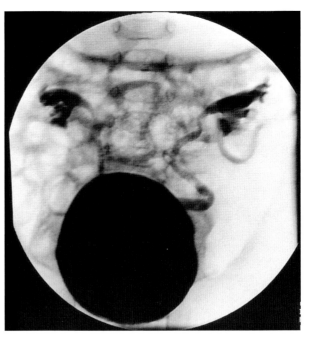

Figure 8.10 Micturating cystogram demonstrating bilateral lower pole vesicoureteric reflux. Note the absence of upper pole calyces and 'drooping flower' appearance of the lower pole pelvi-calyceal systems. On the left there is lateral displacement of the kidney and 'scalloping' of the ureter, owing to the presence of a grossly dilated upper pole ureter terminating ectopically.

almost always restricted to the *lower* renal pole (Figure 8.10). Reflux to *both* poles is indicative of *incomplete* duplication. Where the reflux differs in severity between the two moieties and is more marked in the lower pole (Figure 8.11), the ureteric confluence is likely to be very low and immediately adjacent to the ureteric orifice. Cystography is also routinely advisable in patients with duplex-system ureterocoele in view of the high incidence of reflux, both ipsilaterally and contralaterally. Similarly, in girls with suprasphincteric ectopia the cystogram may demonstrate reflux to the upper pole during voiding.

Intravenous urography (IVU)

The IVU retains a useful role in the evaluation of duplex systems, particularly in the detection of 'cryptic duplication', the radiological signs of which may include an 'absent' upper calyx, lateral and downward displacement of the lower moiety, and a 'scalloped' appearance of the lower polar ureter (Figure 8.12). With the exception of the 'absent' upper pole calyx these radiological signs are caused by the presence of a dilated drainage system arising from the upper renal pole. In addition, the discovery of an incomplete duplication anomaly on one side may raise the possibility of 'cryptic duplication' contralaterally.

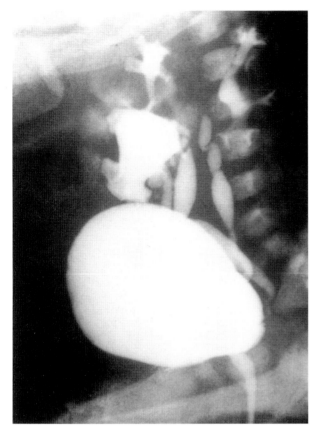

Figure 8.11 Micturating cystography demonstrating bilateral vesicoureteric reflux. Incomplete duplication on the right. (The disparity between the upper and lower pole reflux on the right is indicative of ureteric confluence just proximal to the ureteric orifice.)

Cystoscopy and examination under anaesthetic

Cystoscopy is routinely advisable for the assessment of duplex-system ureterocoeles, principally in order to determine whether or not the lesion is ectopic (Figure 8.13). In girls with a suprasphincteric ectopic ureter the examination usually readily locates the ectopic ureteric orifice immediately below the bladder neck. Examination under anaesthetic may also reveal an ectopic orifice in girls with infrasphincteric ectopia, but failure to identify an ectopic orifice by no means excludes this diagnosis.

Methylene blue test

This may be employed in girls suspected of having infrasphincteric ectopia but in whom the duplication is 'cryptic' and examination under anaesthetic has been negative. Methylene blue is instilled into the bladder

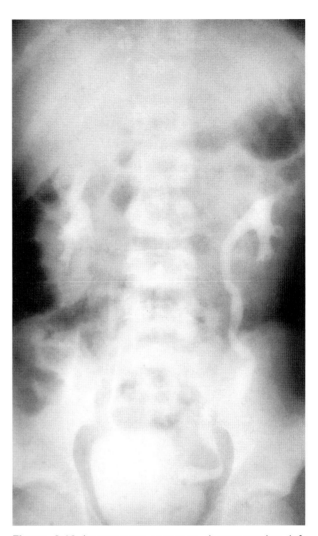

Figure 8.12 Intravenous urogram demonstrating left duplication with non-functioning upper pole. A left upper calyx is not visualised, the lower pole is displaced laterally and downwards ('drooping flower') and the lower pole ureter is deviated ('scalloped') by the presence of the grossly dilated upper pole ureter.

via a catheter, which is then removed, and a pad is placed upon the vulva. If subsequent wetting of the pad is 'blue' the incontinence is due to a bladder problem, but if the fluid on the pad is 'clear' the diagnosis of infrasphincteric ectopia is confirmed.

Management

Duplex-system ureterocoele

Management of this anomaly is influenced by a number of factors, including the mode of presentation, and the presence of any associated or secondary effects of the ureterocoele on the upper renal pole, the

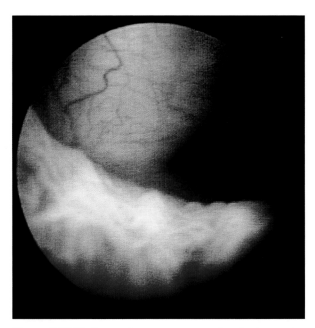

Figure 8.13 Endoscopic appearances of a duplex urete-rocoele at the level of the bladder neck.

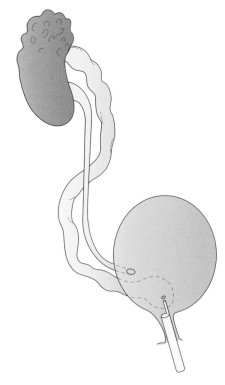

Figure 8.14 Diagrammatic illustration of the simplest form of intervention – endoscopic puncture.

ipsilateral lower renal pole, the bladder and the contralateral upper renal tract.

Unquestionable indications for surgical intervention are:

- Symptoms
- Well-preserved ipsilateral upper polar function
- Ipsilateral lower polar reflux, if complicated by urinary infection
- Ipsilateral lower polar obstruction
- Bladder outflow obstruction
- Ureterocele prolapse.

In an appreciable proportion of cases detected by prenatal ultrasonography, none of these considerations applies as the affected infants are asymptomatic and the urinary tract is normal, with the exception of an affected upper pole with minimal function. Whether any surgical intervention is called for in such cases remains open to debate.

Options for surgical intervention comprise:

- **Endoscopic ureterocoele incision** (Figure 8.14) Although it represents the least invasive form of intervention, endoscopic incision runs a risk of inducing upper polar reflux. Although the risk can be reduced by making the incision as close to the bladder wall as possible, there remains an appreciable chance that

further, more definitive, surgery will be required. The long-term results of endoscopic incision have yet to be fully assessed. Encouraging medium-term results have been reported by some authors, suggesting that endoscopic incision alone may be adequate definitive treatment in selected cases. However, many paediatric urologists continue to regard endoscopic incision as a temporising measure, best employed in patients presenting acutely with gross upper polar sepsis.

- **Upper pole nephrectomy** (Figure 8.15a) This procedure (sometimes termed the 'simplified approach') is the first choice in cases where upper polar function is severely compromised. The upper moiety is excised, together with as much of the ureter as can be safely mobilised and excised through the same incision. The ureterocoele is aspirated and drained via the ureteric stump, which is left in situ. The 'simplified approach' is usually sufficient, with subsequent excision of the ureteric stump and ureterocoele and reimplantation of the lower polar ureter being required in only some 20% of cases.

- **Pyelopyelostomy** (Figure 8.15b) is appropriate for cases having useful upper polar function accom-

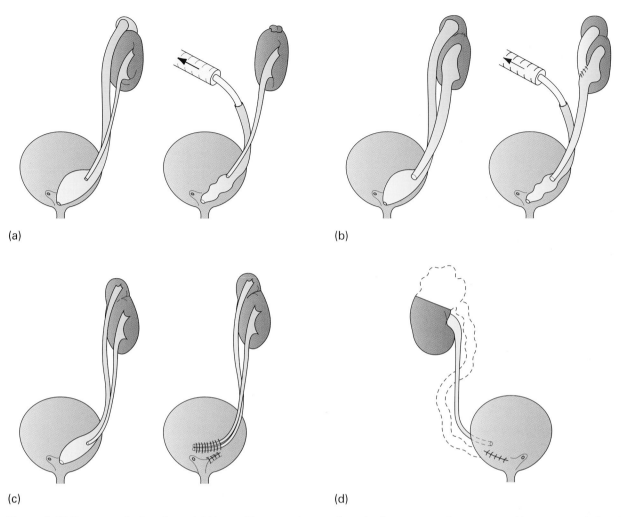

(a)

(b)

(c)

(d)

Figure 8.15 Open surgical options. (a) Normal lower pole, non-functioning upper pole – managed by upper pole heminephrectomy, excision of the proximal ureter via the same incision, and aspiration of the residual upper pole ureteric stump ('simplified approach'). (b) Functioning upper pole, dilated lower pole – management by pyelopyelostomy. Excision of proximal upper pole ureter and aspiration of ureteric stump. (c) Functioning upper pole, non-dilated lower pole – management by excision of ureterocoele and reimplantation of conjoined duplex ureters. (d) Heminephroureterectomy with excision of ureterocoele (often necessitating lower pole ureteric reimplantation). Definitive surgical treatment, but a major procedure requiring two separate incisions.

panied by a degree of dilatation of the lower renal pole. The defunctioned upper ureter and ureterocoele should be aspirated at the time of surgery.

● **Ureterocoele excision and reimplantation** (Figure 8.15c), is employed when there is useful upper polar function and no dilatation of the lower pole. In these circumstances the ureterocoele is usually orthotopic and the upper polar ureter only moderately dilated, thereby enabling straightforward reimplantation of the conjoined ureters once the ureterocoele has been excised.

● **Nephrectomy** is required when the function of both renal poles is severely compromised. Reflux-

ing ureters should be excised, but a non-refluxing ureteric stump may be left in situ provided the ureterocoele is aspirated.

● **Upper pole nephrectomy, ureterectomy and ureterocoele excision** (Figure 8.15d) This, the most extensive operation for a duplex system, requires the use of two incisions and is a potentially lengthy and technically challenging surgical undertaking. Particular care is required when excising a caecoureterocoele in view of the risk of damage to the bladder neck and striated sphincter mechanism. Other possible iatrogenic complications include vesicovaginal fistula. To minimise the risk of complications the bulk of the ureterocoele should be excised from above, the detrusor and mucosal defect closed, and any remaining distal lip resected endoscopically from below. Reimplantation of the ipsilateral lower pole ureter is often required, and care is needed when mobilising the dilated upper pole ureter to avoid damaging or devascularising the healthy lower pole ureter.

Suprasphincteric ectopic ureter

Indications for surgical intervention are relative, not absolute, and principally comprise recurrent urinary infection resulting from the presence of the ectopic ureter. In the great majority of cases, with negligible upper polar function, heminephrectomy suffices. In girls with upper polar reflux the affected ureter should also be excised, via a separate lower abdominal incision, as close to the urethra as is practicable. In the occasional case with useful upper polar function the ectopic ureter may be reimplanted into the bladder. If, as is usual, the distal ureters are conjoined, it is necessary to reimplant them both together *en bloc*.

Infrasphincteric ectopic ureter

As previously indicated, the main problem with this complaint is diagnostic rather than therapeutic. It is always worth bearing in mind that in some 10% of cases the lesion is bilateral, and a detectable duplex system may be accompanied by a cryptic contralateral upper pole associated with an ectopic ureter. Excision of the affected upper renal pole(s) invariably cures the presenting complaint. Ureteric reimplantation may be considered for the very occasional case having useful function in the upper pole.

Vesicoureteric reflux

As a rule, management of vesicoureteric reflux in the presence of a duplication anomaly runs along the same lines described for reflux generally (Chapter 5). There are, however, two particular features pertaining to complete duplication anomalies which may influence management:

- **Persistent reflux** Lower polar reflux, especially if severe, is less likely to resolve spontaneously than is the case with single-system reflux. For this reason antireflux surgery is more commonly required (although only where there are positive indications,

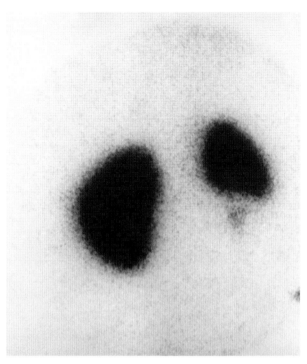

Figure 8.16 DMSA scintigraphy of right lower pole reflux into a virtually non-functioning, dysplastic lower pole moiety.

such as breakthrough infections while on antibiotic prophylaxis, or infections following discontinuation of prophylaxis). As a rule, STING procedures are ineffective in the presence of complete duplication, and open antireflux surgery is needed. The adjacent ureteric orifices are circumcised together and the underlying ureters mobilised *en bloc* and then reimplanted in their common sheath.

- **Lower polar dysplasia** In a proportion of cases DMSA scintigraphy demonstrates grossly impaired function in the affected lower pole (Figure 8.16) which, with few exceptions, represents congenital dysplasia rather than acquired reflux nephropathy. When surgical intervention is indicated this should take the form of lower polar nephrectomy, along with excision of the ureter down to the point where it enters a common sheath with the upper polar ureter.

Single-system ureterocoele

These anomalies, which affect boys more commonly than girls, almost always lie entirely within the bladder (orthotopic ureterocoeles). Some are detected by prenatal ultrasonography and others come to light by way of symptoms. Urinary infection is the most common mode of clinical presentation, but very occasionally they present with bladder outflow obstruction causing intermittent retention, or symptoms related to calculi. In addition, a sizeable proportion are picked up on ultrasonography or intravenous urography as a more or less incidental finding. In the majority of cases obstructive changes in the affected upper renal tract are absent or minimal, and renal function is normally preserved (Figure 8.17).

Indications for surgical intervention comprise:

● Symptoms.
● Upper renal tract obstruction: although treatable by endoscopic incision this risks subsequent reflux, and

as a rule it is usually preferable to excise the ureterocoele and to reimplant the underlying ureter.

Opinion is divided on the management of small asymptomatic orthotopic ureterocoeles, and although some paediatric urologists advocate endoscopic incision others simply advise no more than watchful observation.

Single-system ectopic ureter

Single vaginal ectopic ureter (Figure 8.18)

Although less well recognised than duplex-system ectopia as a cause of urinary incontinence in girls, this anomaly is not so very much less common. The ureter terminates ectopically in the vagina, usually around the junction of the middle and distal thirds, and the clinical presentation is the same as for infrasphincteric duplex-system ectopia, namely continuous dribbling of urine superimposed upon otherwise normal micturition. Similarly, this condition presents diagnostic rather than therapeutic difficulties, partly because the affected kidney, being small and dysplastic, is difficult to image, and partly because it may lie ectopically anywhere from the lumbar region to the pelvis.

An initial ultrasound examination often reports 'unilateral renal agenesis', but a more purposeful search

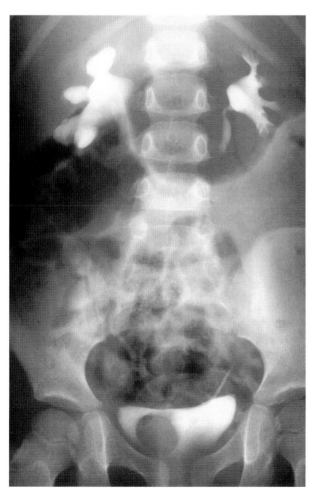

Figure 8.17 Intravenous urogram demonstrating a right-sided orthotopic (single-system) ureterocoele with brisk uptake of contrast, indicating good preservation of renal function.

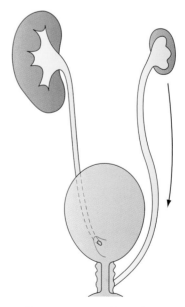

Figure 8.18 The anatomy of a single-system infrasphincteric ectopic ureter. The arrow indicates that the affected kidney may be sited ectopically.

may locate the kidney. DMSA scintigraphy and MRI may be helpful in locating a small kidney which cannot be visualised by ultrasound. The diagnosis may also be confirmed by identification of the ectopic orifice and retrograde contrast studies. Nephrectomy is curative.

Unilateral urethral ectopic ureter

In this rare anomaly, which is virtually confined to girls, the single ureter terminates ectopically in the proximal urethra. The function of the overlying kidney is usually impaired – sometimes severely so – presumably as a result of congenital dysplasia. The ureter is usually sufficiently dilated to be detectable by ultrasonography.

When not picked up by prenatal ultrasonography the anomaly generally presents with urinary infection. In symptomatic cases with useful renal function the ureter can be reimplanted into the bladder, if necessary with trimming when the ureter is markedly dilated. Otherwise, nephrectomy is indicated.

Bilateral single ectopic ureters

This rare anomaly affects girls more often than boys. Both single ureters terminate ectopically in the proximal urethra; the bladder neck and external urethral sphincter are incompetent, and the bladder itself is usually small (Figure 8.19). Both kidneys often demonstrate a degree of dysplasia (which is sometimes severe), while the

ureters tend to be dilated and are thus detectable by ultrasonography. Presentation may be either with continuous dribbling incontinence in childhood or with symptoms of renal insufficiency in infancy.

Treatment requires reimplantation of the ectopic ureters into the bladder, plus augmentation cystoplasty when the bladder is small. Finally, it is necessary to deal with the sphincteric incompetence, either by bladder neck repair or by bladder neck closure along with a Mitrofanoff procedure.

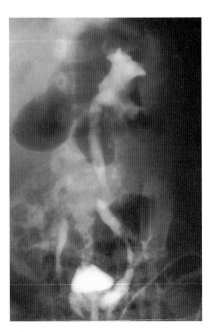

Figure 8.19 Intravenous urogram in a child with bilateral single ectopic ureters. Both ureters drain infravesically and the bladder is of small capacity.

Key points

- In contrast to incomplete duplication anomalies, complete duplications are rarer and more frequently of clinical significance as a cause of symptoms, impaired renal function or both.
- On the basis of their embryology, complete duplication anomalies are classifiable as those principally affecting the upper renal pole (ureterocoele, suprasphincteric or infrasphincteric ectopic ureter) and those affecting the lower renal pole (notably vesicoureteric reflux).
- Renal dysplasia of the upper or lower pole is common in all forms of complete duplication.
- In addition to upper polar dysplasia, duplex-system ureterocoeles may be further complicated by problems affecting the lower renal pole, the bladder and the contralateral upper renal tract.
- Infrasphincteric ectopic ureter in girls, leading to urinary incontinence, often presents problems with diagnostic imaging because the affected upper renal pole tends to be severely dysplastic.

Further reading

Johnston JH, Davenport TJ. The single ectopic ureter. *Br J Urol* 1969; 41: 428

Lee JD, Rickwood AMK, Anderson PAM, Williams MPL. Experience with duplex-system anomalies detected by prenatal ultrasonography *J Urol* 1995; 149: 808

Mackie GG, Stephens FD. Duplex kidneys: a correlation with renal dysplasia with position of the ureteric orifice. *J Urol* 1975; 114: 274

Rickwood AMK, Reiner I, Jones M, Pournaras C. Current management of duplex-system ureterocoeles; experience with 41 patients. *Br J Urol* 1992; 70: 196

Shankar KR, Vishwanath N, Rickwood AMK. Outcome of patients with prenatally detected duplex system ureterocoele: natural history of those managed expectantly. *J Urol* 2001; 165: 1226

Posterior urethral valves and other urethral abnormalities

9

Patrick G Duffy

Topics covered
Posterior urethral valves
    Anatomy/pathophysiology
    Presentation/investigation
    Treatment

Prognosis
Long-term management
Anterior urethral diverticulum
Urethral duplication
Other urethral pathology

Introduction

With the exception of strictures, urethral obstruction in childhood is congenital in origin and of the various causes of urethral obstruction only posterior urethral valves commonly give rise to secondary changes in the upper renal tracts – sometimes with devastating consequences. There is increasing evidence to indicate that the consequences of outflow obstruction are due as much to secondary effects upon bladder function as to the underlying obstruction itself. Moreover, the earlier the obstruction develops the worse the impact on the upper tracts, to the extent that obstruction dating from early fetal life is commonly complicated by renal dysplasia.

Posterior urethral valves

First accurately described by Young in 1919, this condition carried a mortality of almost 100% during the early years of the 20th century and the mortality rate remained as high as 50% until the 1950s. By contrast, the mortality reported in one recent series was only 0.3%, but this improvement has come at the expense of a greater proportion of young patients in chronic renal failure.

Posterior urethral valves occur only in males, in whom the incidence is of the order of 1 in 4000–8000. Although a few familial cases have been recorded, including in siblings, there is no established genetic predisposition. In some series boys with Down's syndrome are disproportionately represented. Posterior urethral valves are not a component of the VACTERL spectrum of anomalies (Chapter 15), nor are they consistently associated with any other congenital anomaly.

Anatomy

Although Young's long-standing classification describes three forms of valvular obstruction, recent studies point to a single common configuration comprising an obliquely orientated membrane with a small eccentric aperture (Figure 9.1), which arises from the verumontanum, extends through the zone of the external urethral sphincter and attaches anteriorly to the urethral wall. Partial rupture in utero or urethral instrumentation, including catheterisation, may disrupt the membrane in the midline to result in the appearance of two separate, side-by-side valvular leaflets (Figure 9.2). Recent anatomical and endoscopic studies provide little support for Young's distinction between type I valves (the most common variety) and type III valves. Moreover, type II valves, which extend upwards from the verumontanum, are not obstructive, and nowadays their very existence is questioned.

Pathophysiology

The valvular obstruction develops at approximately 7 weeks' gestation as a result of abnormal embryogenesis at the confluence of mesonephric ducts and the

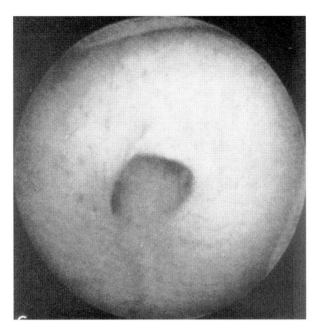

Figure 9.1 Endoscopic appearances of intact valve membrane in an infant prior to any form of urethral catheterisation or instrumentation.

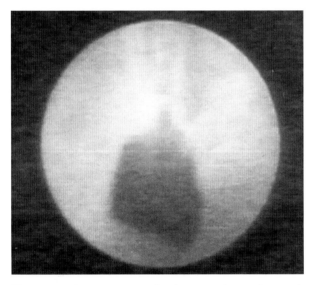

Figure 9.2 Appearances of valve membrane in previously catheterised urethra. Artefactual changes creating appearance of cusp-like 'valves'.

urogenital sinus membrane. When the degree of obstruction is severe the consequent dilatation of the fetal urinary tract may be detectable by ultrasonography as early as the 14th week of gestation.

Studies of experimentally induced fetal bladder outflow obstruction in animals have established the following:

- Early outflow obstruction leads to an abnormal bladder wall with an increased collagen component, and to renal dysplasia (renal dysplasia is characterised by distinctive histological features, including primitive tubules and the persistence of abnormal mesenchymal derivatives such as cartilage).
- Obstruction in later gestation gives rise to the sequelae typical of chronically raised intravesical pressure, but without renal dysplasia.

Clinical experience indicates that the consequences of obstruction by posterior urethral valves in man may exist at these extremes or at any point between them, and hence that the long-term prognosis is determined by an interplay of:

- early abnormal development of the urethra, bladder, kidneys and, possibly, the ureters;
- later secondary effects of bladder outflow obstruction.

The relative contributions made by these different factors to the functional outcome in any individual case is often difficult to determine, and this difficulty may be compounded by the effects of bladder dysfunction persisting after relief of the valvular obstruction itself.

Presentation

The fetus

The proportion of cases detected by fetal ultrasonography continues to increase, and currently more than 80% are detected prenatally. Although the underlying urethral anomaly dates from the seventh to the ninth week of gestation, dilatation of the urinary tract may not develop until much later in pregnancy. Only 55% of cases of prenatally detected posterior urethral valves are picked up on routine maternal ultrasonography performed between 16 and 20 weeks. In the remaining prenatally detected cases the appearances of the fetal urinary tract are normal in the second trimester, and the condition is only detected as a result of scans in later pregnancy performed for obstetric indications.

Functional outcome is closely linked to the gestational age at which dilatation first becomes apparent, and in those detected at 16–20 weeks a poor prognosis is certain if oligohydramnios is also present at this

Table 9.1 Ultrasound features of posterior urethral valves in the fetus

> Male fetus
> Bilateral upper tract dilatation
> Persistently distended full bladder
> **Predictors of poor functional outcome and early-onset renal failure**
> Detection before 24 weeks' gestation
> Bladder wall thickening
> Echo-bright kidneys (renal dysplasia)
> Oligohydramnios

stage. In pregnancies proceeding to term the affected infant often demonstrates features of Potter's syndrome at birth (characteristic facies, skeletal 'moulding' deformities), and death supervenes in the early newborn period as a result of pulmonary hypoplasia. In the absence of second-trimester oligohydramnios the functional prognosis is linked to the severity of the dilatation and a number of other prognostic features of the second-trimester ultrasound findings (Table 9.1). A number of biochemical constituents of fetal urine (sodium, calcium, β_2-microglobulin, osmolality) have been studied as possible prognostic markers, but there is considerable overlap with normal values and predictive sensitivity is poor.

In cases where dilatation develops later in gestation, the prognosis is generally good. In addition to dilatation and renal dysplasia, other complications of urethral valves detectable by fetal ultrasonography are urinary ascites and perinephric urinoma.

The neonate

Symptoms in this age group usually relate to the bladder outflow obstruction itself or, less often, to the effects of impaired renal function. Listlessness, poor feeding and irritability are common. The urinary stream, if witnessed, is usually poor, although this is not always so. The bladder is palpably enlarged in most instances; the kidneys can also be palpated. Urinary ascites occurs as an occasional complication.

The infant

When the condition presents for the first time in infancy it is generally with urinary infection (Chapter 4) without any preceding symptomatology. Gram-negative septicaemia and gross electrolyte disturbance

were once common forms of presentation, but with increasing detection by fetal ultrasonography and heightened awareness of urinary infection among infants they have become unusual. Chronically impaired renal function is usually manifest as poor growth. In a majority of cases localising physical signs are absent.

The older child

Presenting features may include manifestations of renal failure, such as growth retardation, urinary infection or voiding symptoms (typically prolonged voiding, rather than a poor urinary stream as such). In addition, the diagnosis of posterior urethral valves is occasionally made during the investigation of diurnal or nocturnal enuresis. Localising physical signs are unusual.

Investigation

Prenatal

The presence of posterior urethral valves can only be inferred from the ultrasound appearances of a distended fetal bladder and dilated upper tracts (Figure 9.3), as the alternative diagnoses include urethral atresia (always lethal), prune-belly syndrome, megacystis–microcolon intestinal hypoperistalsis syndrome, and marked primary vesicoureteric reflux.

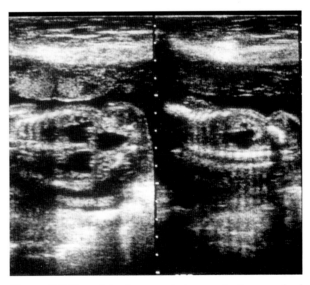

Figure 9.3 Prenatal ultrasound demonstrating marked dilatation of both fetal kidneys and the fetal bladder. The fetal spine and thorax are clearly visible in both these longitudinal images.

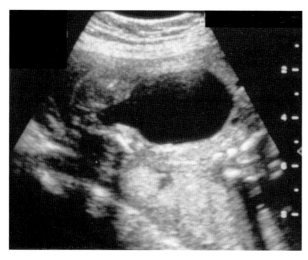

Figure 9.4 Ultrasound appearances illustrating the diagnostic 'keyhole sign'. Dilated (thick-walled) bladder and dilated posterior urethra.

However, the diagnosis can be made with more certainty if there is dilatation of the posterior urethra – the so-called 'keyhole sign' (Figure 9.4).

Postnatal

Ultrasonography is the initial investigation, the relevant findings comprising upper tract dilatation (which is

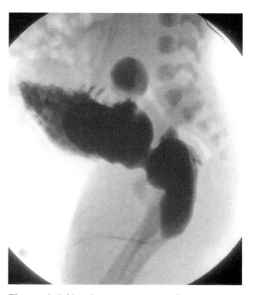

Figure 9.6 Newborn preterm infant, prenatal diagnosis. Heavily trabeculated bladder with diverticulum, prominent bladder neck, and demarcation between dilated posterior urethra and non-dilated distal urethra at the site of the valve membrane.

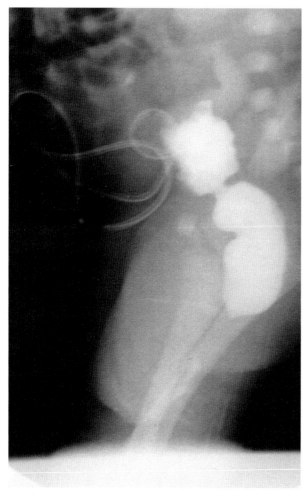

Figure 9.5 Newborn infant: micturating cystourethrogram (MCU) findings. Grossly dilated posterior urethra, indentation by prominent bladder neck, small trabeculated bladder.

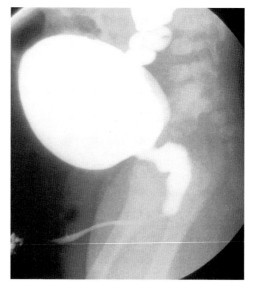

Figure 9.7 MCU in a boy presenting in the first year of life with urinary infection. Smooth-walled non-trabeculated bladder, unilateral grade IV reflux.

sometimes only unilateral), perinephric urinoma (occasionally), thickening of the bladder wall, with or without residual urine, and, if voiding views can be obtained, dilatation of the posterior urethra. Micturating cystourethrography (MCU), rather than endoscopy, provides the definitive diagnosis, with a range of findings, as illustrated in Figures 9.5, 9.6 and 9.7. Vesicoureteric reflux is present in 40–60% of cases at the time of initial evaluation and is unilateral in approximately two-thirds of cases. Initial assessment also includes measurement of electrolyte balance and renal function (although it should be noted that in the first 48 hours of life serum creatinine levels reflect maternal renal function rather than that of the neonate).

Treatment

The fetus

The rationale for fetal intervention derives from experimental studies which demonstrated that experimentally induced obstructive renal damage could be ameliorated by intrauterine decompression of the obstructed fetal bladder. However, the extent to which these experimental findings can be translated to humans remains unclear. In clinical practice prenatal intervention, in the form of vesicoamniotic shunting, has a chequered history and the weight of published experience indicates that, it may have a limited role.

- Termination of pregnancy is the most widely undertaken form of intervention, particularly when marked dilatation and maternal oligohydramnios are detected in early pregnancy. In these circumstances decompression of the obstructed urinary tract is of no benefit, as the die is cast and irreversible renal dysplasia is almost invariably present.
- Elective preterm delivery represents another form of intervention, and there is some anecdotal evidence that it may be beneficial in cases of later-onset dilatation which shows evidence of rapid progression.

Between these extremes vesicoamniotic shunting may have a role in the presence of early obstruction and preserved renal function. However, the procedure carries an appreciable risk of fetal morbidity which, although only 5% in skilled hands, is considerably higher in some published series.

Evaluating the possible benefits of vesicoamniotic shunting in the management of posterior urethral valves is subject to the following limitations:

- Posterior urethral valves (as opposed to other causes of bladder and upper tract dilatation) can be difficult to diagnose with certainty in the fetus.
- Because renal failure may not supervene until late childhood or adolescence, long-term follow-up is required to assess the true impact of intervention.
- No controlled trials have been undertaken to compare the outcome in boys who were treated in utero against those who were not.

Although the role of fetal intervention remains controversial there is universal agreement that prenatal diagnosis has been beneficial by ensuring that the treatment of posterior urethral valves can be undertaken promptly following delivery, and that the risk of serious sepsis can be minimised.

The neonate

To minimise risk of electrolyte disturbances or of urinary infection the bladder outflow obstruction should be relieved promptly, the options being:

- Urethral or suprapubic bladder drainage is the usual primary treatment. This will remain for 2–7 days to obtain base-line renal function.

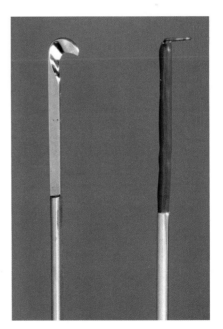

Figure 9.8 Cold knife and cutting resectoscope loop for use with neonatal resectoscope. The availability of instruments designed for neonatal use has simplified management and greatly reduced the incidence of instrumentation-induced urethral trauma.

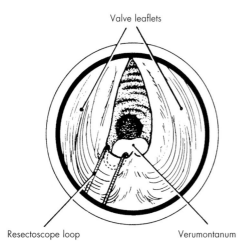

Valve leaflets

Resectoscope loop   Verumontanum

Figure 9.9 Position of the cutting loop prior to ablation of the valve membrane.

- **Endoscopic valve ablation.** With modern miniaturised endoscopes (Figure 9.8), this is usually practicable even in small premature neonates. The valve leaflets are incised from margin to base (rather than fully resected), conventionally at the 4 and 8 o'clock positions (Figure 9.9). In the absence of significant bleeding post operative catheterisation is unnecessary.
- **Vesicostomy.** This may be undertaken when a suitable endoscope is unavailable, or as the procedure of first choice where it is thought essential to provide particularly effective drainage for the upper tracts. The stoma is created at the apex of the bladder to minimise the risk of subsequent mucosal prolapse. Closure is undertaken after subsequent valve ablation – and usually within an interval of 6–18 months, depending on the initial indication for vesicostomy and the child's level of renal function.
- When endoscopic valve ablation is feasible within a few days of birth, preliminary urethral catheterisation is unnecessary in infants with satisfactory and stable renal function. Conversely, vesicostomy drainage may be preferred in those with markedly impaired renal function, especially if deteriorating despite catheterisation, and/or in those with gross bilateral vesicoureteric reflux. In the past ureterostomies were often employed to manage these situations but are now rarely used, partly because of evidence that defunctioning the bladder may adversely affect its later performance, and partly because vesicostomy provides equally effective drainage and is more easily managed by parents.

Urinary ascites usually responds to a short period of catheter drainage of the bladder and, similarly, perinephric collections or 'urinomas' resolve following relief of the bladder outflow obstruction. Large or persistent perirenal collections may require ultrasound-guided percutaneous aspiration or open drainage (in combination with open nephrostomy).

The infant

Urinary infection in infants with previously undiagnosed posterior urethral valves is often complicated by septicaemia and gross disturbances of electrolyte and acid–base balance, of which hyperkalaemic acidosis is the most serious form. The metabolic disturbances and underlying sepsis demand vigorous treatment, preferably in cooperation with a paediatric nephrologist. Surgical treatment of the bladder outflow obstruction is best deferred until the general condition has been stabilised – usually 2–7 days. Vesicostomy is only rarely required in infants.

The older child

With few exceptions, no more is needed in the short term than endoscopic ablation of the valves.

Prognosis

Approximately one-third of individuals have impaired renal function in the long term, although this may not become manifest until adolescence. Factors implicated in the aetiology of chronic renal failure include:

- Primary renal dysplasia
- Secondary damage resulting from bladder outflow obstruction; this occurs principally in utero, but may also occur postnatally if undiagnosed obstruction persists after birth
- Urinary infection, often in association with vesicoureteric reflux
- Secondary damage resulting from bladder dysfunction which persists despite relief of the outflow obstruction.

The importance of this last component, which is manifest clinically as impaired continence, has become appreciated only during recent years. Only 25% of boys with this condition have a urodynamically normal bladder, and the remainder have detrusor non-compliance (65%) or detrusor instability (10%) as the major abnormality. Moreover, patterns of bladder dysfunction may change over time, with a tendency for detrusor overactivity to be replaced by detrusor failure, along with increasing residual volumes of poorly concentrated urine.

Although the ultimate outcome is difficult to predict, especially at presentation, immediate and later predictors of a poor prognosis for renal function are:

Prenatal
- A history of maternal oligohydramnios, regardless of the gestational age at onset;
- Early detection on prenatal ultrasonography and other prognostic features of the fetal urinary tract.

Postnatal
- Clinical presentation in the first 6 months of life (if not detected prenatally);
- Proteinuria;
- Bilateral vesicoureteric reflux;
- Impaired continence at 5 years of age upwards.

Apart from the absence of these predictors of poor prognosis, the positive indicators of good prognosis include presentation in later childhood and protection of the upper tracts by a 'pop-off' phenomenon. Of these, the most common is a pattern of unilateral high-grade vesicoureteric reflux in which the affected kidney has negligible or zero function whereas the contralateral kidney is normal.

However, the protective value of unilateral high-grade reflux has probably been overstated, and recent evidence suggests that although this may impart some medium-term benefit for renal function, a proportion of boys do nevertheless progress into later-onset renal failure. Other less common forms of 'pop-off' mechanism include urinary ascites, perinephric urinoma and a large bladder diverticulum.

Follow-up and long-term management

All boys with posterior urethral valves require follow-up through adolescence and into early adulthood. A suggested follow-up protocol is given in Table 9.2. Differential renal function is monitored, by MAG-3 renography or by DMSA scintigraphy, once overall function has stabilised. Although upper tract dilatation often resolves (albeit slowly) following valve ablation, it may persist either unilaterally or, more commonly, bilaterally. Possible explanations include:

Table 9.2 Follow-up protocol for patients with posterior urethral valves

Routine at every visit
Height and weight
Blood pressure
Urinary tract ultrasonography
Serum creatinine and electrolytes
As indicated
Isotope renography (MAG3 or DMSA)
Flow rate
Urodynamics
Formal estimation of GFR

- Incomplete relief of bladder outflow obstruction;
- Persistent vesicoureteric reflux;
- Ureterovesical obstruction secondary to occlusion of the ureterovesical junction by a thick-walled bladder (rare);
- Upper tract obstruction due to high-pressure bladder dysfunction (non-compliance, instability);
- Ureteric decompensation, particularly in conjunction with polyuria. A high obligatory output of dilute urine occurs when the concentrating ability of the kidneys declines with the onset of early chronic renal failure. It is not uncommon for the urinary tract to demonstrate increasing dilatation in response to an unphysiologically large urine output.

Further investigation may occasionally be indicated to exclude a urological complication giving rise to obstruction, but in the absence of symptoms late-onset dilatation is much more likely to be due to 'decompensation' of a previously dilated upper tract in conjunction with increasing polyuria. Investigation should therefore be aimed at reassessing glomerular and tubular renal function.

Vesicoureteric reflux resolves in 30–60% of cases following valve ablation. However, resolution is less likely in the presence of bladder dysfunction and when function in the renal unit is poor. Antireflux surgery (or nephroureterectomy) is occasionally required for boys troubled by breakthrough urinary infections despite antibiotic prophylaxis.

Bladder dysfunction

When this gives rise to diurnal enuresis there is often a good symptomatic response to detrusor antispasmodics such as oxybutynin. Intermittent catheterisation should be considered where incontinence is associated with a impaired voiding and a large volume of residual urine. In practice, urethral self-catheterisation rarely proves acceptable to boys with posterior urethral valves, because, in contrast to patients with neuropathic bladder, their urethral sensation is normal. For this reason, effective long-term intermittent catheterisation is usually dependent on the creation of a continent catheterisable (Mitrofanoff) channel.

The role of augmentation cystoplasty (ideally ureterocystoplasty; see Chapter 14) is controversial. Although continence is usually improved, this is at the expense of impaired voiding in some 40% of individuals, which in turn calls for intermittent catheterisation. Whether the procedure also secures its more important objective, long-term preservation of renal function, remains to be definitively established.

Other urethral abnormalities

Anterior urethral valves, diverticula and megalourethra

These anomalies, which are confined to males, are approximately eight times less prevalent than posterior urethral valves. In many respects they comprise a continuum of urethral pathology while also being distinct entities in their own right. For example, it is difficult to define the point at which the urethral dilatation proximal to anterior urethral valves becomes a diverticulum, and similarly the point at which an extended diverticulum becomes a megalourethra.

Anterior urethral valves

As classically described, these take the form of either a fenestrated diaphragmatic membrane or a mucosal cusp arising from the ventral wall of the urethra. In 40% of cases the valve is sited at the bulbar urethra, whereas in 30% it is at the penoscrotal junction and in 30% in the penile urethra. The presentation is usually with obstructive symptoms, such as a poor urinary stream, hesitancy or urinary retention. Secondary changes in the upper urinary tracts are rare. Micturating cystourethrography is required to demonstrate the obstruction prior to treatment by endoscopic incision.

Urethral diverticulum

In the more common wide-mouthed form, usually located in the region of the penoscrotal junction, the distal lip may give rise to a form of valvular obstruction as the diverticulum undergoes progressive distension. Presentation is either with obstructive symptoms or with postmicturition dribbling. The rarer saccular lesions with a narrow neck may occur anywhere along the penile urethra, including in the fossa navicularis. Presentation is with urinary infection and/or, very rarely, arising from stone formation within the diverticulum.

Megalourethra

This rare condition is characterised by marked dilatation of the penile urethra in the absence of any evident obstruction. Megalourethra may be associated with lack of corpus spongiosum or, in its most extreme form, with complete absence of the corpora cavernosa. In such cases the penis amounts to little more than a floppy sac comprised of skin externally and urethral mucosa internally. An association exists between megalourethra and other congenital abnormalities, particularly prune-belly syndrome.

Cowper's gland cysts (seryngocoele)

These paired structures, lying either side of the urethra at the level of the urogenital diaphragm, are each drained by a duct coursing distally through the corpus spongiosum to enter the bulbar urethra. Distension of the ducts, or of the glands themselves, may cause urethral compression or, if the anterior wall of the cyst ruptures into the urethra, may result in an obstructive membrane.

Urethral duplications

These rare anomalies take two principal forms, sagittal and collateral. Of these, the sagittal pattern is more common and takes the form of two channels running one above the other in the sagittal plane, whereas in the collateral form the duplicate urethras run side by side. The most common sagittal configuration comprises an orthotopic principal urethral channel and an epispadiac accessory urethra lying dorsal to it.

Many different variations have been described: for example, in some cases both urethras leave the bladder separately and remain separate throughout their length, whereas in other cases the duplicate urethras unite distally to form a single channel. In the so-called 'spindle' variety the urethra separates into two components before reuniting again more distally, whereas in 'Y' duplications, an accessory urethra diverges from the main channel to emerge in the perianal region or the perineum. Reconstruction is dependent upon individual anatomy but nearly always incorporates excision of the narrower accessory urethra.

Posterior urethral polyps

These fibroendothelial lesions arise from the verumontanum. Small ones are usually discovered quite incidentally during the course of endoscopy for some unrelated purpose, whereas the larger lesions, with a polypoid head floating freely on an extended stalk, tend to obtrude through the bladder neck to give rise to acute, transient episodes of urinary retention. Haematuria or frank urethral bleeding represents another form of presentation. Diagnosis is by cystourethroscopy or MCU (Figure 9.10). Most polyps can be excised endoscopically, although for large lesions an open transvesical approach may be required.

Urethral strictures

The aetiology, investigation and management of post-traumatic strictures is considered in Chapter 23. Occasionally, however, a urethral stricture is discovered in a boy with no antecedent history of external injury, urethral instrumentation or catheterisation. In very young boys the aetiology can be assumed to be congenital, but in the older age group the possibility of previously unrecognised trauma must be entertained. Whether congenital or acquired, such strictures are generally mild and respond well to endoscopic urethrotomy. Formal urethroplasty is rarely required.

Cobb's collar

The clinical status of this anomaly is arguable and its principal significance is as an occasional radiological finding on MCU comprising a short, narrowed segment of urethra immediately distal to the urogenital membrane. On endoscopy the findings consist of little more than a soft, non-obstructing concentric ring. Although Cobb's collar has sometimes been implicated as a possible cause of voiding disorders, notably enuresis, the consensus is that in children it is essentially a radiological finding without clinical significance.

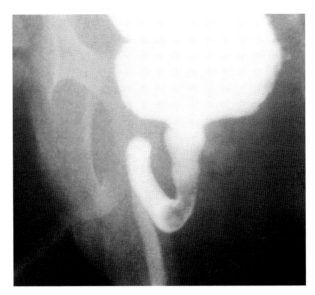

Figure 9.10 MCU outlining a posterior urethral polyp prolapsing from its point of origin into the membranous and bulbar urethra.

Urethritis

Although the existence of this condition in boys is recognised by paediatric urologists it has received little attention in the literature, the clinical features are non-specific and the aetiology is poorly understood. The condition is uncommon but occurs in boys aged 6 years and upward, with presenting features that include dysuria, penile discomfort and urethral discharge or urethral bleeding – usually consisting of no more than spotting on the underclothes. Attempts to culture a specific organism are unrewarding. In the absence of other features cystourethroscopy is not indicated, as it rarely makes a practical contribution to clinical management. However, when urethroscopy is performed the findings are characterised by erythema of the anterior and bulbar urethra, with a granular appearance and strands of fibrinous exudate. There is no specific treatment and the condition is self-limiting, although it sometimes runs a protracted course.

Key points

● The original classification devised by Young is outdated. Congenital urethral obstruction generally conforms to a uniform anatomical pattern, although there is considerable variability in the severity of obstruction and the degree of congenital damage to the upper tracts.

- The majority of cases are now detected prenatally. The time-scale and characteristics of the prenatal ultrasound findings provide a guide to the prognosis for renal function. Published results of fetal intervention are disappointing.
- Despite relief of the urethral obstruction in infancy, ongoing bladder dysfunction in childhood may contribute to deteriorating upper tract function and the onset of renal failure.
- Approximately one-third of individuals with posterior urethral valves are destined to develop chronic renal failure. Careful follow-up should be maintained throughout adolescence and into early adulthood.

Further reading

Cuckow PM. Posterior urethral valves. In: Stringer MD, Oldham KT, Mouriquand PDE, Howard ER (eds) *Paediatric surgery and urology: long term outcomes.* London: WB Saunders, 1998; 487–500

Dinneen MD, Duffy PG. Posterior urethral valves. *Br J Urol* 1996; 78: 275–281

Holmdahl G, Sillen U, Hanson E et al. Bladder dysfunction in boys with posterior urethral valves before and after puberty. *J Urol* 1996; 155: 694–698

Hutton KA, Thomas DFM, Arthur RJ et al. Prenatally detected posterior urethral valves: is gestational age at detection a predictor of functional outcome? *J Urol* 1994; 152: 698–701

Cystic renal disease

10

David FM Thomas

Topics covered
Prevalence of different forms of cystic renal diseases in childhood
Autosomal recessive polycystic kidney disease

Autosomal dominant polycystic kidney disease
Multicystic dysplastic kidney
Multilocular renal cyst
Simple renal cyst

Introduction

Cystic pathology of the kidney is relatively common across the age range from childhood into late adulthood. The pattern of renal cystic disease in infancy and childhood differs from that encountered in adults, with multicystic dysplastic kidney (MCDK) and the autosomal recessive form of polycystic kidney disease assuming greater importance than autosomal dominant polycystic kidney disease.

The introduction of routine ultrasound imaging into obstetric practice has revealed that the true prevalence of asymptomatic unilateral multicystic dysplastic kidney is considerably higher than was previously suspected, but only a small percentage are clinically evident at birth and the majority of unilateral MCDKs clearly remained undetected in the past.

The terminology previously used to describe the different clinical and pathological forms of cystic renal disease has given rise to understandable confusion. In particular, terms such as 'dysplastic', 'hypoplastic', 'shrunken', 'polycystic' and 'multicystic' have often been used loosely or interchangeably in the literature with little regard to differences in histology and developmental biology. In clinical practice, confusion commonly arises from the failure to distinguish between multicystic dysplastic kidney, a sporadic structural abnormality which, when unilateral, carries a good prognosis, and polycystic kidney disease, an inherited disorder characterised by diffuse pathology of the parenchyma of both kidneys.

Embryology and pathology

The different types of cystic renal disease encountered in childhood are so diverse that their embryology, inheritance and pathology are more conveniently summarised under the relevant headings. The Potter classification represented the first systematic attempt to categorise the differing forms of cystic renal pathology, but has been rendered obsolete by advances in molecular biology and genetics which have found little scientific justification for the groupings devised by Potter.

Polycystic renal disease

This important group of disorders is characterised by the presence of microscopic or macroscopic cystic tissue distributed diffusely throughout the parenchyma of both kidneys. There are no histological features of dysplasia.

Two major forms of polycystic renal disease are encountered, i.e. autosomal recessive (the type most commonly encountered in children) and autosomal dominant, which, although sometimes evident on renal ultrasound in childhood, is of little clinical impact until adult life.

Autosomal recessive polycystic renal disease (Figure 10.1)

Incidence

1:10 000–1:40 000.

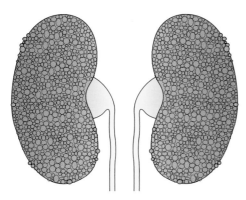

Figure 10.1 Autosomal recessive polycystic renal disease. Diffuse bilateral renal enlargement.

Pathology

Typically the kidneys retain their normal outline but are considerably enlarged. The pelves, calyces and ureter are normal in morphology. The renal parenchyma is extensively replaced by cylindrical, radially orientated cysts which are usually less than 2 mm in diameter. Liver involvement is almost invariable, with a pattern of bile duct abnormalities termed 'biliary dysgenesis'.

Presentation

Autosomal recessive polycystic kidney disease is associated with characteristic ultrasound appearances of diffuse bilateral renal enlargement (Figure 10.2). Ultrasound findings of oligohydramnios or reduced bladder volume are predictors of severe functional impairment. Termination of pregnancy is an option when the condition is detected in the second trimester, but ultrasound evidence of the disorder is not always apparent at this stage in gestation, or may not be sufficiently diagnostic until later in pregnancy.

Clinical features

In the neonatal period these include readily palpable abdominal masses and, in more severe cases, pulmonary hypoplasia and 'moulding' deformities, e.g. Potter's facies, talipes etc. Occasionally autosomal recessive polycystic kidney disease does not come to light until later childhood, when it presents with hypertension or manifestations of hepatic fibrosis, such as portal hypertension or bleeding oesophageal varices.

Diagnosis is with ultrasound in conjunction with intravenous urography (IVU) and, in some cases, CT. Renal biopsy may also be indicated.

Treatment

Initial ventilatory support may be required for the management of respiratory distress and pulmonary hypoplasia in severely affected infants. The requirement for ventilation does not carry the universally poor prognosis that was once the case. **Medical management** is directed at the treatment of hypertension, prevention of malnutrition, and measures designed to minimise anaemia and renal bone disease. Children progressing to end-stage renal failure are managed by dialysis and transplantation, with native nephrectomy being indicated to control hypertension or create space for the transplanted kidney. Specific treatment may be required for the complications of hepatic disease.

Prognosis

In the absence of severe pulmonary hypoplasia most affected infants can now be expected to survive beyond the neonatal period. The survival rate has been documented as 86% at 3 months, 79% at 1 year, 51% at 10 years and 46% at 15 years.

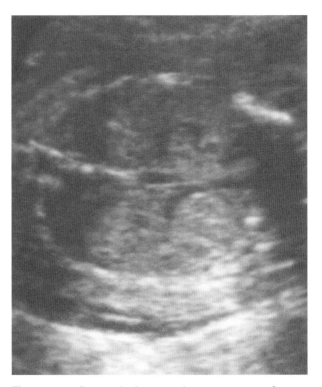

Figure 10.2 Prenatal ultrasound appearances of autosomal recessive polycystic kidney disease

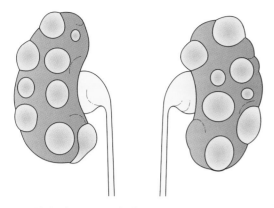

Figure 10.3 Autosomal dominant polycystic kidney disease. Discrete cysts of varying size interspersed between areas of normal renal parenchyma.

Autosomal dominant polycystic kidney disease (Figure 10.3)

Incidence

The most commonly inherited form of renal disease, autosomal dominant polycystic kidney disease has a reported prevalence ranging from 1:200 to 1:1000. It is essentially a disorder of adult life, accounting for approximately 5–10% of adults on end-stage renal replacement programmes.

Pathology

Histologically, the cysts are lined by tubular epithelium and the intervening renal parenchyma may be normal or show evidence of glomerulosclerosis. Extrarenal manifestations include hepatic cysts and cerebral aneurysms.

Genetics

The defective gene responsible for 80–90% of cases was first identified in 1994. Located on chromosome 16, the *PKD1* gene encodes for a glycoprotein believed to play an important role in cell matrix interaction. A second gene defect affecting the *PKD2* gene on chromosome 4 is thought to account for the majority of the remaining cases.

Presentation

Autosomal dominant polycystic kidney disease is occasionally identified during routine prenatal ultrasound examination. In addition, asymptomatic individuals can sometimes be diagnosed on ultrasound screening of the offspring or other young family members of patients known to have the disorder.

Clinical presentation is usually in adult life, with hypertension, abdominal pain, palpable abdominal masses, haematuria or other urinary symptoms.

Management

The condition is managed expectantly, with follow-up aimed at the detection and early treatment of complications, notably hypertension. Cyst drainage or nephrectomy are occasionally indicated in the management of severe hypertension, or to control pain or urinary infection.

Prognosis

When the autosomal dominant form of polycystic kidney disease is diagnosed on ultrasound in childhood, either incidentally or during family screening, the prognosis for renal function is generally good, with 80% of children maintaining normal levels of renal function into adult life. In contrast, when detected prenatally or in the neonatal period, autosomal dominant polycystic kidney disease carries a poor prognosis.

Multicystic dysplastic kidney (MCDK) (Figure 10.4)

Prior to the introduction of routine ultrasound examination in pregnancy MCDK was regarded as a relatively rare anomaly which generally presented as an abdominal mass in the neonatal period. Nephrectomy was routinely undertaken in such cases. It is now

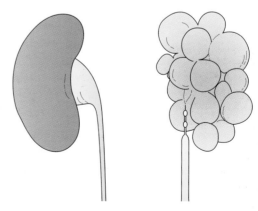

Figure 10.4 Multicystic dysplastic kidney. Kidney replaced by collection of cysts of varying size. Ureteric atresia.

evident that the true prevalence of MCDK is far higher than was previously suspected, but in the majority of cases the lesion is clinically undetectable and the affected infant is entirely asymptomatic and outwardly normal. The management of prenatally detected MCDK and the arguments surrounding 'prophylactic' removal of asymptomatic kidneys remain a source of controversy.

Incidence

Current evidence from a number of sources indicates a prevalence for unilateral MCDK in the range 1:2500–1:4000 live births. Bilateral MCDK, a lethal anomaly, has an estimated incidence of 1:20 000 pregnancies.

Aetiology/embryology

Proximal ureteric atresia (or, more rarely, distal ureteric obstruction) is almost invariably found in association with MCDK (Figure 10.5). Complete ureteric obstruction at an early stage in embryonic development has therefore been invoked as the cause of the MCDK malformation.

Faulty development of the ureteric bud and metanephric mesenchyme may also be implicated (see Chapter 1). The incidence of vesicoureteric reflux (VUR) in children with MCDK is around 30% and is thus comparable to that in the siblings of children with known VUR. Moreover, MCDK is closely linked to renal agenesis, which is also associated with a far higher than expected incidence of VUR. The familial basis of VUR and renal agenesis is well established and it seems likely that MCDK belongs within the same spectrum of embryonic ureteric bud anomalies, which in some instances may be genetically determined.

The familial occurrence of MCDK has been reported in the literature, and although MCDK generally appears to behave as a sporadic anomaly, in some families it may be inherited as an autosomal dominant trait with variable penetrance (Figure 10.6).

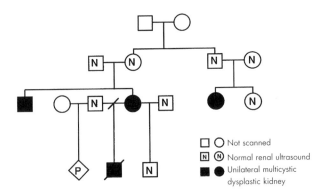

Figure 10.6 Familial occurrence of MCDK. Pedigree of affected family. Probable autosomal dominant pattern of inheritance. Most MCDKs occur as a sporadic anomaly.

Pathology

MCDK comprises an irregular collection of tense non-communicating cysts of varying size lined by cuboidal or flattened tubular epithelium. Renal parenchyma, where present, is dysplastic and consists of small islands or flattened plates of abnormal tissue interposed between cysts.

Presentation

MCDKs present in one of three ways:

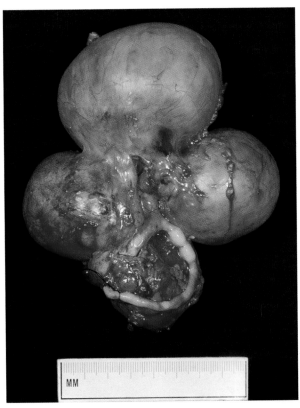

Figure 10.5 Nephrectomy specimen. Multicystic dysplastic kidney. (Courtesy of Mr P G Ransley).

- **Clinically** – usually as an abdominal mass in the neonatal period. Only a small proportion of all

MCDKs now present clinically. Typically the surface of a palpable MCDK is 'knobbly' and irregular in contour, contrasting with other neonatal renal masses, e.g. hydronephrosis or polycystic kidney, which have a smoother surface on palpation.

- **Incidental postnatal ultrasound finding** in an infant with coexisting congenital anomalies, e.g. oesophageal atresia.
- **Prenatal ultrasound.** The majority of prenatally diagnosed MCDKs (> 80%) are small and clinically undetectable at birth.

Diagnosis

Although the prenatal ultrasound appearances of MCDK can occasionally be difficult to distinguish from those of marked hydronephrosis, most experienced radiologists can make the diagnosis with a high degree of accuracy. Postnatally the diagnosis is confirmed by a combination of ultrasound and isotope imaging. MCDKs are characterised by a total absence of isotope uptake (0% differential function) on **DMSA**. In some centres **MAG3** is favoured, as this yields additional information on drainage in the contralateral kidney.

The role of the micturating cystourethrogram (**MCU**) in the evaluation of infants with prenatally detected MCDK is controversial. When performed routinely, it reveals a 20–40% incidence of low-grade contralateral or ipsilateral VUR. However, the clinical significance of this finding is uncertain, as in these infants the low-grade VUR rarely gives rise to symptomatic infection and is mostly destined to resolve in early life. In the author's experience less than 3% of children with MCDK have required ureteric reimplantation for the correction of reflux, and it is therefore the author's preference to reserve MCU for those infants in whom there is ultrasound evidence of ureteric or contralateral renal dilatation. However, it is essential that parents and general practitioners are aware that otherwise normal ultrasound appearances do not exclude the possibility of low-grade VUR, and the occurrence of a documented urinary tract infection (UTI) or an unexplained febrile illness is an indication to proceed to MCU.

Natural history

A number of studies have now documented the potential for prenatally detected MCDKs to involute – i.e.

disappear on ultrasound – both pre- and postnatally. Approximately 30% of MCDKs involute in the first 12 months of life, and 50% are no longer visible on ultrasound at 5 years of age. Further follow-up data are awaited. Those that remain detectable on ultrasound are either smaller or unchanged in size, and thus relatively smaller in relation to the growing child.

The documented tendency for MCDKs to involute spontaneously, coupled with the relative rarity with which unilateral renal agenesis is diagnosed in utero, has been interpreted as evidence that a proportion of cases of apparent renal agenesis diagnosed in adult life or at postmortem may in fact represent the legacy of involuted MCDKs.

Complications

Hypertension is a rare but well documented complication of MCDK. Nephrectomy is undoubtedly warranted in these circumstances.

Is the risk of hypertension sufficient to justify routine 'prophylactic' nephrectomy for asymptomatic prenatally detected MCDKs? In a recent literature review spanning 30 years, Manzoni and Caldamone identified 13 reported cases of hypertension attributed to MCDK. Blood pressure reverted to normal following nephrectomy in the 11 cases for which follow-up information was available. Closer scrutiny of these case reports reveals one in which the diagnosis of MCDK was incorrect, and two in which the original diagnosis of hypertension is at the very least arguable

Viewed in the context of the prevalence of MCDK (1:2500–1:4000) the published data on hypertension would point to a very low order of risk. But do the published cases simply represent the tip of the iceberg, with the majority of instances of hypertension going unreported? Unpublished data emerging from the ongoing American Registry of MCDKs suggests that the incidence of hypertension may genuinely be higher than previously reported – although still less than 1%.

The possible link between MCDK and hypertension can be studied from a different angle. If hypertension occurs on an appreciable scale this should be reflected in the published literature on renal hypertension in childhood, but this is not the case. No cases of MCDK were encountered in 454 children with hypertension presenting to the paediatric nephrology unit at the Hospital for Sick Children, Great Ormond Street. Similarly, two published series of children in Glasgow and Boston with 'surgical' forms of renal hypertension undergoing nephrectomy did not include a single MCDK.

On the basis of evidence currently available it therefore appears that the risk of hypertension associated with MCDK is probably very low (of the order 0.01–0.1%) and does not justify 'prophylactic' nephrectomy in asymptomatic infants and children.

Malignant potential

Reviewing the literature over a 30-year period, Manzoni and Caldamone identified six published cases of Wilms' tumour in children with MCDK. A further five cases of renal cell carcinoma had been reported in association with MCDK in adults ranging from 15 to 68 years of age. As with hypertension, it is likely that the number of published cases understates the risk. However, as with hypertension it is also possible to view the question from a different angle by asking 'How commonly does MCDK figure in published series of Wilms' tumours?' In the United States detailed data on 7500 Wilms' tumours were collected over an 18-year period as part of the National Wilms' Tumor Study. Out of these 7500 tumours only five arose in MCDKs. On current estimates of the true prevalence of MCDK this represents an individual lifetime risk of the order 1:2500. Given that Wilms' tumour is now largely curable, the lifetime risk of dying from a Wilms' tumour arising in an MCDK has been calculated to be comparable to the risk of mortality associated with general anaesthesia. **Although opinion remains divided, the available evidence does not justify submitting asymptomatic infants or children to nephrectomy as a prophylactic measure.**

Other complications

Symptoms such as pain or haematuria have been ascribed to MCDKs in rare cases reported in the adult literature. These symptoms are rarely, if ever, seen in association with MCDK in the paediatric age group. When urinary infection occurs in children with MCDK it is more likely to be due to underlying vesicoureteric reflux or some coexistent anomaly rather than the MCDK itself (which by virtue of ureteric atresia does not communicate with the rest of the urinary tract).

Management

Coexisting anomalies

Contralateral PUJ obstruction is present in 5–10% of cases and is managed conservatively or surgically according to its severity. Vesicoureteric reflux is generally low grade and is usually managed conservatively by antibiotic prophylaxis and urine surveillance.

Multicystic dysplastic kidney

Nephrectomy is indicated for those rare instances when MCDK presents in the neonatal period as a large, clinically evident abdominal mass. Depending on factors including the size of the mass and the presence or absence of other anomalies, surgery can usually be deferred until 4–6 weeks of age or later.

The arguments for the 'prophylactic' removal of asymptomatic MCDKs centre principally on the perceived risks of malignancy and hypertension, and have already been considered. Specialist opinion in the UK generally favours conservative management. Genuine indications for nephrectomy include hypertension, increasing size, or the appearance of unusual or worrying features on ultrasound follow-up.

Ultrasound follow-up is maintained on an annual basis until 5 or 6 years of age. Although some paediatric urologists insist on the disappearance of the MCDK before discharging the child, this has not been the author's practice. Measurement of blood pressure in infants or fractious young children can be difficult but becomes easier as the child grows. At the time of discharge from surgical follow-up it is prudent to arrange for blood pressure to be checked by a paediatrician or GP on an annual basis thereafter, continuing into adult life.

Nephrectomy

MCDKs can be removed safely either through a small incision anterior to the tip of the 12th rib or via a posterior lumbotomy approach. Aspiration of cyst fluid facilitates removal through a limited incision. Laparoscopic nephrectomy for MCDK has also been reported, although the benefit seems arguable in view of the established safety and low level of morbidity when open nephrectomy is performed through a small lumbotomy incision.

Multilocular renal cyst (Figure 10.7)

This rare renal lesion, also described as cystic nephroma, benign multilocular cystic nephroma etc., may give rise to diagnostic difficulty, typically being misdiagnosed as a cystic Wilms' tumour.

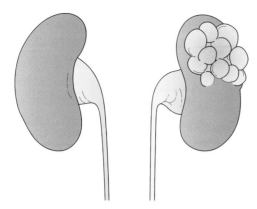

Figure 10.7 Multilocular renal cyst.

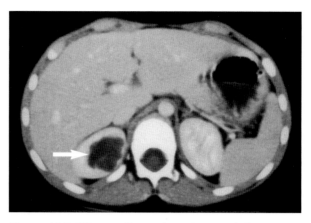

Figure 10.8 CT scan illustrating characteristic appearances of a multiloculated space-occupying lesion within the right kidney (arrowed).

Aetiology

It remains unclear whether multilocular renal cyst should be regarded as a neoplasm or a developmental anomaly. Although malignancy ascribed to this lesion has been reported in adult life, multilocular renal cyst is not generally considered a premalignant lesion. It occurs sporadically with no evidence of an inherited basis.

Incidence

Experience in the Yorkshire region would put the incidence at approximately 1:200 000–1:250 000. The condition demonstrates a bimodal age distribution, with one peak in infancy and a second peak in early adult life, separated by an unexplained hiatus in distribution. Children account for 30–50% of cases.

Presentation

Most cases present with haematuria, loin pain or an abdominal mass, although multilocular cyst can occasionally come to light as an incidental finding on ultrasound during the investigation of unrelated symptoms.

Diagnosis is by ultrasound complemented by CT (Figure 10.8) and possibly MRI. Typically the multilocular cystic lesion is localised within the renal parenchyma, but may extend into the collecting system or distort the renal capsules. An experienced paediatric radiologist should be able to distinguish multilocular renal cyst from other forms of renal pathology, but even with sophisticated imaging it may be difficult to distinguish from a cystic variant of Wilms' tumour.

Management

Nephrectomy is the accepted form of treatment. In view of the benign nature of the lesion nephron-sparing surgery, i.e. partial nephrectomy, might be considered in certain circumstances, such as a multilocular renal cyst in a solitary kidney.

Simple renal cyst (Figure 10.9)

Although a common finding in adults, simple or 'solitary' renal cysts are only occasionally encountered in childhood and are thus likely to be acquired rather than congenital in aetiology A simple cyst rarely gives rise to problems in this age group, and it is important that an incidental ultrasound finding is not misinterpreted as the cause of some unrelated symptom, such as non-specific abdominal pain. Dilatation of the upper pole of a duplex kidney is sometimes mistaken

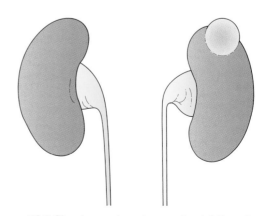

Figure 10.9 Simple renal cyst – rare in childhood.

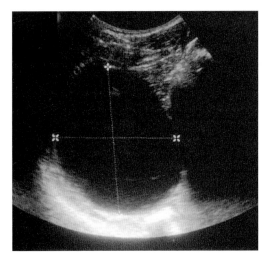 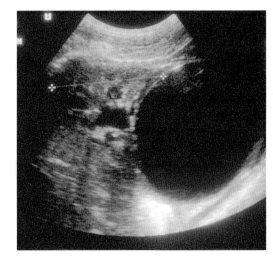

Figure 10.10 Ultrasound appearances of large simple cyst in the lower pole of the left kidney of a 7-year-old boy presenting with abdominal pain and a palpable mass.

on ultrasound for a simple cyst by radiologists unfamiliar with paediatric urology. Very rarely a child may present with abdominal pain or other symptoms which are genuinely attributable to the presence of a large, tense simple renal cyst (Figures 10.10). Management is the same as for symptomatic renal cysts in adults, and comprises percutaneous cyst aspiration and injection of alcohol, or laparoscopic or open deroofing and subtotal excision of the cyst wall. Recurrence is uncommon.

Further reading

Gabow PA. Autosomal dominant polycystic kidney disease. In: Gardner KD, Bernstein J (eds) *The cystic kidney*. Dordrecht, Netherlands: Kluwer, 1990; 295–326

Manzoni GM, Caldamone AA. Multicystic kidney. In: Stringer MD, Oldham KT, Mouriquand PDE, Howard ER (eds) *Paediatric surgery and urology: long-term outcome*. London: WB Saunders, 1998; 632–641

Thomas DFM, Fitzpatrick MM. Cystic renal disease in childhood. In: Thomas DFM (ed) *Urological disease in the fetus and infant*. Oxford: Butterworth-Heinemann, 1997; 237–249

Key points

- Despite the potentially confusing terminology it is important to have a clear understanding of the various patterns of cystic renal disease in view of the important differences in clinical significance and prognosis.
- Autosomal recessive polycystic kidney disease is detected prenatally or presents in the newborn period.
- Autosomal dominant polycystic kidney disease does not generally come to light until adulthood.
- Multicystic dysplastic kidney (MCDK) is a developmental abnormality of the kidney which is more prevalent in the general population than was previously recognised.
- Current evidence suggests that the risks of hypertension and malignancy are very low in relation to the true prevalence of MCDK and do not justify routine 'prophylactic' nephrectomy in asymptomatic infants.

Prenatal diagnosis

11

HK Dhillon

Introduction

The first few examples of fetal uropathies, detected by prenatal ultrasound, were reported in the mid 1970s but it was not until the early to mid 1980s that maternal ultrasound was fully incorporated into routine obstetric practice in the United Kingdom. Since then, a substantial body of experience has accumulated and the management of infants with prenatally detected uropathies currently constitutes a major component of paediatric urological practice. However, it is important to recognise that our knowledge of the long term clinical outcome of prenatally detected uropathies remains very limited since comparatively few children have so far even reached their teens. Prospective follow up studies would be highly desirable to determine the long term prognosis and natural history of these conditions. Only then will it be possible to resolve some of the controversies surrounding early surgical intervention or conservative management of prenatally detected conditions such as pelvi-ureteric junction obstruction, multicystic dysplastic kidney and vesicoureteric reflux.

Those Paediatric Urological units which manage a large number of infants with prenatally detected uropathy have a responsibility to undertake prospective studies in order to identify prognostic criteria, which will serve to identify sub-populations at risk of later functional deterioration or clinical complications. Conversely, the evidence of long term follow up studies should also make it possible to identify which forms of prenatally detected uropathy are not destined to pose any threat to health and which may indeed, not warrant any investigation.

Until this information becomes available the management of infants with prenatally detected urinary tract abnormalities must be guided by two important considerations:

- **The majority of infants with prenatally detected urinary tract abnormalities are outwardly normal and healthy at birth.** As such they cannot be considered as patients in the conventional sense. This is particularly true of infants with isolated unilateral anomalies, in whom relevant clinical findings are present in fewer than 5% of cases. Bilateral renal pathology is more likely to be associated with relevant physical signs or coexisting syndromes but, nevertheless, the majority of infants with prenatally detected bilateral uropathy are asymptomatic and seemingly normal.
- Only a very small proportion of infants with prenatally detected uropathies (< 5%) have renal insufficiency of sufficient severity to require nephrological support and, overall, the majority of affected infants do not require any form of early surgical intervention.
- **The prenatal detection of a fetal urinary tract abnormality is often a source of disproportionate parental anxiety during the pregnancy.** Parents, who have been told that their unborn child has a kidney abnormality, tend to assume the worst, including a scenario involving dialysis and renal transplantation. In our experience, only 10% of parents receive accurate counselling on the prognosis of the urological abnormality diagnosed in utero. Ideally, Paediatric Urologists would play a far greater role in prenatal counselling but the

pressure of heavy clinical workloads in many centres makes this a difficult goal to achieve.

Obstetric ultrasound, current practice

In the United Kingdom, virtually every pregnant mother is routinely scanned at least once – usually between weeks 14 and 19 of gestation. The timing of this fetal anomaly scan is designed to ensure that severe congenital malformations are diagnosed with sufficient accuracy to permit an informed decision on termination of pregnancy. The fetal urinary tract is routinely visualised as part of the anomaly scan and amniotic fluid volume (an indicator of fetal urinary output) is also assessed. In addition to the routine second trimester fetal anomaly scan, many women are also scanned in later pregnancy, for a variety of obstetric indications.

The sensitivity and specificity of ultrasonography in the detection urinary tract anomalies is influenced by a number of technical factors including the image resolution of the equipment used, the experience of ultrasonographer or radiologist performing and interpreting the scan and by maternal size and obesity.

Abnormalities such as renal ectopia or renal agenesis, which are not associated with dilatation, are considerably more difficult to detect than those characterised by dialatation such as uropathy and cystic disease. Although virtually every major, potentially lethal, urinary tract malformation is detectable in the second trimester it has become increasingly apparent that most cases of pelviureteric junction obstruction, vesicoureteric reflux, duplication and mild to moderate urethral obstruction, are not associated with dilatation at this stage in gestation and are only be picked up on scans performed later in pregnancy. Thus **gestational age at the time of scanning is the most important factor determining the sensitivity of prenatal urological diagnosis.**

Incidence

The incidence of prenatally detected urinary tract abnormalities encountered in different centres varies considerably, depending on the gestational age at which ultrasound screening is routinely performed and local practice relating to the scanning in later pregnancy. The incidence of significant prenatally detected uropathies reported from a number of European centres averages around 1:500–1:600 pregnancies. One UK study found that mild dilatation (generally defined as an antero posterior diameter of the renal pelvis of less than 1 cm) was a feature of 1:100–1:200 pregnancies.

Management

Prenatal

The scope for influencing the clinical outcome of a prenatally detected uropathy by active intervention during pregnancy is limited to the severe end of the spectrum and comprises fetal surgery (generally vesicoamniotic shunting) or termination. However, there is also some anecdotal evidence that preterm delivery and early postnatal treatment may favourably modify the outcome for some males with posterior urethral valves.

In the overwhelming majority of cases the pregnancy is allowed to progress normally to term and medical input consists of monitoring (where appropriate) and counselling of the parents.

Counselling should ideally include:

- The differential diagnoses – insofar as this can be ascertained with the ultrasound information available.
- An explanation of the investigations, which are likely to be advised following delivery.
- A broad outline of prognosis.

Where the need for surgery is envisaged, parents should be reassured that this is rarely of a serious or life-threatening nature. Unfortunately, it is often impossible to provide a detailed account of what the future holds since the prenatal ultrasound findings are non-specific in approximately 70% of cases. For example, the discovery of unilateral ureteric and renal dilatation at 34 weeks gestation would require a discussion encompassing megaureters, vesicoureteric reflux and duplex kidneys.

For logistical reasons, counselling for mild to moderately severe prenatally detected uropathies, particularly those detected in later pregnancy, is mostly undertaken in the hospital where the mother is receiving her routine obstetric care. However, for more severe urinary tract abnormalities, particularly when detected on second trimester fetal anomaly scanning it may be appropriate to consider termination of pregnancy. In this situation, prompt referral to a specialist centre is indicated for more detailed investigation and specialist counselling.

Fetal intervention

The question of whether to intervene during the pregnancy only arises at the severe end of the pathological spectrum where the ultrasound findings and results of any additional investigations point to the likelihood of intrauterine death or early postnatal death. Termination of pregnancy may also be sought following the discovery of a major, non lethal, malformation which nevertheless carries grave implications for the affected individual's quality of life.

Bilateral renal agenesis or bilateral multicystic dysplastic kidneys are clear examples of anomalies which are incompatible with survival. In one study renal agenesis and multicystic dysplasia (or combinations thereof), accounted for more than 60% of terminations of pregnancy for urological anomalies.

By contrast, the prognosis of urethral obstruction (usually in male fetuses), is more difficult to predict since it spans a broader spectrum of severity ranging from urethral atresia with oligohydramnios and pulmonary hpoplasia to milder forms of urethral valve obstruction in which renal function is largely unaffected. However, the high overall level of morbidity associated with congenital urethral obstruction is reflected in the statistic that males comprise 90% of children undergoing treatment for renal failure in the first 4 years of life. The rationale of intervention aimed at modifying this outcome is considered below and in Chapter 9.

Fetal intervention is subdivided into diagnostic procedures intended to assess functional prognosis and detect chromosomal abnormalities, termination of pregnancy and therapeutic intervention (most commonly vesicoamniotic shunting).

Karyotype

Chromosomal analysis can be performed by examining exfoliated cells in amniotic fluid or by sampling blood from the umbilical cord ('cordocentesis'), or chorionic villus sampling.

Fetal urine sampling

Urine is aspirated from the fetal bladder by percutaneous puncture under ultrasound guidance with further imaging to determine whether the bladder refills and if so, how long this takes (an indicator of fetal urinary output). A number of urinary constituents have been studied as possible markers of fetal urinary function and prognostic indicators of longer term functional outcome. Of these, fetal urinary sodium, chloride and osmolality have proved the most useful. Fetal urinary calcium and Beta 2 microglobulin have also been evaluated as prognostic indicators. Unfortunately, a considerable overlap exists between pathological and normal values, and there are limited data on normal values to serve as a reference range at different gestational ages. Fetal urinary biochemistry, therefore, provides only an approximation of fetal renal function.

Fetal blood sampling (usually in conjunction with cordocentesis)

Levels of urea and creatinine in the fetal blood provide no indication of fetal renal function since these excretory metabolites cross the placenta and fetal blood levels are identical to those in the maternal circulation. However, Beta 2 microglobulin does not cross the placenta and may prove to be of more value as an indicator of potential glomerular function independently of maternal renal function.

Vesicoamniotic shunting

The rationale for this therapeutic intervention is based on the premise that decompression of the obstructed urinary tract in utero will avert progressive renal damage and prevent further functional deterioration. Although hysterotomy, open fetal surgery, fetoscopy and valve ablation have been reported the technique most widely practised comprises ultrasound guided percutaneous insertion of a pigtail shunt catheter to drain urine from the fetal bladder into the amniotic fluid. Since congenital urethral obstruction represents the sole indication, vesicoamniotic shunting is also considered in Chapter 9.

With few exceptions, the published results of fetal intervention (either open fetal surgery or vesicoamniotic shunting) have been disappointing. In the mid 1980s, the Fetal Surgery Registry published a series of 73 cases, with an overall mortality rate of 60%. A subsequent review of the literature noted a 45% incidence of procedure-related morbidity, including premature labour. The most authoritative, recent data on fetal intervention are those published from Detroit, in which 34 fetuses were treated in the period from 1987 to 1996. Despite treatment, 13 (38%) died in utero or postnatally and of the survivors assessed after 2 years of age, 57% had renal insufficiency – of whom the majority had already required early renal transplantation.

Whilst the published results of vesicoamniotic shunting do not appear to support its use in routine clinical practice it is important to note that shunting has generally been confined to a population of fetuses characterised by oligohydramnios and other evidence of grossly impaired renal function. In the cases comprising most published series there was very little potential for improving the prognosis and it is hardly surprising that shunting was of no benefit. However, one cannot dismiss the possibility that shunting might prove beneficial where bladder distension and bilateral upper tract dilatation is not accompanied by oligohydramnios or severely deranged urine biochemistry. The outcome of fetal intervention in this population is not known since shunting has been performed so rarely. Ideally a controlled trial would resolve some of these questions, but for a number of practical reasons, it is now unlikely that a statistically meaningful controlled trial could ever be undertaken.

Termination of pregnancy

With the increasing prevalence and accuracy of prenatal diagnosis, parents are increasingly opting for termination of pregnancy following the discovery of a urological abnormality which is inconsistent with survival – or which carries grave implications for quality of life.

At this highly stressful time in parents' lives it is essential that they receive sympathetic counselling and are given all the information they need to make an informed (and often very difficult) decision about their unborn child.

For example, it is important that they have a realistic picture of what is entailed in the management of renal failure in childhood, in terms of hospital visits, in-patient stays, medication, surgery and the difficulties inherent in dialysis and transplantation.

Unfortunately, even with benefit of detailed information provided by ultrasound and other diagnostic modalities, it may not be possible to provide parents with an accurate prediction of the prognosis and timescale of clinical events in infancy and early childhood.

Termination of pregnancy is also being increasingly requested following the discovery ,on prenatal ultrasound of major anomalies such as cloacal and 'classic' bladder exstrophy. As a result, many paediatric urologists have already noted decreasing referral numbers of newborns with these abnormalities and conditions such as prune belly syndrome.

Post natal management

Antibiotic prophylaxis

As a rule, antibiotic prophylaxis (usually Trimethoprim 2 mg per kg nocte) should be commenced for all newborn infants with prenatally detected uropathies pending the outcome of postnatal investigations (notably a micturating cystogram).

Exceptions include:

- Infants with mild, isolated renal dilatation with an AP diameter of 10 mm or less.
- Multicystic dysplastic kidney with an entirely normal contralateral kidney.
- Ectopic kidney without evidence of dilatation.

Postnatal ultrasound

Urinary output is often reduced in the first day of life with the result that an abnormal urinary tract may appear less dilated when not subjected to a representative diuretic load. For this reason, the initial postnatal scan should ideally be deferred until 24–48 hours of age, i.e. when normal diuresis has been established. However, this optimal timing may be difficult to achieve since many mothers now opt for early discharge from hospital. The timing of the initial ultrasound scan is, therefore, best guided by the prenatal findings.

- Prompt postnatal ultrasound and referral to a specialist unit is essential for fetuses with suspected lower urinary tract obstruction – as signified by bilateral upper tact dilatation, thick-walled bladder, ureteric dilatation, etc.
- Bilateral dilatation without bladder or ureteric involvement also merits early ultrasound – ideally between 3 and 7 days of age.
- In contrast, unilateral dilatation with a normal contralateral kidney carries a low risk of early morbidity and the initial postnatal scan can reasonably be deferred and performed on an outpatient basis at around 2 weeks of age.

In most specialist centres, the antero posterior (AP) diameter of the renal pelvis is now routinely measured. Although this figure is subject to factors such as operator error and the degree of hydration, the measurement of renal pelvic diameter is nevertheless preferable to subjective descriptions such as 'mild', 'moderate', 'gross' hydronephrosis, 'full', or 'baggy' renal pelvis. In addition to documenting the AP diameter of the renal pelvis, the appearances of the calices and parenchyma should also be noted.

Micturating cystourethrogram (MCU)

The role of the MCU in the routine postnatal evaluation of infants with prenatally detected dilatation remains controversial, with practice varying considerably between different centres.

However, as a guideline it is agreed that the following represent **definite indications for a post natal MCU**:

- Abnormal bladder (particularly a thick-walled bladder or other evidence of outflow obstruction).
- Bilateral upper tract dilatation.
- Ureteric dilatation demonstrated either on pre or postnatal ultrasound.
- Duplex kidneys (in view of the high incidence of lower pole reflux).

The main controversy centres on whether infants with mild dilatation (less than 15 mm antero posterior diameter) should routinely be investigated by micturating cystourethrography.

The value of mild pelvic dilatation as a possible marker of vesicoureteric reflux is inadequately documented. Moreover, when reflux is detected, it tends to be low grade (Grades I–III), is generally associated with two good kidneys and usually resolves spontaneously in the first 2 years of life. The clinical significance of a low grade reflux detected on prenatal ultrasound is, therefore, largely unknown. Micturating cystourethrography is an invasive, potentially distressing procedure, which carries some risk of morbidity (predominantly infection). For these reasons, many paediatric urologists do not advocate routine micturating cystourethrography if dilatation is confined to the renal pelvis (i.e. no evidence of ureteric and/or caliceal dilatation), and the AP diameter of the pelvis is less than 15 mm. Some cases of low grade VUR will be missed by this approach, but this is outweighed by the

benefit of a greatly reduced burden of unnecessary investigation into healthy infants.

If an MCU is not undertaken parents should, nevertheless, be aware of the importance of having their child's urine checked for possible infection in the event of an unexplained febrile illness or more specific features of urinary infection.

Isotope imaging

The choice of imaging is determined largely by the findings on the postnatal ultrasonography (and micturating cystourethrography when this has been performed.) ^{99m}Tc-DMSA is best suited to confirming total absence of function in a multicystic kidney and for studying differential function and renal damage associated with congenital vesicoureteric reflux. ^{99m}Tc-MAG3 is the isotope most widely used for the diagnosis of obstruction. It is important to note, however, that drainage curve data cannot be relied upon in young infants, even following the administration of Frusemide. Since the information derived from DMSA scintigraphy or diuretic renography rarely influences practical management in the first few weeks or months of life isotope imaging is best deferred until 1–3 months of age.

A rational approach to diagnosis and management

Diagnostic pathways

Suggested diagnostic pathways for the postnatal investigation of different prenatally detected urinary tract abnormalities are illustrated in Figures 11.1, 11.2, 11.3 and 11.4. These are intended as broad guidelines but it may be necessary to take additional factors into account when planning the timing and nature of postnatal investigation in an individual case.

At its best, prenatal diagnosis constitutes an effective form of preventative medicine, which affords an opportunity to identify children, who would benefit by intervention before they develop renal functional deterioration or complications resulting from infection. However, such cases only represent a small percentage of the total and many healthy children with asymptomatic prenatally detected urinary tract anomalies are still being subjected to needless investigation. In particular, the prenatal diagnosis of mild

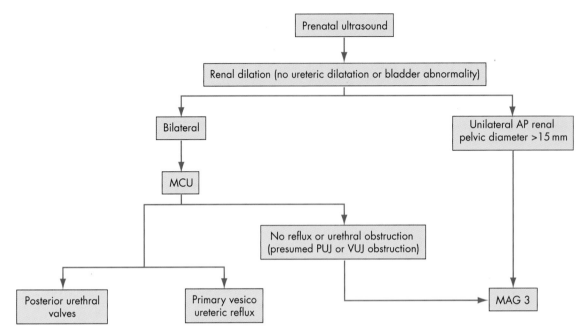

Figure 11.1 Diagnostic pathway for postnatal investigation of prenatally detected dilatation confined to the renal collecting system(s).

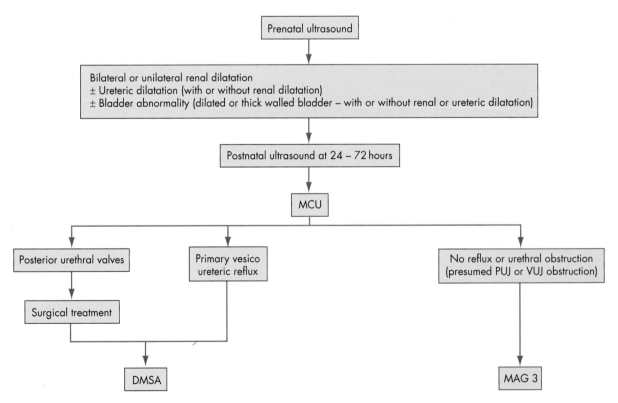

Figure 11.2 Diagnostic pathway for postnatal investigation of renal dilatation which is accompanied by ureteric dilatation and/or a bladder abnormality.

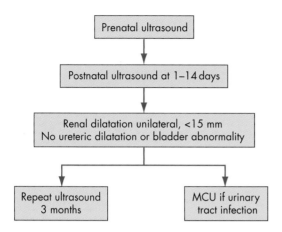

Figure 11.3 Diagnostic pathway for postnatal investigation of mild unilateral dilatation (renal pelvic anteroposterior diameter < 15 mm), without coexisting ureteric dilatation or bladder abnormality.

dilatation has often been a source of unwarranted parental anxiety and has generated a burden of investigation which is wholly disproportionate to the risk of morbidity. Put simply, too much is still being done for very little real benefit.

Ideally, DGH paediatric units should work to clear diagnostic and management guidelines established in collaboration with their local paediatric urological centres. In this way, the need for unnecessary invasive investigations can be avoided and the duplication of investigations kept to a minimum.

Further reading

Lind T. The Biochemistry of amniotic fluid. In: Sandler M (ed). *Amniotic fluid and its clinical significance*. New York: Marcel Dekker, 1979; 1–25

Tassis BMG, Trespidi L, Tirelli AS et al. Serum (3 2-microglobulin in fetuses with urinary tract anomalies. *Am J Obstet Gynaecol* 1997; 176: 54–57

Freedman AL, Johnson MP, Smith CA, Gonzalaez R, Evans M. Long-term outcome in children after antenatal intervention for obstructive uropathies. *Lancet* 1999, 354: 374–377

Benacerraf BR, Mandell J, Estroff JA, Harlow BL, Frigoletto FD. Fetal pylectasis: a possible association with Down's syndrome. *Obstet Gynaecol* 1990; 76: 58–60

Cortville JE, Dickie JM, Crane JP. Fetal pyelectasis and Down's syndrome: is genetic amniocentesis warranted? *Obstet Gynaecol* 1992; 79: 770–772

Yeung CK, Goldey ML, Dhillon HK, Gordon I, Duffy PG, Ransley PG. The characteristics of primary vesicoureteric reflux in male and female infants with prenatal hydronephrosis. *Brit J Urol* 1997; 80: 319–327

Thomas DFM (ed). *Urological disease in the foetus and infant: diagnosis and management*. Oxford: Butterworth-Heinemann, 1997.

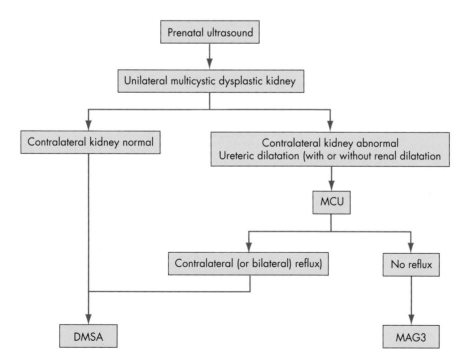

Figure 11.4 Diagnostic pathway for the investigation of prenatal ultrasound appearances suggesting multicystic dysplastic kidney (see also Chapter 10).

Key points

- The sensitivity of ultrasound for the prenatal detection of urinary anomalies is dependant upon a number of factors – most importantly gestational age at scanning.
- The majority of infants with prenatally detected uropathies are entirely asymptomatic and outwardly normal at birth.
- The long-term outcome and natural history of asymptomatic prenatally detected uropathies is unknown. Surgical intervention is generally unwarranted unless there are clear cut indications.
- The published results of vesicoamniotic shunting relate to fetuses with a severe degree of renal impairment. There is a need to reappraise the possible benefits of fetal intervention in less severely affected cases where there is a better prospect of improving the functional outcome.

- The combination of prenatal diagnosis and termination of pregnancy is resulting in declining numbers of referrals of severe but non-lethal urological malformations such as prune-belly syndrome, cloacal and classic bladder exstrophy.
- Prenatal diagnosis is beneficial for individuals at risk of functional deterioration or severe sepsis-related complications. At the mild end of the spectrum, however, prenatal diagnosis has generated needless parental anxiety and created a burden of investigation which is disproportionate to the risk of morbidity
- Investigation and management of prenatally detected uropathies should ideally be undertaken according to locally agreed protocols. An integrated approach between District General Hospitals and specialist paediatric urology centres can help to avoid unnecessary invasive investigations and minimise the risk of duplication.

Stone disease in children

12

David FM Thomas

Introduction

Urinary calculi (stones) are rare in children, who are estimated to account for only 2–3% of all patients with stone disease. Infection is the major aetiological factor in children, whereas in adults stones are largely multifactorial or metabolic in aetiology. Other important differences include the lower stone recurrence rate in children and the differing role of minimally invasive treatment. Although an estimated 90% of stones in adults are now managed by lithotripsy or endourological treatment, more than 50% of children's stones are still managed by open surgery.

Incidence and epidemiology

Geographical variations in the incidence of stone disease in children reflect differences in the prevalence of environmental, dietary and genetic factors. In the UK the estimated incidence of urinary calculi in children is approximately 3 new cases per million of the population per year. A comparative review of the aetiology of children's stones published from different centres found that in children in the UK urinary infection accounted for 60% of urinary calculi, in France 74%, and in the northeastern states of the USA 40%.

The greater frequency of urinary infection in uncircumcised infants and differing cultural attitudes to neonatal circumcision may help to explain the higher incidence of urinary stone disease in certain European countries compared to the United States.

A geographical 'stone belt' extending from the Balkans across Turkey, Pakistan and northern India is characterised by a high incidence of endemic bladder stones in children. Chronically inadequate dietary intake of protein has been implicated, but relative dehydration associated with the climate and diarrhoeal illness may also be a contributory factor.

Pathology/aetiology

Urinary calculi are composed of crystalline and matrix components in varying proportions. Matrix, a gelatinous glycoprotein, is a particular feature of infective stones, which are typically soft and crumbly in composition. Metabolic stones, e.g. cystine and xanthine, are predominantly crystalline and correspondingly harder The terminology historically used to describe the crystalline structure of urinary calculi ('struvite', 'brushite', 'wedellite' etc.) is uninformative, and in this chapter stones are categorised by reference to their chemical composition.

Factors involved in stone formation

- **Urinary concentration, ionic activity and solubility of stone-forming constituents** Stone formation is initiated by the precipitation of urinary constituents from solution, followed by crystal formation. In turn, this process is influenced by the urinary excretion rate of the stone-forming substance, the level of hydration and the urinary pH.
- **Presence of abnormal urinary metabolites or pathologically elevated concentration of normal urinary constituents** When a metabolite is excreted in high concentrations its saturation point

in the urine is exceeded and crystal deposition occurs, progressing to stone formation. Reduced urinary output leading to a higher urinary concentration of the metabolite and unfavourable pH will accelerate this process.

- **Urinary infection** Certain bacterial species, notably *Proteus*, *Klebsiella* and *Pseudomonas*, are capable of the enzymatic splitting of urea to produce NH_3, with consequent elevation of the urinary pH and precipitation of ammonium salts. Infection is also a key factor in the production of the proteinaceous matrix component of calculi.
- **Anatomical abnormalities of the urinary tract** Urinary infection associated with underlying urological abnormalities predisposed to stone formation by the mechanisms outlined above. Stasis of urine within an obstructed or dilated urinary tract creates an environment in which stone-forming substances are more likely to precipitate out of solution and thus initiate stone formation. This process can occur in sterile urine, but not uncommonly infection and stasis coexist.
- **Foreign materials** Non-absorbable foreign bodies, usually surgical in origin (stents, fragments of catheters, non-absorbable sutures or staples) act as a nidus of encrustation and stone formation.

Aetiology: clinical aspects

Infective calculi

It is estimated that 75% of children with urinary calculi are under 5 years of age at the time of diagnosis. Of these, 70–80% are boys with infective calculi. Infective stones initially comprise a combination of magnesium, ammonium phosphate and glycoprotein matrix in varying proportions. Calcium phosphate and other inorganic constituents then become incorporated into the expanding stone mass. Their consistency is variable, with areas of hard calcified material embedded within softer, less densely calcified matrix. Calcified areas are radio-opaque but the softer matrix component, which may extend throughout much of the collecting system, is radiolucent or only faintly apparent on plain X-ray. The descriptive term 'staghorn' refers to a an infective calculus that has adopted the configuration of the renal pelvis and calices (fancifully likened to the antlers of a stag). Rarely, the infective process progresses to involve the entire renal parenchyma in a chronic inflammatory mass – xanthogranulomatous pyelonephritis (see below).

Metabolic calculi

Calcium

Abnormalities of calcium metabolism and excretion play an important aetiological role in adult stone disease but are much less commonly implicated in children. Isolated hypercalciuria is usually the result of an inherited renal tubular defect of calcium reabsorption. Major disorders of calcium metabolism which are associated with hypercalcaemia and hypercalcuria tend to give rise to calcification of the renal parenchyma (nephrocalcinosis), as well as the formation of calculi within the collecting system. Hypercalcaemia and stone formation are also occasionally seen as a consequence of bone demineralisation resulting from immobilisation or neoplastic deposits.

Oxalate

Two rare genetically determined metabolic disorders are expressed as excessive production of oxalic acid: urolithiasis and nephrocalcinosis. The infantile form of primary hyperoxaluria is rapidly progressive and is characterised by the deposition of oxalate throughout the tissues. A second form presents with calculi in adult life. A combination of renal and orthotopic liver transplantation has been advocated for severe forms, with the aim of treating not simply the renal complications but also the underlying hepatic enzyme deficiency.

Cystine

Cystine is one of four amino acids affected by a recessive inherited disorder of renal tubular reabsorption (the others being lysine, arginine and ornithine). The solubility of cystine is relatively poor and its elevated concentration within the collecting system results in crystal deposition and stone formation.

Although cystine itself is only weakly radio-opaque the incorporation of calcium within the aggregation of amino acid crystals forms hard stones which are clearly visualised on plain X-ray.

Uric acid

Metabolic disorders of uric acid metabolism are rare in children, but acute deposition of uric acid crystals within the urinary tract can occur as a result of massive cell breakdown, e.g. following the introduction of cytotoxic treatment for leukaemia or lymphoma. In these conditions uric acid crystalline debris 'silts up' the collecting systems, leading to anuric renal failure. Uric acid is radiolucent and thus cannot be directly visualised on plain X-ray.

Xanthine

Xanthine oxidase deficiency, a rare autosomal recessive disorder, results in the deposition of insoluble non-opaque xanthine stones within the urinary tract.

Underlying urological conditions

Predisposing urological abnormalities can be identified in approximately 20–30% of children with urinary calculi, a far higher figure than in adults. Although vesicoureteric reflux may play an aetiological role by promoting urinary infection it may represent a secondary phenomenon, particularly following the passage of ureteric calculi. Reflux should therefore be reassessed some months after stone clearance if antireflux surgery is envisaged.

The role of obstruction and stasis is generally easier to establish. Although uncommon, stones associated with primary pelviureteric junction (PUJ) obstruction are characteristically small and multiple (fancifully likened to melon seeds). Stones forming within megaureters can occasionally present acutely with complete upper tract obstruction following impaction at the vesical junction.

The use of intestinal segments for bladder reconstruction (enterocystoplasty) is accompanied by a significant risk of stones, amounting to 30–40% in some series. A combination of factors includes stasis, the presence of intestinal mucus within the urine acting as a nidus for crystalline deposition, and chronic low-grade bacteruria. Regular bladder washouts reduce the risk, principally by ensuring more effective clearance of urinary mucus than intermittent catheterisation alone.

Clinical presentation

Urinary infection

Although older children may present with recognisable symptoms of urinary infection the clinical picture in infants may be deceptively non-specific, consisting of vague ill-health, low-grade fever and failure to thrive. The isolation of *Proteus* from a child's urine should always prompt investigation for underlying stone disease.

Haematuria

Macroscopic or microscopic haematuria is a common feature of calculi, but there is only a poor correlation between the severity of haematuria and the extent and distribution of stones within the urinary tract. Absence of blood on microscopy or reagent strip testing does not exclude the possibility of stones.

Passage of stone material per urethram

Occasionally stones come to light when a fragment or some softer matrix material is passed per urethram. In infants the presence of unusual material and streaks of blood in the nappy may be incorrectly ascribed to balanitis.

Pain

Acute renal colic of the pattern and severity encountered in adults is not a prominent feature of the symptomology in children. When pain does occur it is often a poorly localised symptom in a fractious, unwell child.

Abdominal mass

Xanthogranulomatous pyelonephritis (see below) presents with general ill-health which may be accompanied by palpable abdominal mass – a clinical picture resembling Wilms' tumour.

Diagnosis

The role of diagnostic imaging can be considered at two levels.

Initial screening for possible calculi
Ultrasound

In experienced hands ultrasound is a sensitive modality for the detection of renal calculi. Depending on their physical characteristics (chemical composition, hardness etc.), calculi can be directly visualised on ultrasound. In addition, solid stones cast a so-called 'acoustic' shadow which serves to distinguish calculi from other echogenic lesions within the renal collect-

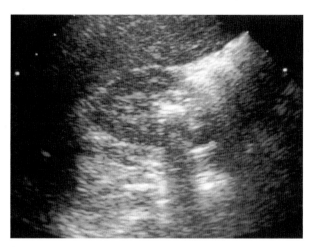

Figure 12.1 Ultrasound appearances of renal calculus, illustrating 'acoustic shadow'.

ing system (Figure 12.1). Ureteric calculi and small bladder calculi may be difficult to detect on ultrasound.

Abdominal X-ray

A plain abdominal radiograph to look for possible calculi should be undertaken in any child undergoing investigation for haematuria. Similarly, the investigation of urinary infection in boys under 5 years of age should always include a plain abdominal X-ray (Figure 12.2). A documented *Proteus* urinary infection, at any age, also merits a plain abdominal X-ray, but in an older girl presenting with uncomplicated urinary infection of mild or moderate severity the plain X-ray can reasonably be omitted from the initial investigation.

Unenhanced spiral CT

This is rapidly being adopted as the initial investigation of choice for adults with suspected stone disease. Spiral CT provides an accurate diagnosis within minutes, avoids the potential risk of adverse reaction to contrast media, and will positively demonstrate the presence of radiolucent calculi that cannot be directly visualised by conventional radiology. However, the radiation dosage is estimated to be three to five times greater than that of an IVU (although this nevertheless amounts to only a quarter of the recommended limit of medical radiation exposure for a child in a year). Other drawbacks include the requirement for more complex equipment than intravenous urography, and greater difficulty in interpreting the images

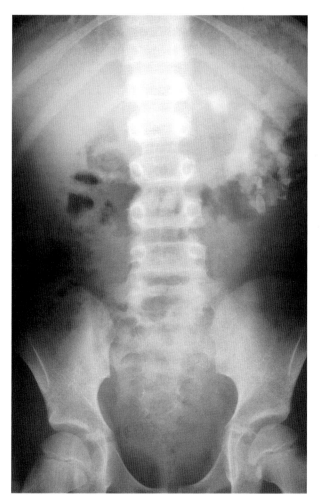

Figure 12.2 Plain X-ray revealing multiple infective calculi in the left kidney.

of the collecting system. The role of spiral CT as front-line diagnostic modality in children requires further evaluation.

Evaluation prior to treatment of proven stone disease

DMSA

Regardless of whether open surgery or minimally invasive treatment is planned, differential function in the affected kidney(s) should be documented on DMSA – and re-evaluated after treatment.

IVU

For a number of reasons the IVU retains a valuable role in the diagnostic evaluation of stones, for example by permitting visualisation of non-opaque stones and

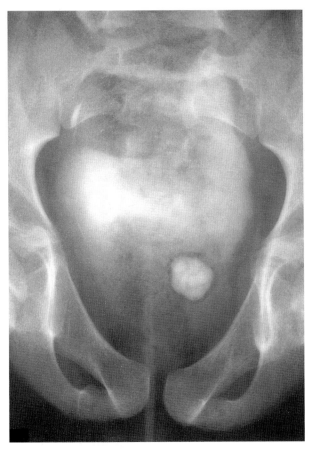

Figure 12.3 Intravenous urogram demonstrating a calculus in a single (orthotopic) ureterocoele. The IVU is also useful in helping to establish the nature of the predisposing anatomical abnormality.

the matrix component of infective staghorn calculi. Information on calyceal anatomy is important in planning percutaneous nephrolithotomy (PCNL) and external shockwave lithotripsy (ESWL). Ureteric calculi are best localised by intravenous urography (Figure 12.3). Finally, the IVU may be helpful in identifying any underlying anatomical abnormality predisposing to urolithiasis.

Additional investigations

- **Micturating cystography (MCU)** is not routinely required. Infection and the passage of stone material to the bladder may result in transient vesicoureteric reflux, which resolves once the infection has been treated and stone clearance achieved. However, when ureteric dilatation persists postoperatively, or in the event of further infection, an MCU should be performed.

Table 12.1 Metabolic screening protocol

Fasting blood sample for plasma levels of urea, electrolytes, creatinine, calcium, phosphate, uric acid
Early morning urine sample (pH to exclude renal tubular acidosis)
'Spot', i.e. untimed, urine sample 2–5 ml (divided in the laboratory into two aliquots)
First aliquot acidified and analysed for creatinine, calcium, magnesium, cystine, oxalate
Second aliquot alkalinised and analysed for creatinine and uric acid

- **Dynamic renography**, e.g. MAG3, DTPA is undertaken if obstruction is suspected either pre- or postoperatively
- **Computed tomography (CT)** As already indicated, the potential role of unenhanced spiral CT in the initial diagnosis of stone disease is still undergoing evaluation in children. However, CT has a well established role in the diagnosis of xanthogranulomatous pyelonephritis and for visualising non-opaque calculi.
- **Metabolic investigations** Underlying metabolic disorders are not always reliably reflected in the chemical composition of the stones they give rise to. For this reason urinary biochemistry is more useful than the the time-honoured practice of sending stones for laboratory investigation. The presence of urinary infection does not exclude the possibility of metabolic stones, as the two aetiologies may coexist. Every child with stone disease, regardless of the perceived aetiology, should therefore undergo metabolic screening after the eradication of infection (Table 12.1).

Stone screening can be reliably undertaken on a random 'spot' sample of 2–5 ml of urine, although an early morning specimen may be preferable for some studies. Twenty-four hour urine collections are impracticable in children and are only required for the specific investigation of rare metabolic disorders.

Management

Some form of intervention is almost invariably required to physically remove the stone(s) or reduce them to fragments which can then be passed spontaneously. The advent of minimally invasive modalities has transformed the management of stone disease in adults, but its impact has been more limited in paediatric practice for the following reasons:

- In adults the majority of stones are discrete, relatively small and non-infective in aetiology. In contrast, more than 60% of paediatric stones are infective in origin, bulky, and comprised of soft or 'crumbly' matrix material which is less amenable to external shock wave lithotripsy (ESWL).

- Current-generation lithotripters cause far less pain and bruising than their predecessors. Nevertheless, general anaesthesia is still necessary for younger children in view of the discomfort and the need to ensure they remain still and suitably positioned during treatment.

- Until recently, the role of percutaneous nephrolithotomy (PCNL) and ureteroscopy has been limited in children by the lack of suitable miniaturised instruments. However, this limitation is likely to be resolved by the availability of new instruments designed for paediatric use.

Open stone surgery

Kidney

Following exposure and mobilisation of the kidney, isolated stones within the collecting system can usually be removed with stone forceps via an incision in the renal pelvis without undue difficulty (Figure 12.4). The bulk of a staghorn calculus can also be removed by this approach, but the subsequent removal of fragments impacted in the the calyces, necessary to achieve total stone clearance, often proves time-consuming and frustrating. Some of the manoeuvres that can facilitate this task are illustrated in Figure 12.5. With the advent of ESWL it is often preferable

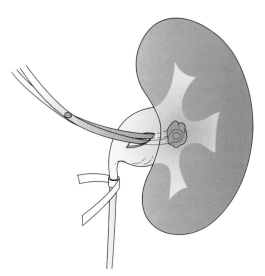

Figure 12.4 Pyelolithotomy. Open removal of a calculus from the renal pelvis.

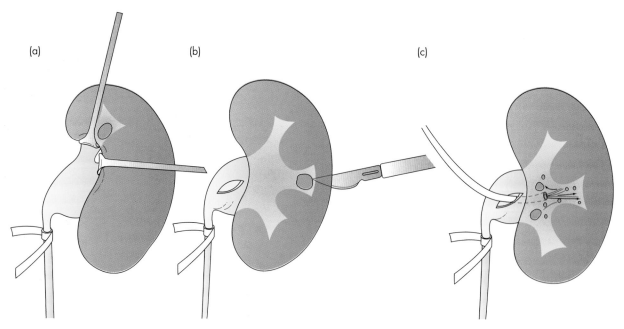

Figure 12.5 Additional intraoperative manoeuvres for the clearance of calyceal calculi or fragments. (a) Surgical exposure of calyceal neck by dissection at the renal hilum. (b) Nephrolithotomy. (c) High-pressure saline irrigation.

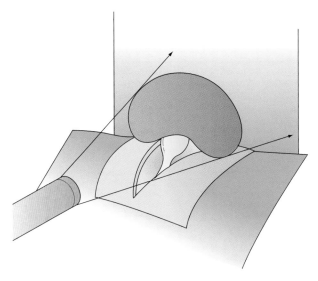

Figure 12.6 Intraoperative 'on-table' X-ray to confirm stone clearance.

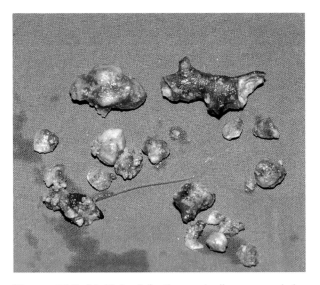

Figure 12.7 Multiple infective calculi, removed by pyelonephrolithotomy from the patient illustrated in Figure 12.2.

to treat any small residual fragments by ESWL at a later date, rather than incur the haemorrhage and parenchymal damage associated with multiple incisions in the renal cortex.

Techniques dating from the days of extensive open stone surgery in adults (anatrophic nephrolithotomy, renal cooling etc.) have only a very limited application in paediatric practice.

To minimise the risk of unsuspected retained fragments, intraoperative 'on-table' X-rays of the kidney are mandatory to confirm that stone clearance has been achieved (Figure 12.6). Intraoperative X-rays may also help the surgeon decide when to abandon nephrolithotomy in favour of postoperative ESWL.

Extrarenal drainage is essential in view of the considerable leakage of urine that may occur from the incision sites in the kidney postoperatively. Following extensive renal surgery a short period of nephrostomy or indwelling JJ stent drainage may also be indicated (Figures 12.7, 12.8).

Ureter

In the absence of obstruction, severe pain or infection a small stone (e.g. < 5 mm) can be managed expectantly in the hope that it will pass spontaneously into the bladder, from where it will be passed by voiding or will be accessible to endoscopic removal. If the stone fails to pass or is accompanied by symptoms or obstruction, the options include:

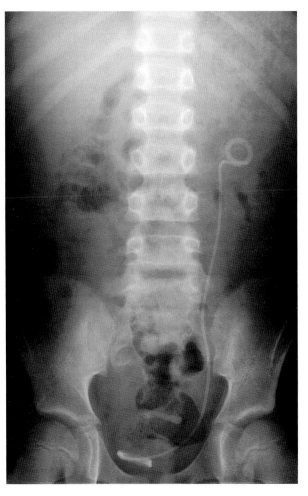

Figure 12.8 Plain abdominal X-ray of the patient illustrated in Figures 12.2 and 12.7. Total stone clearance achieved, indwelling JJ stent in situ.

- **Ureteroscopy** For an isolated ureteric stone in a child aged 3 years upwards ureteroscopy and lithotripsy probably now represent the best form of first-line treatment (see below).
- **Stone basket** Despite the availability of stone baskets designed for paediatric use the risk of ureteric damage is considerable and their use should only be attempted for small stones (< 5 mm) located in the distal third of the ureter. Screening with an image intensifier is essential.
- **Ureterolithotomy** Stones in the distal ureter can be removed via a Pfannenstiel incision. Midureteric stones are best approached transperitoneally via an oblique muscle-cutting incision. The ureter is closed loosely with a few interrupted absorbable sutures to minimise the risk of stricture formation.

Bladder

Stones which have recently passed into the bladder from the upper tracts can be managed conservatively in the expectation that they will be passed from the bladder by voiding, but stones arising de novo within the bladder, or bladder stones forming around the nidus of an upper tract fragment, are often too large to pass spontaneously by the time they are diagnosed.

Open surgery (cystolithotomy) remains the preferred option for very large stones, particularly those forming within augmented bladders. Where the bladder neck has been formally closed in conjunction with augmentation and the creation of a Mitrofanoff stoma, open cystolithotomy is the simplest and most effective surgical option.

Urethra

Urethral calculi are rare in children and result from impaction of a calculus (or post-ESWL fragments) during its passage through the urethra, or in situ stone formation within an anatomical abnormality, such as a müllerian remnant or the urethral stump of a rectourethral fistula following surgery for an anorectal anomaly.

Urethral calculi can be removed or crushed using rigid endoscopic biopsy forceps. Meatotomy may be required to release a stone impacted within the fossa navicularis.

Minimally invasive treatment

Kidney

External shockwave lithotripsy (Figure 12.9)

Shockwaves generated either by high-tension spark or by piezoelectric energy are transmitted through a fluid to the patient. Using ultrasound or X-ray linked to the shockwave generator, this energy is focused on the renal stone(s). General anaesthesia is not generally necessary in older children or adults, but is required for younger or uncooperative children to ensure their position is maintained throughout the duration of treatment.

The limitations of ESWL in children centre principally on:

- the physical characteristics of infective calculi, which tend to be bulky, partially comprised of soft proteinaceous matrix and unsuited to shockwave treatment;
- the drawbacks associated with repeated general anaesthetics if multiple ESWL sessions are needed to achieve stone clearance.

However, ESWL is proving increasingly valuable for the treatment of small or non-infective stones in older children, and for 'mopping up' residual fragments following open stone surgery.

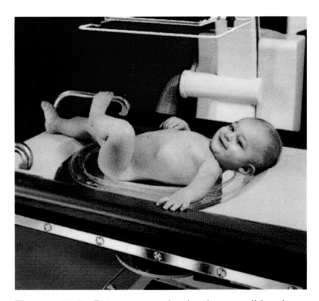

Figure 12.9 Extracorporeal shockwave lithotripsy. General anaesthesia is usually required in infants and young children. Reproduced with permission from Storz Medical AG, Kreuzlingen, Switzerland.

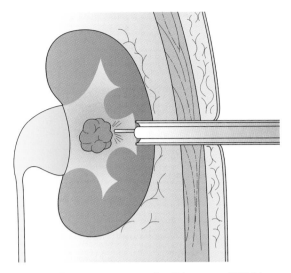

Figure 12.10 Percutaneous nephrolithotomy (PCNL).

Percutaneous nephrolithotomy (PCNL)

A percutaneous track is established to permit the introduction of an endoscope into the renal collecting system. Under direct vision the stone is removed percutaneously or disintegrated with a lithotripter probe (Figure 12.10). Although PCNL has so far been largely limited to older children and adolescents, the availability of instruments designed specifically for paediatric use will extend the role of this modality.

Ureter

Ureteric stones, once visualised by semirigid or flexible ureteroscopy (Figure 12.11), are fragmented by pulsed dye laser, electrohydraulic lithotripsy or lithoclast. A JJ stent is generally left in situ.

Bladder

Endoscopic treatment is now feasible for the majority of bladder stones. The stone is shattered using a lithoclast (employing the principle of a pneumatic drill) passed down the channel of a paediatric cystoscope (Figure 12.12). Larger fragments are removed by vigorous irrigation and suction, whilst small fragments can be left to pass spontaneously.

Complications of open stone surgery

These include haemorrhage, particularly after multiple nephrotomies, retained or displaced stone fragments, prolonged urinary leakage, and parenchymal damage resulting in loss of renal function.

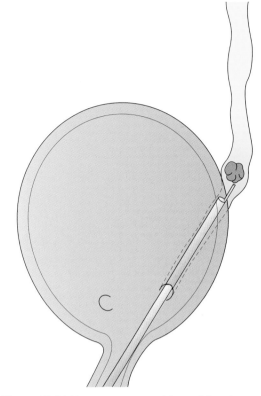

Figure 12.11 Ureteroscopy and laser lithotripsy.

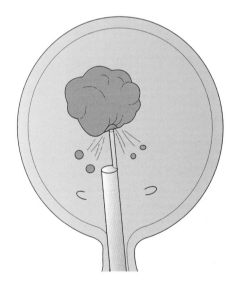

Figure 12.12 Endoscopic fragmentation of bladder calculus by lithoclast.

Open ureterolithotomy carries a risk of ureteric stricture. Ureteric damage (perforation, avulsion) may also result from injudicious attempts at ureteric basket extraction.

Complications of minimally invasive modalities

These have yet to be adequately documented in children, but the available evidence indicates that anxieties surrounding the risks of parenchymal damage and hypertension are likely to prove unfounded.

The injudicious use of adult PCNL instruments in children poses a considerable threat of renal trauma and haemorrhage. Ureteroscopy may result in transient reflux and carries a possible risk of fibrosis and vesicoureteric junction obstruction, but in the hands of an experienced endourologist the risk of complications appears to be low.

Results

A historical review of 270 children treated in Liverpool for stone disease over a 28-year period reported a recurrence rate of 14% for infective stones and 30% for metabolic stones. In a recently published series of 43 children treated by different minimally invasive modalities at the author's centre, 88% were rendered stone-free on a minimum of 3 months' follow-up. Metabolic disorders accounted for most cases of residual calculi.

High stone clearance rates have also been reported in a sizeable series of children treated at the Institute of Urology in London.

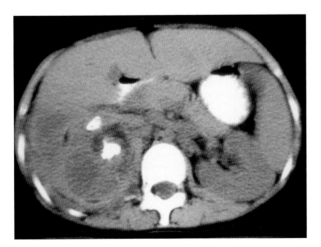

Figure 12.13 CT scan. Xanthogranulomatous pyelonephritis of the right kidney, illustrating calculi embedded within a non-functioning inflammatory renal mass. Normal left kidney.

Recurrence

Infective calculi

The recurrence risk can be minimised by correcting any underlying predisposing anatomical abnormality and by maintaining infection-free urine with antibiotic prophylaxis for 12 months following surgery.

Metabolic calculi

A high fluid intake is essential. In addition, a number of specific measures can be employed, e.g. pyridoxine in primary hyperoxyaluria, D-penicillamine in cystinuria, and allopurinol in conjunction with a low-purine diet for xanthinuria.

Xanthogranulomatous pyelonephritis

This rare manifestation of stone disease is characterised by features of chronic sepsis (weight loss, anaemia, elevated ESR) and the presence of an inflammatory mass which may extend to involve adjacent viscera. The diagnosis is confirmed by a combination of ultrasound, CT (Figure 12.13) and DMSA, which reveals absent or minimal function in the affected kidney. Treatment consists of nephrectomy.

Key points

- Urinary calculi are rare in childhood. Urinary infection is the most important aetiological factor.
- Every child presenting with calculi should be thoroughly evaluated to identify any underlying metabolic disorder or urological malformation.
- Urine biochemistry is more reliable for the diagnosis of metabolic disorders than is stone analyis.
- Minimally invasive modalities such as ESWL, PCNL and endoscopic lithotripsy are rapidly acquiring an important role in the treatment of children's stones. The availability of specialised instrumentation will hasten this process. However, open pyelolithotomy seems likely to retain an important place in the primary management of bulky staghorn calculi in young children.
- Careful follow-up, with maintenance of sterile urine and appropriate treatment of any metabolic disorder, is essential to minimise the risk of stone recurrence.

Further reading

Adams MC, Newman DM, Lingeman JC. Paediatric extracorporeal shockwave lithotripsy: long-term results and effects on renal growth. In: Lingeman JE, Newman DM (eds) *Shock wave lithotripsy 2: urinary and biliary lithotripsy*. New York: Plenum, 1990; 233

Diamond DA. Clinical patterns of paediatric urolithiasis. *Br J Urol* 1991; 68: 195–198

Fraser M, Joyce AD, Thomas DFM, Eardley I, Clark PB. Minimally invasive treatment of urinary tract calculi in children. *Br J Urol* 1999; 84: 339–342

Ghazali S. Childhood urolithiasis in the United Kingdom and Eire. *Br J Urol* 1975; 47: 739–743

Henderson MJ. Renal stone disease – investigative aspects. *Arch Dis Chil* 1993; 68: 160–163

Henderson MJ. Stone analysis is not useful in the routine investigation of renal stone disease. *Ann Clin Biochem* 1995; 32: 109–111

Kroovand RL. Urinary calculi in childhood. In: O'Donnell B, Koff SA (eds) *Paediatric urology*. Oxford: Butterworth-Heinemann, 1997; 629–645

Mor Y, Elmasry YET, Kellett MJ, Duffy PG. The role of percutaneous nephrolithotomy in the management of paediatric renal calculi. *J Urol* 1997; 158: 1319–1321

Sperling O. Inherited metabolic stone disease. In: Whitfield HN, Hendry WF, Kirby RS, Duckett JW (eds) *Textbook of genito-urinary surgery*. Oxford: Blackwell Science, 1998: 757–770.

Thomas R, Ortenberg J, Lee BR, Harmon EP. Safety and efficacy of paediatric ureteroscopy for management of calculus disease. *J Urol* 1993; 149: 1082–1084

Urinary incontinence

13

AMK Rickwood

Topics covered
Development of bladder control
Patient assessment

Organic urinary incontinence
Functional diurnal incontinence
Nocturnal enuresis

Introduction

Urinary incontinence – by day, by night, or both – is extremely common during childhood and may be a cause of major social morbidity in affected individuals. A simple classification of the complaint, used in this chapter, is shown in Figure 13.1. Although organic causes of incontinence are rare, accounting for well under 1% of referrals from general practice, they must always be excluded as a first priority as active treatment is almost always necessary and sometimes there is also a risk to the upper renal tracts. Only when an organic cause has been excluded can the complaint be assumed to be functional in aetiology. At this point the problem becomes essentially social rather than medical, and because the natural history of almost all these disorders is benign, with spontaneous resolution occurring during the course of childhood, active treatment is called for only should the family wish it.

With few exceptions, the various clinically recognisable forms of functional diurnal enuresis are associated with detrusor instability, the nature of which, in children, requires an understanding of the normal development of bladder control.

Developmental of bladder control

During infancy voiding is an entirely reflex act, mediated and coordinated at brainstem level, although the arousal characteristic of premicturition indicates that sensory input percolates to higher centres. Indeed, at this time of life voiding rarely, if ever, occurs during sleep.

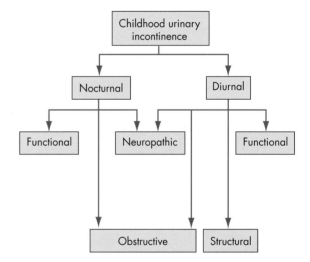

Figure 13.1 Simple classification of childhood urinary incontinence.

Whereas such reflex voiding contractions are by definition 'unstable', true instability during the filling phase is exceptional and micturition occurs with detrusor–sphincter synergia and with the detrusor contraction sustained until the bladder is empty. This pattern of normal reflex voiding is disturbed in infants with bladder outflow obstruction. Furthermore, studies of boys with high-grade vesicoureteric reflux have shown high-pressure dysfunctional voiding even in the absence of demonstrable urethral obstruction. During the first year of life the number of voidings remains fairly constant, at approximately 20 per day, declining over the next 2 years to around 11 per day, and by the age of 7 years settles to an average of five per day. This decreased frequency is due to a growth-related increase in bladder capacity which is disproportionately greater than the volume of urine produced.

Successful toilet training is dependent upon several factors, the most important being the development of voluntary inhibition of the voiding reflex. Once fully established, volitional voiding at any degree of bladder filling sets humans apart from all other mammals bar the dog. In some young children – perhaps even a majority – there is a transitional phase wherein this ability to inhibit the voiding reflex is related to filling volume, with the result that there is only a modest interval between the first perception of a desire to void and the necessity to do so. Beyond this phase, and usually by 5 years of age, a mature filling/voiding cycle exists, with detrusor stability even in the face of a strong desire to void and with voiding to completion by sustained detrusor contractions and with detrusor–sphincter synergia.

Patient assessment

Clinical

The exclusion of organic disease (Table 13.1) is the first priority, and this is usually possible on the basis of history and physical examination, supplemented, in selected individuals, by ultrasonography of the urinary tracts. More invasive investigations, including urodynamics, are only occasionally required, principally when there is suspicion of neuropathy or, in girls, of ureteric ectopia.

History

When dealing with a child with urinary incontinence there are always three fundamental questions to be addressed: Does the wetting occur principally or entirely by night or, similarly, by day? Is the problem primary (i.e. dating from the time of toilet training) or secondary. And, in the case of daytime wetting, does this occur continuously or only intermittently?

- **Purely night-time wetting** which is primary and unaccompanied by any daytime symptoms (primary monosymptomatic nocturnal enuresis) for practical purposes *never* has an underlying organic basis. Although nocturnal enuresis has a functional basis in the great majority of cases, bedwetting of secondary onset or which is associated with daytime symptoms can very occasionally be related to bladder outflow obstruction or to neurological disease. Polyuric states (e.g. diabetes mellitus) typically cause nocturia and only very rarely nocturnal enuresis, primary or secondary.

- **Primary and secondary wetting** are both compatible with either a functional disorder or organic disease, but whereas secondary wetting is compatible with bladder outflow obstruction or with neurological disease, a congenital structural anomaly can be virtually discounted as a cause of wetting in a child who was previously dry.

- **Continuous daytime wetting always** has an underlying organic cause, either structural or neurological. Intermittent daytime wetting, although compatible with both bladder outflow obstruction and neurological disease, is functional in the great majority of cases, particularly when the wetting occurs infrequently.

Physical examination

Abdomen

A palpably enlarged bladder, with or without palpable kidneys, is indicative of bladder outflow obstruction, either functional or organic. An expressible bladder is virtually pathognomonic of neurological disease, a diagnosis which is also suggested by the presence of gross constipation.

Male genitalia

Relevant findings comprise epispadias, pathological phimosis and meatal stenosis (including, occasionally, stenosis of a hypospadiac orifice).

Table 13.1 Organic causes of childhood urinary incontinence

Urinary infection (Intermittent leakage)	Structural (Continuous leakage)
Neuropathic (Continuous/intermittent leakage)	Exstrophy/epispadias
Bladder outflow obstruction (Intermittent leakage)	Ureteric ectopia (girls)
	Congenital short urethra (girls)
	Urovaginal confluence (girls)

Female genitalia

Conditions to be excluded are epispadias, common urogenital sinus and imperforate hymen. An ectopic ureteric orifice is only very rarely evident on gross inspection, although in some affected individuals urine may be seen leaking from the introital area.

The spine

The spine should always be inspected for the presence of hairy patches, swellings, cutaneous haemangiomata and sinuses which may be indicative of underlying spinal dysraphism (although blind-ending pits overlying the tip of the coccyx are of no neurological significance). Sacral agenesis is detectable clinically by a palpable absence of the lowermost sacral segments and, in most cases, by flattening of the upper buttocks.

Neurology

Neurological disease is suggested by exaggerated lower limb reflexes (or frank clonus) or by wasting of the calves or deformities of the feet, especially if asymmetrical. The lowermost sacral segments should be examined for motor and sensory integrity.

Investigations

Ultrasonography

This examination is advisable for all children troubled by daytime wetting and should, whenever practicable, include estimation of residual urine. Ultrasound findings of possible significance include:

- **Duplication anomalies** These are relevant only in girls. Uncomplicated duplication is unlikely to be significant, but a finding of upper polar dilatation or dysplasia points to ureteric ectopia. Occasionally, a dilated ectopic ureter is visualised behind the bladder in the absence of any detectable renal anomaly.
- **Upper tract dilatation** This is indicative of organic bladder outflow obstruction or, more commonly, of neuropathic bladder. Although dilatation is usually present bilaterally, unilateral dilatation does not exclude these diagnoses.
- **Bladder wall thickening** Although this finding is suggestive of bladder outflow obstruction or neuropathy, it is also commonly found to a minor extent in children with idiopathic detrusor instability and/or detrusor–sphincter dyssynergia.

- **Residual urine** within the bladder after voiding is suggestive of bladder outflow obstruction or neuropathy, but this finding should be viewed sceptically in children. This is particularly true of younger children, even when there is a significant postvoid residual exceeding 10% of expected bladder capacity. In the absence of any other positive finding, ultrasonography is best repeated before considering a more invasive examination.

Urine examination

Despite being routinely advisable, urine culture is only rarely positive. An exception exists in the case of a few children with asymptomatic bacteriuria. Here, although antibiotic treatment scarcely ever benefits the presenting complaint, the wetting and the infection may have some common underlying basis (e.g. bladder outflow obstruction).

Urodynamics

This examination should be employed sparingly and selectively, specific (but not mandatory) indications comprising:

- suspicion of neuropathic bladder;
- suspicion of genuine stress incontinence;
- failure to respond to empirical treatment based on a clinical diagnosis;
- failure to arrive at a clinically based diagnosis.

The key features of the equipment used in videourodynamic investigation are illustrated in Figure 14.2.

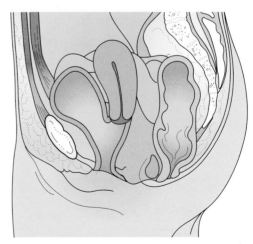

Figure 13.2 Anatomy of common urogenital sinus with urovaginal confluence. (see also Chapter 15, Cloacal anomalies).

Organic urinary incontinence in children (Table 13.1)

Urinary infection

Although it is by far the commonest organic cause of urinary incontinence in children, this complaint deserves merely a passing mention. The patient, nearly always a girl and otherwise with normal bladder control, develops symptoms typical of lower urinary tract infection and becomes incontinent at the same time. Investigation for any cause of the infection is merited (Chapter 4), but no more than that.

Spinal neurological disease

In children presenting with daytime wetting, only rarely will spinal or neurological examination reveal some evident abnormality which has previously been overlooked. In the absence of such signs, clinical features suggestive of neurological disease are:

- Urinary incontinence of unusual severity, especially if accompanied by constant dribbling of urine;
- Marked disturbance of bowel habit, particularly if associated with faecal soiling;
- A bladder that is expressible.

A spinal X-ray is advisable in the presence of one or more of these features, or of positive signs of neurological disease. Significant findings comprise abnormalities of one or more vertebral bodies, or laminal defects at two or more levels (isolated laminal defects at L5 or S1 represent mere variations of normal anatomy). Ultrasonography may disclose upper tract dilatation or marked thickening of the bladder wall.

A neurological opinion should be sought whenever signs or other clinical features positively point to spinal neurological disease, or if there remains suspicion of such a lesion.

Exstrophy/epispadias (see Chapter 16)

Urogenital sinus anomalies

Isolated lesions which are not associated with anorectal or cloacal anomalies sometimes present with urinary incontinence. This may be due either to neuropathic bladder resulting from a spinal anomaly, or to a form of urogenital sinus anomaly (urovaginal confluence) associated with an incompetent sphincteric mechanism (Figure 13.2). In such cases there is always constant urinary leakage. All urogenital sinus anomalies are characterised by a single vulval orifice which resembles neither vagina nor urethra.

Congenital short urethra

Again, the history is one of continuous urinary leakage and the urethral meatus is typically both wide and patulous. The diagnosis is confirmed by endoscopy.

Bladder outflow obstruction

This is encountered far more commonly in boys than in girls. Its causes in boys include posterior urethral valves, urethral stricture (including post hypospadias repair), meatal stenosis and, exceptionally, pathological phimosis. In girls haematocolpos or hydrocolpos due to imperforate hymen may present with bladder outflow obstruction, generally at or after puberty, and with an accompanying history of primary amenorrhoea. Causes affecting both sexes are pelvic tumours and severe constipation, although these conditions more often present with urinary retention than with incontinence.

The urinary stream is usually impaired but many boys are unaware of this (as are their parents). If there is suspicion of bladder outflow obstruction it is often helpful to observe the child voiding, where this is possible, or alternatively to obtain a measurement of flow rate. With few exceptions, incontinent episodes are associated with urgent micturition, which in turn is the consequence of obstructive detrusor instability. Residual urine, if not detectable clinically, is nearly always to be found on ultrasonography, often in conjunction with thickening of the bladder wall. The upper renal tracts, however, usually remain undilated, even in some cases of posterior urethral valves. In girls, hydro- or haematocolpos is always demonstrable by ultrasonography.

All patients suspected of having bladder outflow obstruction deserve examination under anaesthetic, cystoscopy, or both. It is important to be aware that the clinical picture may resemble primary detrusor instability and, for a while at least, there may be a symptomatic response to detrusor antispasmodics. After relief of obstruction it is not uncommon for the incontinence to persist, occasionally even for years, and treatment with antispasmodics is entirely appropriate during this time.

Genuine stress incontinence and the wide bladder neck anomaly

A small percentage of girls, most of at least prepubertal age, prove to have genuine stress incontinence, which can be demonstrated urodynamically. The clinical history is that to be expected of this complaint. The 'wide bladder neck anomaly' is periodically described in the literature, but whether this is a genuine entity remains open to doubt. During videourodynamic examination of girls it is not uncommon to find the bladder neck slightly open, but rarely, if ever, is it possible to demonstrate stress urinary leakage. In doubtful cases an empirical trial of an α-adrenergic agonist (e.g. ephedrine) may be employed, and in the event of a clear-cut clinical response genuine stress incontinence may be assumed, even if this has not been confirmed urodynamically.

Ureteric ectopia (see Chapter 8)

Occult neuropathic bladder

See under 'Functional diurnal urinary incontinence'.

Functional diurnal urinary incontinence

Among 7-year-olds, 3% of girls and 2% of boys experience functional daytime wetting at least once a week. Some 30% of the former and 50% of the latter are also troubled by nocturnal incontinence. Functional diurnal enuresis in children is distinguishable in several forms (Table 13.2), almost all of them

Table 13.2 Functional diurnal enuresis

Detrusor instability
Urge syndrome
  uncomplicated
  dysfunctional voiding
Deferred voiding
Lazy bladder
Occult neuropathic bladder

?Detrusor instability
Giggle incontinence

Non-detrusor instability
Diurnal frequency syndrome
Sensory urgency

with a benign natural history and most with a common underlying basis, detrusor instability.

The urge syndrome
Aetiology

More than of 80% of children who are troubled by daytime wetting experience urgent micturition. In the great majority this is due to detrusor instability, typically end-stage rather than during the filling phase. The cause is unknown and may be multifactorial. It is, however, plausible to suppose that in most instances the phenomenon represents no more than delayed maturity of bladder control, namely that affected children remain at that transition phase wherein detrusor inhibition is still volume related. Why this should occur is seldom evident, as with few exceptions they are otherwise well-adjusted individuals who have experienced nothing out of the ordinary by way of toilet training. In contrast to monosymptomatic nocturnal enuresis, there is no familial predisposition to this complaint.

Clinical features

Incontinence associated with urgency of micturition is the universal feature of this complaint, and as the majority of affected children experience only the briefest interval between the first desire to void and the necessity of doing so.

Affected children attempt to counter the consequent urinary leakage by contraction of the striated urethral sphincter and pelvic floor muscles, and may reinforce this process by various manoeuvres – classically by crouching and the heel pressed into the perineum (Vincent's curtsey sign). Sometimes urinary leakage is considerable, but is mostly relatively slight. However, urinary leakage of as little as 2 ml will be sufficient to stain boys' trousers, and a similar amount will embarrass girls by the resulting urinary malodour. Symptoms of provoked instability are uncommon, but some children find their problem worse in cold weather and others that it may be precipitated by certain drinks, particularly fizzy drinks. A measure of diurnal frequency exists in a majority of cases and, as previously indicated, a proportion – more boys than girls – are also troubled by nocturnal enuresis.

The urge syndrome has two subcategories:

- **Uncomplicated urgency** is clinically distinguishable by a normal, smooth, uninterrupted urinary stream, and is urodynamically characterised by detrusor–sphincter synergia and, usually, by voiding to completion. Girls and boys are almost equally affected and there is only seldom a history of urinary infection. Minor degrees of constipation are common, although whether more so than among children generally is open to doubt. It has been suggested that an appreciable proportion exhibit features of the attention-deficit disorder.

- **Dysfunctional voiding** is clinically recognisable by a urinary stream which is fluctuant or interrupted ('staccato' voiding), and the urodynamic picture during intentional micturition is one of detrusor–sphincter dyssynergia, either with incomplete relaxation of the sphincter or with alternating phases of contraction and relaxation. Incomplete voiding is common. It may be supposed that these children, having learned to ameliorate the consequences of detrusor instability by voluntary contraction of the urethral sphincter, subsequently and behaviourally come to lack sphincter inhibition during deliberate voiding. Girls are affected almost exclusively, and upwards of 90% experience recurrent urinary infections. Some 30% have vesicoureteric reflux, with or without associated renal scarring, and there is evidence that such reflux develops secondarily as a result of repetitive episodes of abnormally high intravesical pressure consequent upon a combination of detrusor instability and detrusor–sphincter dyssynergia. Major degrees of constipation are sometimes found, but these children only rarely exhibit features of any psychological disorder.

Prognosis

Spontaneous resolution is the rule, with only 2–3% remaining troubled by the complaint into adult life. Among those who are more intractably affected, coming to live independently away from home tends to effect the final cure. The chance of spontaneous resolution during any one year is of the order of 1 in 6.

Investigation

Urine culture and ultrasonography are the only investigations routinely advisable, although children also troubled by urinary infections merit other investigations appropriate to that complaint (Chapters 3 and 4). Ultrasonography commonly demonstrates minor thickening of the bladder wall, and the finding of

significant residual urine (> 10% of expected bladder capacity) is suggestive of dysfunctional voiding.

If necessary, uncomplicated urgency can be distinguished from dysfunctional voiding by flowmetry. Urodynamic examination is seldom needed for diagnostic purposes, as the alternative diagnosis of genuine stress incontinence is very rare in girls (as opposed to adult women). Similarly, bladder outflow obstruction is a very rare cause of urgency in boys (unlike adult males).

Management

Active measures are seldom effective before 5 years of age. Thereafter the options comprise:

- **Ameliorative measures** The complaint should be made known to school authorities so that the child is allowed to go to the toilet as necessary. Inconspicuous incontinence pads are available in children's sizes.
- **Simple bladder retraining** Strategies include a fluid intake evenly distributed through the day, the avoidance of drinks known to precipitate bladder misbehaviour, and a regimen of timed voiding, beginning at hourly intervals and, if successful, slowly extendimg these by degrees. Significant constipation should be treated.
- **Detrusor antispasmodics** Oxybutynin is immediately and unequivocally effective in 60–70% of cases, and troublesome side-effects are less common than in adults. As a rule, treatment must be continued for at least 3 months, and in a few instances for more than a year. Tolterodine is an alternative for those unable to tolerate oxybutynin.
- **Cognitive bladder retraining** Although it is effective in as many as 80% of cases, including those unresponsive to detrusor antispasmodics, this technique is an elaboration of simple retraining and is unsuitable for children under 8 years of age. Because it is also both time-consuming and expensive, it is best employed on a selective basis, being most useful in well-motivated girls troubled by dysfunctional voiding. Conducted by a trained urotherapist, children in age- and sex-matched pairs undergo a structured programme, first introducing them to the elements of bladder anatomy and physiology and next using non-invasive biofeedback techniques to teach them to recognise and then control their bladder signals.

Lazy bladder

This condition, confined to girls, typically comes to light at 8–10 years of age. Presentation may be with diurnal incontinence, with urinary infection or with incidental detection of the defining physical sign, a palpably and usually visibly distended bladder post micturition.

The upper renal tracts are always undilated and the urodynamic picture is one of low-pressure retention with detrusor–sphincter dyssynergia and non-sustained detrusor contractions. Detrusor instability is a further feature in most cases. The complaint is almost certainly behavioural in origin, resulting from excessive reliance on hold manoeuvres over a prolonged period of time. It is ultimately self-limiting, characteristically resolving quite suddenly during the course of puberty. In the interim, only those troubled by symptoms need treatment, supplemented by antibiotic prophylaxis in the case of urinary infection. Diurnal incontinence represents a more difficult problem as, for obvious reasons, detrusor antispasmodics must be used with caution. Intermittent catheterisation serves well, but may not be tolerated. Cognitive bladder retraining represents the most effective remedy.

Giggle incontinence

Largely confined to girls, this complaint typically presents prepubertally at 9–12 years of age. The history is unmistakably one of urinary leakage occurring with giggling or laughing but at no other time. In most cases there is otherwise an entirely normal pattern of micturition. Urodynamic examination may disclose detrusor instability, either spontaneous or provoked, but is more often wholly unremarkable, even during giggling. The aetiology is unknown. Whether the complaint is truly self-limiting is open to doubt, and the apparent improvement that usually occurs through puberty and into adult life may, in reality, represent no more than adaptation to avoid the precipitating circumstances.

Frequent episodes call for treatment. Oxybutynin is helpful in some cases and imipramine in others. Ritalin, the most consistently effective agent, is a controlled drug and should be reserved for severely affected patients.

Deferred voiding

This complaint is very commonly encountered in 4–6-year-olds of both sexes, but only occasionally in older individuals, most of whom have a manifest behaviour disorder. Urgent micturition, owing to presumed detrusor instability, is a consistent feature, but the problem arises principally because the child defers micturition until it is too late. In most cases it is apparent that pleasurable distractions, notably playing outdoors, take precedence over the social desirability of continence. Treatment is unnecessary for youngsters as the complaint is quickly self-limiting. Older children with behavioural disorders require the attention of a clinical psychologist.

Occult neuropathic bladder

In children with this rare disorder the bladder behaves as though 'neuropathic' yet there is no identifiable neurological disease. The condition is distinguishable from severe dysfunctional voiding or lazy bladder by the radiological features of sacculation and elongation of the bladder ('fir-tree' bladder), which in most instances are accompanied by secondary changes in the upper renal tracts.

In the classic form, Hinman's syndrome, there is almost always a background of domestic turmoil or a history of severe physical or psychological upset occurring at, or shortly after, the time of toilet training.

It is likely that affected children, because they are far more than usually fearful of wetting themselves, grossly overuse their external urethral sphincter to counteract unstable detrusor contractions in a desperate attempt to stay dry. This leads to excessive intravesical pressures, to detrusor hypertrophy and, ultimately, to detrusor non-compliance, with secondary upper renal tract complications.

Presentation, typically at 5–8 years of age, is with unusually severe urinary incontinence, which is compounded in most cases by urinary infections and marked disturbance of bowel habit. A few children have symptoms of renal insufficiency. The natural history is variable but, if untreated, the condition carries a very real threat to the upper tracts. Expectant management is not a safe option and treatment should be instituted along the lines described for neuropathic bladder proper (see Chapter 14).

In the other form of this complaint it would appear that there is some genuine but unidentifiable neurological lesion. There is never any background of psychological disturbance and presentation is often with episodic urinary retention, sometimes dating back to early infancy. Somewhat curiously, bowel habit is usually normal. So far as treatment is concerned, any distinction between these two categories of occult neuropathic bladder is academic.

Sensory urgency

A few children, mostly girls with clinical features typical of the urge syndrome yet which are wholly unresponsive to treatment, are found on urodynamic examination to have sensory rather than motor urgency. Apart from a very small number of cases with chronic or interstitial cystitis, the aetiology of this complaint is no less obscure than is that of its adult counterpart. Bladder overdistension under general anaesthesia produces symptomatic relief in some individuals.

Diurnal urinary frequency of childhood

More commonly affecting boys than girls, and principally those aged 4–7 years, this complaint is characterised by the sudden onset of gross diurnal urinary frequency – as often as every 10–15 minutes – which, pathognomonically, is unaccompanied by any corresponding degree of nocturia. Once asleep affected children wake to void not more than once or twice a night, and most of them not at all. Bedwetting may occur during the first few days, and occasionally diurnal enuresis also, but otherwise incontinence is not a feature of the condition and all other urinary symptomatology is conspicuous for its absence. Urine culture and ultrasonography are normal and the frequency is wholly unresponsive to detrusor antispasmodics. The aetiology is unknown, although the discrepancy between bladder behaviour awake and that asleep is compatible with a behavioural origin. The complaint is always self-limiting, usually over 3–12 weeks. A minority of children experience recurrent cycles over a period of 1–2 years.

Primary monosymptomatic nocturnal enuresis

Some 5–10% of 7-year-olds bed wet three or more times a week. This figure comprises some children with secondary nocturnal enuresis and a slightly higher proportion who have both nocturnal and daytime symptoms, with or without actual wetting. However, the substantial majority who wet the bed have primary monosymptomatic nocturnal enuresis and, of these, two-thirds are boys.

The aetiology of this complaint is multifactorial and in any individual one or more factors may apply. The established aetiological factors include:

- A positive family history (upwards of 75% of cases);
- Impaired functional bladder capacity, which is clinically manifest by a degree of daytime frequency;
- Uninhibited nocturnal detrusor contractions, which occur in approximately a third of patients (although this also occurs in asymptomatic children). Diurnal urgency of micturition is a clinical indicator of such detrusor activity;
- Sleep arousal difficulty. Nocturnal enuresis does not, as is commonly supposed, result from deep sleep, as bed wetting occurs at all stages of the sleep cycle, but many affected children lack the normal arousal from sleep that should occur as functional bladder capacity is approached;
- Absence of a circadian rhythm of vasopressin release. This normally increases nocturnally, but in as many as 75% of bed wetters and a still higher proportion of those with a positive family history the normal increase in vasopressin release is absent or diminished. This leads to a nocturnal urinary output that exceeds the functional bladder capacity.

Young infants do not void when asleep, and the age at which nocturnal micturition becomes established is unknown. Similarly, the age at which a circadian rhythm of vasopressin release is established is not known, although by inference both phenomena develop before the usual time of toilet training. Although nocturnal enuresis is sometimes a manifestation of psychosocial problems or of behavioural disorders, the great majority of bed wetters are normally adjusted children.

The **clinical features** vary from one patient to another. Some wet every night or almost so, whereas others are troubled less often and tend to experience alternating spells of wet and dry nights. Some children wet more than once a night, and the time of wetting varies between individuals. With only occasional exceptions, the wetting does not wake the child. As previously indicated, secondary enuresis should prompt suspicion of organic disease. However, this is most unlikely when, as is often the case, the onset has coincided with some physical or emotional upset.

Except for those with daytime symptoms also or with 'suspicious' secondary enuresis, **investigation**, beyond the exclusion of urinary infection, is unnecessary. The **prognosis** is excellent, with spontaneous resolution by the time of physical maturity occurring in 97–99% of affected individuals. The probability of cessation in any one year is approximately 1 in 6.

Treatment, if sought, should not commence before 5 years of age. The type of treatment depends in some measure on the clinical features, and its success is heavily dependent on the motivation of the child and the family. It should be emphasised that all medications represent treatment rather than cure, although symptomatic treatment may help to expedite cessation of the underlying problem earlier than would otherwise have been the case. The parents should be encouraged to take a positive attitude towards the problem, and scolding and punishment are to be condemned. Active measures comprise the following:

- **Star charts**, combined with rewards, are particularly suited to the younger patient.
- **Enuretic alarms**, in alerting and sensitising the child to respond appropriately to a full bladder during sleep, serve to convert this signal from one of micturition to one of inhibition of urination and waking (Figure 13.3). The success rate with this measure, which is best avoided before 7 years of age, varies from 60 to 75% and, unlike treatment

with medication, subsequent relapse is uncommon. Failures tend to occur in those least motivated and in those with a background of domestic disharmony or a history of daytime symptoms.

- **Desmopressin** has a vasopressin-like action and, whether administered intranasally (Desmospray) or orally (Desmotabs), is effective in upwards of 70% of patients. The relapse rate after cessation of treatment is high – 30–50% – and is to some extent dependent on the duration of treatment. Desmopressin may be used for short periods, to cover special occasions, or for a more extended duration, up to 12 months. In the latter instance dosage should be periodically reduced or stopped in order to determine whether the treatment need be continued. Predictors of success include a positive family history or of early wetting; and of failure, concurrent daytime symptoms.
- **Detrusor antispasmodics**, such as oxybutynin, are principally of value in children who are also troubled by daytime urgency and frequency. When given on this selective basis these drugs are effective in up to two-thirds of cases.
- **Imipramine** is nowadays considered an unfashionable treatment of last resort. Nevertheless, its efficacy has been confirmed in several well controlled trials. Its mode of action is unknown.
- **Combination treatments** In some patients, treatments that are unsuccessful individually may prove effective when used in combination. Examples are desmopressin with oxybutynin, and desmopressin and an enuretic alarm. Imipramine should never be prescribed in conjunction with desmopressin.

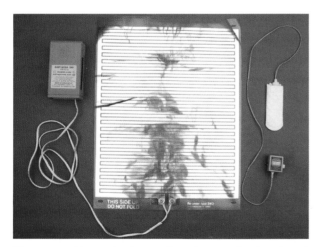

Figure 13.3 Enuresis alarms. Pad designed to be placed under the bed sheet, with bedside battery-powered buzzer. Compact alternative shown on the right. Sensor pad worn within underclothes, vibrating alarm. This device is also suitable for ambulatory treatment of diurnal enuresis.

Key points
- The initial priority is to exclude organic causes of urinary incontinence, although these are rare.
- Primary monosymptomatic nocturnal enuresis seldom, if ever, has an underlying organic basis.
- Most organic causes of daytime wetting can be excluded on the basis of history, examination and ultrasonography.
- Organic causes of daytime wetting are classifiable as neurological, obstructive and structural, the last category being confined almost exclusively to girls.
- Functional diurnal enuresis is due to detrusor instability in the great majority of cases, and the natural history of this complaint in children is one of spontaneous resolution.

Further reading

Chandra M. Nocturnal enuresis in children. *Curr Opin Pediatr* 1998; 10: 167–173

Koff SA. Relationship between dysfunctional voiding and reflux. *J Urol* 1992; 148: 1703–1705

Norgaard JP, van Gool JD, Hajlmas K, Djurhuus JC, Hellstrom AL. Standardization and definitions in lower urinary tract dysfunction in children. *Br J Urol* 1988; 81 (Suppl 3): 1–16

van Gool JD. Dysfunctional voiding: a complex of bladder/sphincter dysfunction, urinary tract infection and reflux. *Acta Urol Belg* 1995; 63: 27–33

van Gool JD, Vijversberg MA. Functional daytime incontinence: clinical and urodynamic assessment. *Scand J Urol Nephrol* 1992; 141: 58–69

Neuropathic bladder

14

AMK Rickwood and Padraig S Malone

Topics covered
Aetiology
Pathophysiology
Patient assessment

Investigation
Management
Bowel management

Introduction

Until the late 1950s, when the development of shunting devices to treat hydrocephalus enabled the survival of large numbers of patients born with myelomeningocoele, children with neuropathic bladder were few and received little attention. It soon became apparent, however, that they posed a variety of problems over and above those encountered in adults with spinal cord injuries. Their urological features included:

- A preponderance of females, with evident implications for the management of incontinence;
- A high incidence of secondary upper renal tract complications which, despite being more common in boys, were also encountered in girls.

Conduit urinary diversion quickly became established as the means of managing neuropathic bladder in children with spina bifida, and this remained in vogue until the mid-1970s, by which time its limitations were apparent and alternative strategies had become available. The first of these, clean intermittent self-catheterisation (CISC), remains the mainstay of treatment today. CISC alone, however, even when practicable, achieves continence in only a minority of patients (10–20%), and does not always protect the upper renal tracts. Subsequent developments circumventing these problems have comprised more effective medication, augmentation cystoplasty, sphincter-enhancing procedures and the Mitrofanoff principle.

Aetiology (Table 14.1)

Myelomeningocoele

Although for several reasons its incidence has declined considerably in recent years, myelomeningocoele remains the most common cause of congenital neuropathic bladder. The condition results from partial failure of tubularisation of the neural crest. Because the normal process proceeds caudally the conus medullaris is almost always involved, with only some 6% of patients escaping neuropathic bladder and bowel. The untubularised neural crest (neural plaque) contains grossly disorganised tissue, and consequently the extent of the plaque determines the degree of paralysis. Regardless of the neurological level, 25–30% of patients retain positive conus (anocutaneous, glans–bulbar) reflexes, and among these a minority with low-level sacral or

Table 14.1 Aetiology of childhood neuropathic bladder

Congenital	Acquired
Myelomeningocoele	Cord trauma
Spina bifida occulta	Cord infarction
Diastematomyelia	Prematurity
Lumbosacral lipoma	Cardiac surgery
Intraspinal cysts	Tumours
Tethered cord	Neuroblastoma
Sacral agenesis	Tranverse myelitis

lumbosacral myelomeningocoele have incomplete cord lesions with sensory sparing and, occasionally, sparing of motor function. Other features of relevance to urological management include:

- **Hydrocephalus** Although almost invariably present this does not always require shunting. The severity of hydrocephalus broadly matches the extent of the neural plaque and because, with some exceptions, the severity of hydrocephalus also reflects the level of intelligence, myelomeningocoele patients are unique in that increasing physical and intellectual disabilities tend to go hand-in-hand. The effects of hydrocephalus on the central nervous system are skewed, with verbal performance being usually relatively well preserved whereas manipulative skills tend to be more severely affected. In some patients CISC, or the manipulation required to manage an artificial urinary sphincter, may be precluded by their limited dexterity.
- **Mobility** Almost all patients with a neurological level above L3 (i.e. lacking normal quadriceps function) ultimately come to lead a wheelchair existence, no matter what they may have achieved during childhood.
- **Spinal deformity** The incidence and severity of such deformities relates to the extent of the neural plaque. Kyphoscoliosis which is so severe that patients of either gender may find it physically impossible to perform urethral CISC, is largely limited to those with thoracolumbar lesions.
- **Congenital upper urinary tract anomalies** Despite being more prevalent than in the population at large, the nature of these anomalies (typically unilateral renal agenesis, or anomalies of position or fusion) is such that they only rarely influence practical management. Vesicoureteric reflux is also prevalent, although it is often secondary rather than primary.

Other congenital cord lesions

Because these are not associated with hydrocephalus nor, as a rule, with major neurological deficits or spinal deformities, urological management is rarely influenced by factors other than the nature of the bladder dysfunction. Most affected patients have negative conus reflexes, including those with incomplete cord lesions.

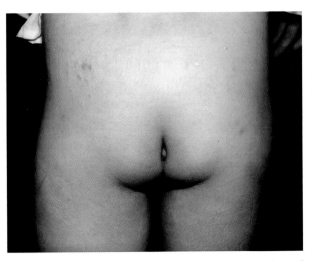

Figure 14.1 Sacral agenesis – characteristic wasting of the buttocks.

Sacral agenesis (Figure 14.1)

This may occur as a feature of anorectal anomalies or as an isolated lesion and, if the latter, the mother is often an insulin-dependent diabetic. The implications of sacral agenesis in children with anorectal malformations are considered in Chapter 16. Regardless of whether it is an isolated or a coexisting anomaly the cord lesion associated with sacral agenesis is invariably incomplete and, uniquely, any peripheral neurological deficit bears no predictable relation to bladder or sphincter dysfunction.

Acquired cord lesions

These are rare. Cord trauma may occur at any level but is most common in the mid-dorsal region. Patients affected by transverse myelitis usually make an excellent recovery except for the bladder, which remains affected in upwards of 50% of cases. Other causes include spinal artery thrombosis (occurring in sick or premature infants) and spinal tumours.

Because of the small numbers the risk of secondary upper renal tract complications is unquantifiable, although they undoubtedly occur more commonly than in adults with spinal cord injury. Girls and boys appear to be at equal risk.

Basic considerations

Management aims to replicate, so far as possible, normal bladder function, namely:

- **Filling and storage**, i.e. by ensuring adequate low-pressure functional capacity (the definition of 'adequate' hinging upon the individual patient's mobility);
- **Emptying**, i.e. to maximise effective bladder capacity and minimise the risk of stasis-related infection;
- **Voiding at will** In patients with neuropathic bladder normal voluntary control of voiding is absent and some unphysiological or artificial means must be employed. This may take the form of abdominal compression or straining (possible only when there is some element of sphincteric incompetence) or CISC.

Some neuropathic bladders fill well – albeit sometimes at the expense of raised intravesical pressure – but do not empty, whereas others empty readily but do not fill. In addition, many neuropathic bladders function imperfectly in both respects. With the near-universal adoption of CISC as the means of achieving both 'emptying ' and 'voiding at will', attention correspondingly focuses on the filling phase of bladder function.

Classification

As with acquired forms, congenital neuropathic bladder dysfunction is largely determined by the siting of the cord lesion, but with the difference that an intermediate pattern of dysfunction is commonly seen. The introduction of **urodynamic investigation** greatly advanced our understanding of the different patterns of bladder dysfunction associated with neuropathic bladder. The essential features of the equipment used for videourodynamic investigation (also termed videocystometry) are illustrated in Figure 14.2. In conducting the study, there are some important practical considerations:

- It is best performed by the clinician who is responsible for the patient's management.
- It should, if at all possible, be combined with simultaneous cystography.
- Slow filling is employed, aiming to reach expected bladder capacity over not less than 20 minutes (expected functional capacity in ml is calculated as follows: 0–1 years, capacity = weight (kg) ×7; 1–12 years, capacity = age (yrs) × 30 + 30; for

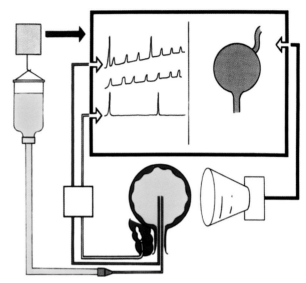

Figure 14.2 Videourodynamic equipment (videocystometry). Two catheters (or a single double-lumen catheter) are inserted into the bladder urethrally or suprapubically to permit filling and simultaneous intravesical pressure recording (TBP = total bladder pressure on the traces illustrated below). Electronic subtraction of intra-abdominal pressure, measured by a rectal balloon catheter (RP = rectal pressure), provides a measurement of true detrusor pressure (IDP = intrinsic detrusor pressure). Anatomical information is obtained by using radiographic contrast for the study, although X-ray screening time should be kept to a minimum.

example, for a 5-year-old child 5 × 30 = 150 + 30 = 180 ml).
- The presence or absence of sphincteric incompetence should be assessed periodically during filling by manoeuvres that raise intra-abdominal pressure (standing, coughing, application of suprapubic pressure).
- In the presence of gross sphincteric incompetence it may be necessary to occlude the bladder neck by a Foley balloon catheter in order to fill the bladder to expected capacity.

In **suprasacral cord lesions** (contractile bladder) the conus medullaris is intact (Figure 14.3) and so too, although isolated from higher centres, is innervation of the detrusor and external urethral sphincter. Conus reflexes are positive. The sphincteric mechanism, usually including the bladder neck (Figure 14.4), is intact and voiding occurs solely by detrusor

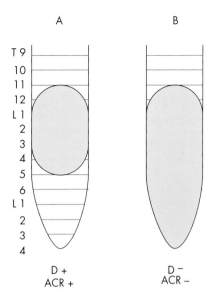

Figure 14.3 Suprasacral (A) and sacral (B) cord lesions: note that bladder innervation is determined by the distal, not the proximal, extent of the lesion (D = reflex detrusor activity, ACR = anocutaneous reflex).

hyperreflexia almost always accompanied by detrusor–sphincter dyssynergia (i.e. loss of the usual coordination between detrusor contraction and sphincter relaxation). Such bladders are typically neither trabeculated nor sacculated, and detrusor non-compliance is uncommon and never sufficient to overcome urethral resistance. None the less, repetitive high-pressure detrusor hyperreflexia may ultimately lead to secondary upper renal tract complications.

In **sacral cord lesions** (acontractile bladder) the conus medullaris is destroyed (Figure 14.3), as is innervation of both detrusor and external urethral sphincter. Conus reflexes are negative, detrusor contractility is absent, but some degree of sphincteric incompetence is always present so that voiding occurs either by overflow or by raising intra-abdominal pressure. During such voiding, any obstruction is located at the level of the external urethral sphincter (Figure 14.5), and is termed **static sphincteric obstruction**. Unlike detrusor–sphincter dyssynergia, a dynamic if inappropriate phenomenon, static sphincteric obstruction represents a fixed urethral resistance that varies unpredictably from one patient to another.

More severe degrees of obstruction result in good functional capacity but at the expense of larger volumes of residual urine (Figure 14.5), whereas minimal obstruction, equating to gross sphincteric incompetence, is associated with greatly reduced

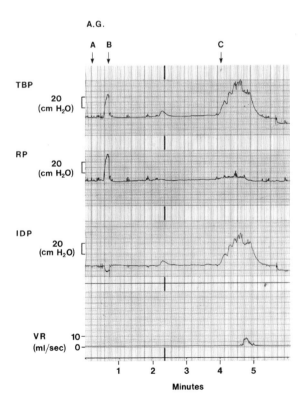

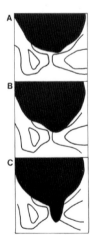

Figure 14.4 Contractile bladder. The bladder neck is closed at rest (A) and remains so despite a rise in intra-abdominal pressure (B). A reflex detrusor voiding contraction is accompanied by detrusor–sphincter dyssynergia and which is initially complete (C) (TBP = total bladder pressure, RP = rectal pressure, IDP = intrinsic detrusor pressure).

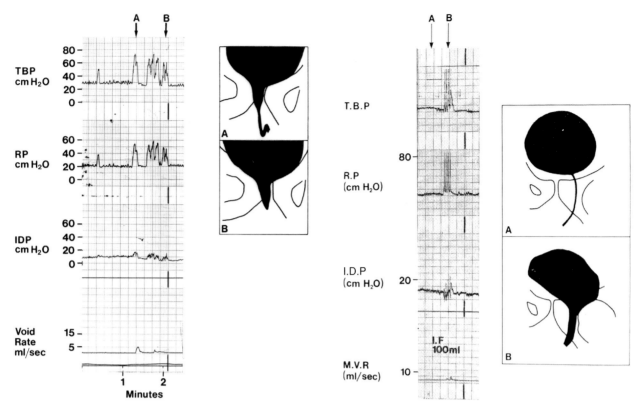

Figure 14.5 Acontractile bladder. During abdominal straining there is persistent narrowing at the level of the external urethral sphincter (A), which ultimately becomes complete (static sphincteric obstruction) despite continued straining (B): baseline intravesical pressure falls following this partial voiding.

Figure 14.6 Acontractile bladder. The bladder neck is closed at rest (A) but the sphincteric mechanism becomes totally incompetent with a rise in intra-abdominal pressure (B).

functional capacity and no residual urine (Figure 14.6). An inevitable consequence of voiding by abdominal straining against a fixed urethral resistance is that functional capacity scarcely exceeds residual urine, and hence effective capacity is virtually zero. Acontractile bladders may be smooth or sacculated. A degree of detrusor non-compliance is common and, when present, serves to further limit functional capacity where urethral resistance is low, or results in excessively raised intravesical pressure where the resistance is high.

Intermediate bladder dysfunction is characterised by a combination of detrusor hyperreflexia, typically generating low pressures, and some degree of sphincteric incompetence (Figure 14.7). Conus reflexes are negative. Sacculation (Figure 14.8) is common, as is detrusor non-compliance. During voiding the appearance of any urethral obstruction more closely resembles that of static sphincteric obstruction than detrusor–sphincter dyssynergia (Figure 14.8).

The factors responsible for impaired bladder capacity are summarised in Table 14.2. In patients with

Table 14.2 Causes of impaired bladder capacity

Contractile bladder	Acontractile bladder	Intermediate bladder
Detrusor hyperreflexia	Sphincteric incompetence Detrusor non-compliance Combinations	Sphincteric incompetence Detrusor non-compliance Detrusor hyperreflexia Combinations

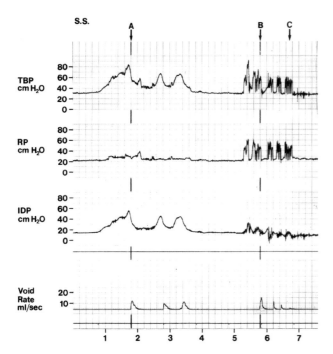

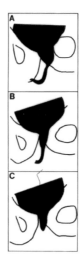

Figure 14.7 Intermediate bladder. Voiding occurs both by detrusor hyperreflexia (A) and by raising extra-abdominal pressure (B).

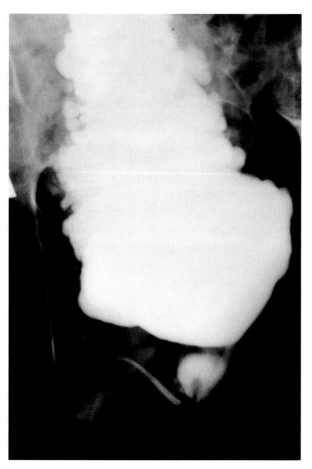

Figure 14.8 Cystographic appearances of neuropathic bladder (intermediate type) showing both sacculation and static sphincteric obstruction.

myelomeningocoele the patterns of dysfunction are: contractile (25%), acontractile (15%) and intermediate (60%). Contractile dysfunction is appreciably rarer with all other forms of congenital cord lesion.

Incomplete cord lesion

Incomplete cord lesions, with sacral sensory sparing (and sometimes motor sparing also), are of clinical significance principally when associated with contractile bladder dysfunction (conus reflexes positive). Such patients are characterised by having some sensation of bladder fullness and experiencing gross urgency of micturition. A proportion achieve spontaneous, if precarious, urinary continence. It is important to note, however, that despite acquiring continence these patients may nevertheless have urodynamic abnormalities that pose a risk to the upper tracts. Urethral sensation may remain largely intact in incomplete cord lesions, to the point that the discomfort experienced during CISC may preclude the urethral route for self-catheterisation.

Secondary upper renal tract complications

Such complications, in the form of obstruction or reflux, are prevalent in all patients with congenital neuropathic bladder and among those with myelomeningocoele some 20% are affected by the age

Table 14.3 Causes of secondary upper renal tract complications

Urinary infection
Vesicoureteric reflux
Bladder outflow obstruction
    Detrusor hyperreflexia
    Detrusor non-compliance

of 2 years. The incidence thereafter is difficult to determine and is influenced (for better or for worse) by the effects of treatment. At an estimate, however, 50% of boys are at risk of upper tract complications by the time they complete puberty; the percentage in girls is somewhat smaller.

Factors responsible for secondary complications are summarised in Table 14.3.

- **Urinary infection** is extremely common and, in the very young, may lead to renal scarring even in the absence of vesicoureteric reflux. Most infections result from bladder dysfunction, and their treatment consequently hinges upon correcting this rather than ceaseless pursuit with antibiotics.
- **Vesicoureteric reflux** may, as previously described, be primary or secondary. In the case of secondary reflux, treatment is aimed principally at correcting the underlying abnormality of bladder function.
- **Bladder outflow obstruction**, whether in the form of detrusor–sphincter dyssynergia or static sphincteric obstruction, is an invariable precursor of secondary upper urinary tract obstruction, but leads to these complications only when associated with raised intravesical pressure due to detrusor hyperreflexia, detrusor non-compliance, or a combination of both. The relative importance of these two factors is a matter of some dispute. Conventional urodynamics tends to point to detrusor non-compliance as the more important factor whereas ambulatory studies have tended to implicate detrusor hyperreflexia. As for detrusor non-compliance, baseline pressures exceeding $20 \, cmH_2O$ within the physiological range of capacity on conventional slow-fill urodynamics should be regarded as 'unsafe'. Whatever the detrusor behaviour, secondary upper renal tract complications never occur in the presence of gross sphincteric incompetence and a permanently empty bladder.

This happy state may, of course, be reversed if sphincteric incompetence is treated without considering the possible subsequent effects of detrusor malfunction.

Natural history of neuropathic bladder malfunction

Neuropathic bladder dysfunction can change over the course of time, in terms of both severity or, less often, the particular pattern of dysfunction. Whatever change occurs, however, is almost invariably for the worse. Although no time of life is free of this problem, the periods of greatest risk are first, during the first 2 years, when some 30% of neonatally 'safe' bladders become 'unsafe', and secondly during the course of puberty. In this age group boys are at greater risk than girls, presumably because prostatic growth increases urethral resistance.

Patient assessment

History

General features comprise mobility, intelligence and social factors, plus the nature and effectiveness of any bowel management. With regard to the urinary tract:

- Continuous dribbling, particularly if exacerbated by coughing, crying or standing, is almost pathognomonic of some degree of sphincteric incompetence.
- A discrete, spontaneous urinary stream is typical of a contractile bladder.
- Urinary infections, especially if febrile, are strongly suggestive of upper renal tract complications, either actual or impending.

Examination: key points

- Bladder distension is indicative of outflow obstruction, whereas an expressible bladder is pathognomonic of both neuropathy and some measure of sphincteric incompetence.
- A bladder that cannot be expressed implies either sphincteric competence or a bladder that is virtually empty by reason of gross sphincteric incompetence.
- Neurological examination, which can be limited to the lowermost sacral segments, is aimed at demonstrating the presence or absence of conus reflexes and the presence of any sensory or motor sparing.

Neonatal assessment

The expressibility of the bladder should be determined in the neonatal period. In addition, a limited neurological examination is performed to test conus reflexes and to look for sensory sparing, as judged by general arousal to perianal pinprick. No matter how slight the neurological deficit, the presence of a neuropathic bladder is certain if the bladder is expressible, *or* the conus reflexes are negative, *or* if there is no sensory sparing. By contrast, bladder function may prove to be normal if the bladder is inexpressible *and* conus reflexes are positive *and* there is sensory sparing.

Investigations

Imaging studies

Ultrasonography of the urinary tracts, with estimation of the volume of residual urine where practicable and relevant, represents the best means of both initial assessment and follow-up. The frequency of ultrasound examinations for the latter purpose is determined by what is known of bladder dysfunction and hence the perceived risk of upper tract complications. Among other imaging studies, DMSA scintigraphy is of value in patients with vesicoureteric reflux or suffering febrile urinary infections; cystography, to confirm or exclude vesicoureteric reflux or bladder outflow obstruction, is best combined with simultaneous urodynamic examination.

Urodynamics

Some of the the technical aspects of urodynamics have been considered above and are illustrated in Figure 14.2. The principal indications for this examination are to:

- identify the 'unsafe' bladder in neonates;
- determine the cause(s) of secondary upper urinary tract complications;
- plan the treatment of incontinence.

Management

Basic considerations

The aims of management are, in order of priority:

- To preserve renal function;

- To provide continence (ideally without dependence on appliances and in a manner the patient may practise independently).

Consequently, all schemes of management incorporate the following basic principles:

- Renal function always takes precedence over continence.
- Treatment must relate realistically to the patient's other characteristics and abilities as a whole (i.e. age, sex, mobility, intelligence, dexterity, deformity, social circumstances).
- Treatment must relate to the nature of the bladder dysfunction.
- When bladder dysfunction is complex its treatment may also need to be more complex (e.g. CISC combined with a measure to improve bladder capacity, or with more than one measure when the reduced capacity is the outcome of two or more factors).
- Measures that are non-invasive and/or reversible take priority over those that are neither (i.e. medical management should always be tried before surgery is considered).

In practice, when CISC proves inadequate any additional measures are invariably directed at securing adequate low-pressure functional bladder capacity.

General management of impaired/high-pressure bladder capacity

Detrusor hyperreflexia

- Medication (anticholinergic)
- Augmentation cystoplasty.

Medical management of hyperreflexia is usually by means of oxybutynin. Because this agent is effective in most cases, augmentation cystoplasty is rarely required for this indication alone. For patients in whom side-effects are not tolerated oxybutynin may be administered, in the same dosage, by the intravesical route. Tolterodine, a recently introduced alternative, is probably equally effective and is claimed to have a lower incidence of side-effects.

Detrusor non-compliance

- Augmentation cystoplasty.

Although the cause of detrusor non-compliance remains disputed, there is general agreement that the phenomenon is unresponsive to any currently available medication.

Sphincteric incompetence

- Medication (α-adrenergic agonists)
- Periurethral injections
- Bladder neck suspension
- Bladder neck slings
- Pippe–Salle procedure
- Artificial urinary sphincter
- Bladder neck obliteration.

Treatment of sphincteric incompetence remains less than satisfactory. Marginal degrees of incompetence may respond to α-adrenergic agonists (e.g. ephedrine), but anything more major calls for surgery. It will be apparent from the length of the list above that there is as yet no single procedure that guarantees success. It must also be re-emphasised that a safe and successful outcome of treatment of sphincteric incompetence is dependent on measures to ensure adequate treatment of any coexisting detrusor hyperreflexia and/or detrusor non-compliance.

Surgery for impaired/high-pressure bladder capacity

Augmentation cystoplasty

Enterocystoplasty

Despite the morbidity inherent in the prolonged exposure of intestinal epithelium to urine (Table 14.4), enterocystoplasty remains the principal means of bladder augmentation as it employs a material that is universally available and, with a few exceptions, secures consistent and satisfactory urodynamic outcomes. Intestinal segments in common usage are ileum, ileocaecum, sigmoid colon, and stomach. With the exception of stomach all require detubularisation to obviate high-pressure peristaltic activity. As a rule, a clam-patch cystoplasty (Figures 14.9, 14.10) is used when the urodynamic problem is principally detrusor hyperreflexia, and a pouched augmentation (Figure 14.11) when the bladder is small and non-compliant. Despite detubularisation, troublesome peristaltic activity may still occur, even to the extent of necessitating further augmentation. As this occurs most commonly following sigmoid cystoplasty, the use of this bowel segment is best avoided where possible.

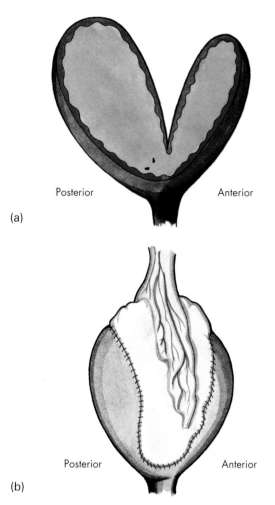

(a)

(b)

Figure 14.9 Clam ileocystoplasty viewed laterally. (a) Bladder opened and incised down to the trigone to create a 'clam' configuration. (b) Segment of ileum isolated on its mesentery, opened (detubularised) and sutured on to the bladder.

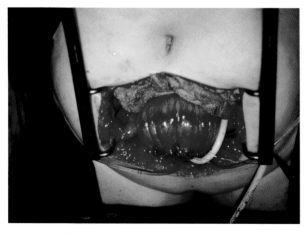

Figure 14.10 Operative photograph showing completed clam ileocystoplasty.

Table 14.4 Complications of enterocystoplasty

Mucus production	**Spontaneous perforation**
Catheter blockage	
Infection	**Metaplasia/malignancy**
Bladder stone	
	Bowel problems
Metabolic changes	Diarrhoea
Hyperchloraemic alkalosis	Vitamin B$_{12}$ deficiency
Electrolyte disturbance	
Systemic alkalosis (gastrocystoplasty)	**Dysuria/haematuria**
	(gastrocystoplasty)

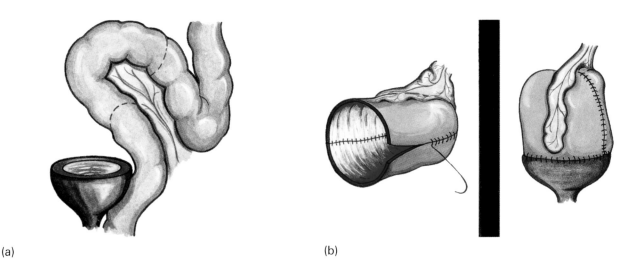

(a)   (b)

Figure 14.11 Sigmoid pouch cystoplasty. (a) Segment of sigmoid colon isolated on its mesentery. (b) Colonic segment detubularised then reconfigured as a pouch. The use of this form of enterocystoplasty is generally limited to small, non-compliant bladders.

Autoaugmentation

Excision of detrusor muscle over the bladder dome creates, in effect, a large, broad-mouthed diverticulum. Although avoiding the potential complications of enterocystoplasty, the urodynamic outcome in terms of increased capacity and reduction of overactivity is rather less impressive or predictable. The long-term results are not encouraging.

Ureterocystoplasty (Figure 14.12)

The dilated ureter, which is opened along its length, is usually anastomosed to the bladder as a clam patch; the overlying kidney is removed if it has no useful function or, if otherwise, is drained by transureteroureterostomy. Ureterocystoplasty provides a urodynamic outcome which equals that of enterocystoplasty, and is thus the procedure of choice whenever a suitably dilated ureter is available. Unfortunately, this is rarely the case.

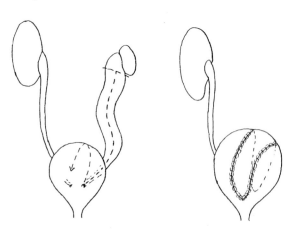

Figure 14.12 Ureterocystoplasty.

Autoaugmentation plus demucosalised enterocystoplasty

The epithelial diverticulum created by a standard autoaugmentation is covered by a demucosalised enteric patch, usually of stomach or colon. Although this technique enjoys the theoretical advantage of creating an augmentation lined by urothelium rather than intestinal epithelium, the long-term outcome has yet to be assessed.

Sphincter-enhancement procedures

These are two general categories of sphincter-enhancement procedure:

- The artificial sphincter, which, because it can be turned 'on' and 'off' at will, enables voiding by abdominal straining;
- Other procedures, which, in creating or enhancing a fixed urethral resistance, necessitate voiding by CISC.

Artificial urinary sphincter (Figure 14.13)

This device has several drawbacks:

- Cost;
- Infection and/or urethral erosion, necessitating device removal;
- Need for revisionary procedures. When the entire device has been inserted, revision is almost always required within 12 years of implantation;
- Although voiding is ideally achieved by abdominal straining in practice some 60% of patients use CISC as the sole or a supplementary means of voiding. This proportion is less if preliminary transurethral sphincterotomy is undertaken, but the effect of this procedure is not always permanent. Conversely, very few patients who have also undergone augmentation can achieve adequate emptying without CISC.

Despite these disadvantages, the artificial urinary sphincter is the best option for boys and renders upwards of 80% reliably dry. Because the device is designed for adults it is not suitable for those under 8 years of age. The sphincter cuff is usually implanted at the bladder neck, although the bulbar urethra is an alternative site after puberty. When augmentation cystoplasty is also required it is best initially to limit

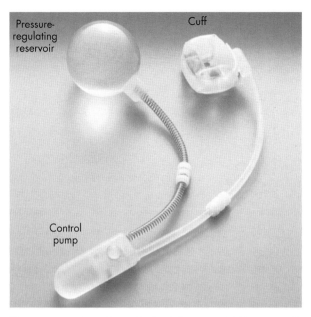

Figure 14.13 American Medical Systems AMS 800 artificial urinary sphincter. Components comprise the cuff, which is implanted around the urethra, the pump which is implanted in the scrotum, and the pressure-regulating balloon which is sited in a plane between the peritoneum and the abdominal wall musculature. (Reproduced with permission from American Medical Systems UK Ltd, Hanwell, Middlesex, UK.)

implantation to the sphincter cuff alone, as this combination will be sufficient to provide continence in some patients, thereby obviating the need to implant the other components of the system.

Periurethral bulking agents (collagen, silicone)

These have limited value, achieving complete continence only in patients with marginal sphincteric incompetence or those already treated by other means and who are no more than damp as a result.

Bladder neck suspension and slings

If combined with simultaneous augmentation cystoplasty, a Marshall–Marchetti bladder neck suspension achieves success in upwards of 80% of girls. The results of bladder neck slings may prove marginally superior.

Pippe–Salle procedure (Figure 14.14)

This urethral lengthening procedure is suitable for girls but not for boys.

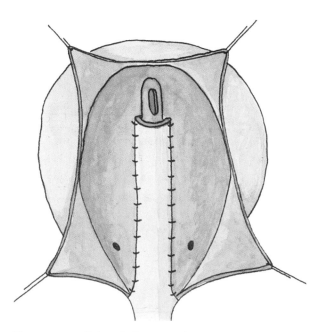

Figure 14.14 Pippe–Salle procedure.

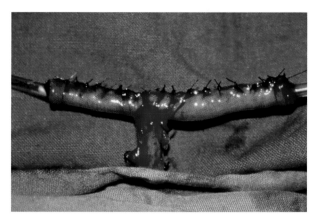

Figure 14.15 Monti tube fashioned from ileum. This is the most satisfactory alternative to the appendix for the creation of a continent catheterisable conduit (Mitrofanoff procedure).

Bladder neck closure

This necessitates a simultaneous Mitrofanoff procedure and, in many cases, an augmentation cystoplasty. Although successful in more than 90% of cases, both boys and girls, bladder neck closure should be considered a procedure of last resort, to be employed only when alternatives have failed or are impracticable. Once the bladder neck has been closed there remains only one, limited, means of endoscopic access to the bladder – an important consideration in view of the incidence of bladder stones following Mitrofanoff procedures and enterocystoplasties.

Other surgical procedures employed with neuropathic bladder

Mitrofanoff procedure

The principal indications comprise:

● Bladder neck closure;
● Patients in whom urethral CISC is impracticable by reason of deformity, or is unacceptable because of urethral sensation.

The appendix, if available and of sufficient length, is the conduit of first choice. The best alternative is a Monti tube (Figure 14.15) which, if constructed of ileum, provides an easily catheterisable conduit some

7 cm long. When necessary, a greater length can be obtained by end-to-end anastomosis of two or more such tubes. The risk of the commonest complication of the Mitrofanoff procedure, stomal stenosis, is minimised by the use of multiple skin flaps or an umbilical siting. In obese patients or those with spinal deformities it is important that the stoma be visible in the sitting position.

Vesicostomy

This is a simple and effective temporising means of reversing established upper renal tract complications. To reduce the risk of prolapse the stoma should be sited as near the apex of the bladder as possible.

Endoscopic urethral sphincterotomy

For boys, sphincterotomy is equally effective in treating detrusor–sphincter dyssynergia and static sphincteric obstruction, but if the bladder neck is incompetent total incontinence ensues. Hence the procedure finds only limited use, as a preliminary to the insertion of an artificial urinary sphincter or, occasionally, for infants and the severely disabled.

Conduit urinary diversion

Although once the mainstay of treatment, this is now limited to the severely disabled. Careful siting of the stoma is critical in patients with spinal deformities. When the ureters are undilated, the best long-term result follows an antirefluxing sigmoid conduit.

Management in neonates and infants

Although the upper renal tracts are the immediate concern, any active treatment should avoid compromising later continence. Neonates identified as having an 'unsafe' bladder are best commenced on intermittent catheterisation at this stage, and oxybutynin may be administered also if there is marked detrusor hyperreflexia. In other circumstances, regular (4-monthly) ultrasound surveillance during the first 2 years of life is usually sufficient.

Despite every effort, major upper renal tract complications may still occur, and these are best managed by a temporising cutaneous vesicostomy. Endoscopic sphincterotomy represents an alternative for male infants with a competent bladder neck (contractile bladder).

Management of the severely disabled

Less ambitious management, limited to protecting the upper renal tracts and securing dryness with a minimum dependence on others, is advisable for patients having impaired intellect, poor dexterity or, most commonly, an inability to balance when sitting without support. A penile appliance is appropriate for boys, and endoscopic sphincterotomy should be performed if there is any element of bladder outflow obstruction. An indwelling urethral catheter, if properly handled, is suitable for long-term management of girls. Where these measures fail or are considered socially unacceptable, a conduit urinary diversion may be offered to patients of either gender.

Bowel management

Bowel management should be addressed at the same time as managing the urinary tract. This will generally involve avoiding gross constipation with the use of appropriate diet or medication, and ensuring colonic emptying by a variety of means: abdominal straining, manual evacuation, purgatives, suppositories or retrograde enemas. If these fail, the antegrade continence enema (ACE) procedure should be considered. This utilises the Mitrofanoff principle to provide continent catheter access to the proximal colon through which the entire colon can be washed out, using a variety of solutions ranging from tap water to phosphate, to produce faecal continence. Since its introduction in 1989, over 1000 ACE procedures have been performed, and for patients with a neuropathy the success rate is in excess of 80%, associated with a significant increase in the quality of life improvement score. The main complication reported is stomal stenosis. The ACE can be performed at the same time as bladder reconstruction, facilitating the achievement of faecal and urinary incontinence at the one operation. If the ACE fails or is deemed not suitable, a permanent colostomy remains an acceptable option.

Key points
- Secondary upper renal tract complications are far more prevalent among children with congenital neuropathic bladder than among adults with acquired lesions, and occur in both boys and girls.
- Bladder function is determined by whether the conus medullaris is intact or destroyed: in the former instance, conus reflexes are positive and the sphincteric mechanism is almost always competent.
- Especially among myelomeningocoele patients, management may be influenced by non-urological considerations (intelligence, mobility, spinal deformity).
- Intermittent catheterisation represents effective management only when there is adequate low-pressure functional bladder capacity. In 80–90% of patients this is lacking.
- Impaired bladder capacity may be the result of detrusor hyperreflexia, detrusor non-compliance or sphincteric incompetence, either singly or in some combination. Of these, sphincteric incompetence is the most difficult to treat.

Further reading

McGuire EJ, Woodside JR, Borden TA, Weiss RM. Prognostic value of urodynamic testing in myelomeningocoele. *J Urol* 1981; 126: 205–209

Mundy AR. *Urodynamic and reconstructive surgery of the lower urinary tract*. Edinburgh: Churchill Livingstone, 1993

Mundy AR, Stephenson TD, Wein AJ (eds) *Urodynamics: principles, practice and application*, 2nd edn. Edinburgh: Churchill Livingstone, 1994

Mundy AR, Shah PJR, Borzyskowski M, Saxton HM. Sphincter behaviour in myelomeningocoele. *Br J Urol* 1985; 57: 647–651

Williams MPL, Katz Z, Escala J, Rickwood AMK. Peripheral neurology as a predictor of bladder dysfunction in congenital neuropathic bladder. *Br J Urol* 1988; 62: 51–53

The urinary tract in anorectal malformations, multisystem disorders and syndromes

15

Duncan T Wilcox

Anorectal anomalies

Anorectal anomalies comprise a spectrum of congenital malformation in which the anus fails to open normally on to the perineum (Table 15.1). At one end of this spectrum are the minor anomalies in which the anal canal is present but the anus is covered by perineal skin (Figure 15.1). The severe forms of anomaly are characterised by a high termination of the rectum and the presence of a congenital fistula connecting the rectum to the lower urinary tract (Figure 15.2). In females the most severe expression of the anomaly is

Table 15.1 Simple classification of anorectal malformations

Male	Female
Anorectal anomaly without fistula	Anorectal anomaly without fistula
Perineal fistula	Perineal fistula
Rectourethral fistula	Vestibular fistula
Rectovesical fistula	Cloaca

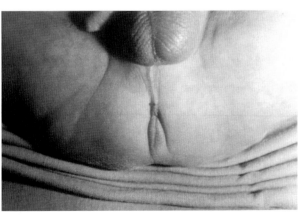

Figure 15.1 Characteristic appearances of the perineum in an infant with low anorectal anomaly.

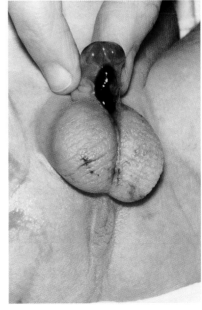

Figure 15.2 Meconium discharging from the urethral meatus of a male infant with rectourethral fistula associated with high anorectal anomaly. Note also the presence of hypospadias.

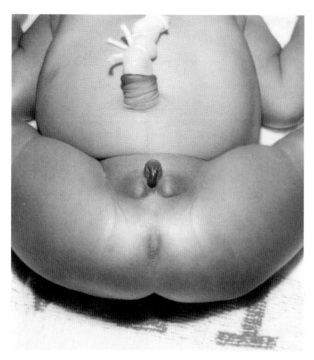

Figure 15.3 Cloacal anomaly. Single perineal orifice draining the urinary, genital and lower gastrointestinal tracts in a female infant.

Table 15.2 Other anomalies associated with anorectal malformations

Anomaly	Incidence (%)
Vertebral	25–40
Cardiac	20
Tetralogy of Fallot	
ASD/VSD	
Gastrointestinal	15
Tracheo-oesophageal fistula	
Duodenal atresia	
Hirschprung's disease	
Genitourinary	60

Associated anomalies (Table 15.2)

Anorectal malformations are frequently associated with abnormalities in other systems with most published series reporting a 50–60% rate of coexisting anomalies. Of these, the most common is the VACTERL association (previously termed the VATER syndrome), which comprises vertebral, anorectal, cardiac, tracheo-esophageal, renal and limb (typically radial) anomalies. Not all components of the VACTERL association are expressed in every patient, the most common being vertebral, anorectal and renal abnormalities.

The anomalies of most relevance to urologists are those affecting the genitourinary tract and spine.

Urinary tract anomalies

Coexisting anatomical anomalies of the upper and lower urinary tract occur in approximately 60% of patients with anorectal malformations. Of these, the most common is vesicoureteric reflux, which in some series has been reported to be present in more than half the patients studied. The pattern of urinary anomalies identified in a recent study from Great Ormond Street Children's Hospital is illustrated in Table 15.3.

Genital anomalies

Abnormalities of the male external genitalia are commonly present, including undescended testes (20%), bifid scrotum (15%), hypospadias (18%) and (rarely) absence of the vas deferens.

Anomalies of the female genital tract are less readily apparent, but vaginal and uterine duplications, as well

the cloacal malformation, in which the rectum, urethra and vagina form a single confluent channel draining by a common opening on the perineum (Figure 15.3).

The incidence of anorectal malformations is approximately 1 in 5000 live births, with a slight male to female preponderance of 3 to 2. The embryological aetiology of anorectal anomalies remains poorly understood. Although the observed association with genetically determined conditions such as Down's syndrome points to a genetic component in some cases, it is most unlikely that the complex spectrum of anorectal malformations will prove to be the outcome of a simple gene mutation.

Approximately two-thirds of girls have the 'low' form of the anomaly, in which the anorectal canal descends through the pelvic floor to terminate at the level of the perineum. Although the anus may end blindly there is frequently a perineal fistula between it and the vaginal vestibule. By contrast, two-thirds of boys have a 'high' anomaly, with the rectum ending above the levator musculature and terminating via a rectourinary fistula. Consequently, the functional outlook for boys is worse. However, cloacal anomalies in girls represent an exception to this general rule and for this reason must be considered separately.

Table 15.3 Pattern of structural anomalies of the urinary tract in 45 children with anorectal malformations treated at the Hospital for Sick Children, Great Ormond Street

Urinary anomaly	Patients (n = 45)
Vesicoureteric reflux	16
Hydronephrosis	6
Crossed fused ectopia	3
Dysplastic kidney	3
Bladder diverticulum	2
Renal agenesis	1
Horseshoe kidney	1
Megaureter	1
Prune-belly syndrome	1

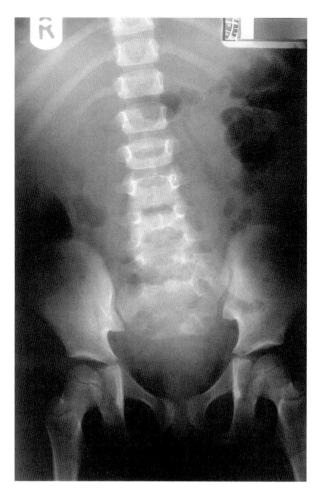

Figure 15.4 Plain radiograph demonstrating sacral agenesis.

as vaginal septae, are well documented and may be present in up to 30% of girls with anorectal anomalies. Cloacal malformations are associated with an even higher incidence of anomalies of the internal genitalia. In addition, clitoral hypertrophy has been reported.

Spinal anomalies

The incidence of vertebral anomalies in children with anorectal malformations has been reported to be as high as 40%. Many of these children have associated intraspinal pathology, carrying a risk of tethered cord syndrome and, in turn, urological, neurological and orthopaedic complications. Because early neurosurgical intervention may be effective in averting progressive neurological deterioration, it is important to identify possible cord tethering at an early stage. Investigation of the spine should therefore be undertaken routinely in all children with anorectal anomalies, with more detailed investigation of the spinal cord in those in whom a problem is identified.

Initial imaging should include both anteroposterior and lateral radiological views of the sacrum to identify sacral anomalies. The most commonly identified lesions are partial and complete sacral agenesis (Figure 15.4), but if the sacrum is radiologically normal intraspinal pathology is unlikely to be present. However, in most centres it is usual to undertake further investigations.

In infants under 4 months of age spinal ultrasound has proved to be very sensitive in identifying intraspinal anomalies (although it is less accurate than MRI for visualising the specific intraspinal pathology). In one recently published series no spinal anomalies

were missed on ultrasound. It is therefore currently recommended that neonates with anorectal malformations should be investigated initially with sacral radiographs and spinal ultrasound, with MRI being reserved for those in whom neurosurgery is being considered.

Lower urinary tract dysfunction

Until recently, relatively little attention has been paid to the problems created by neuropathic voiding dysfunction in children with anorectal anomalies. This is somewhat surprising, given that 22% of affected children suffer from urinary tract infections. Bladder dysfunction may be the result of a congenital neuropathy associated with a coexisting spinal anomaly, or may represent neurological damage acquired during surgical repair of the anorectal malformation. In one large series 25% of children with anorectal anomalies were found to have severe lower urinary tract dysfunction, which in every instance was associated with a demonstrable sacral abnormality. The majority of children with severe bladder dysfunction were incontinent, and a third also had reflux nephropathy, highlighting the importance of investigating the lower urinary tract in children whose anorectal anomaly is accompanied by a sacral abnormality.

In addition to those children with bladder neuropathy associated with a congenital spinal anomaly, a further 20% of children experienced deterioration of bladder function following surgical repair of their anorectal malformation; in half of them this proved to be permanent.

In summary, up to 20% of patients with anorectal malformations suffer from urinary incontinence. Moreover, bladder dysfunction, when present, can lead to renal damage in a third of patients. Consequently, awareness and appropriate investigation of these children is necessary to minimise the risk of ongoing renal damage.

Urological investigation of children with anorectal anomalies

The radiological investigations of the spine and urinary tract in children with anorectal malformations are summarised in Figures 15.5 and 15.6. Whether all children should also be routinely investigated by urodynamics is debatable, although, as might be expected, there is a high incidence of abnormal urodynamic findings in those with sacral abnormalities.

In addition, despite the use of a midline posterior approach for surgical correction of the anorectal anomaly, up to 10% of children develop demonstrable and permanent bladder dysfunction following surgery.

Initial urodynamic assessment and urodynamic follow-up are advisable for all children with sacral anomalies, but those affected should still undergo routine clinical follow-up (including renal and bladder ultrasound) until urinary continence has become established. The onset of new symptoms or a change in the pattern of existing symptoms, both of which might indicate the onset of neurological deterioration, merits formal urodynamic assessment.

Surgical management of anorectal anomalies

A detailed account of the surgical management of anorectal anomalies is beyond the scope of this chapter

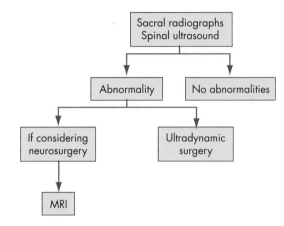

Figure 15.5 Diagnostic algorithm for the investigation of the spine in an infant with an anorectal anomaly.

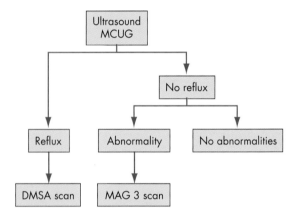

Figure 15.6 Diagnostic algorithm for the investigation of the urinary tract in an infant with an anorectal anomaly.

but is covered in the reading list. In general, these children undergo sigmoid colostomy shortly after birth, followed by formal repair at approximately 3 months of age. The technique most widely employed is the posterior sagittal anorectoplasty originally described and popularised by Pena.

Urological complications of surgery

Although the introduction of the midline posterior sagittal approach has reduced the incidence of neuropathic bladder, approximately 10% of children develop new or increased bladder dysfunction following this procedure. Mobilisation and division of the rectourethral fistula is an integral step in the operation and, as such, may inevitably cause some damage to the immediately adjacent autonomic pelvic nerves.

The urethra itself is also at risk during this dissection. Urethral damage occurred in 12% of patients during the older abdominoperineal operations for anorectal anomalies, but this complication is much rarer with posterior sagittal anorectoplasty. Injuries to the vas deferens have also been reported.

The complexity of the surgery, and hence the risk of complications, is greatest in children with severe anorectal anomalies associated with the presence of a fistula between the rectum and the urinary tract.

Cloacal anomalies

These account for approximately 10% of anorectal malformations in girls. The cloacal malformation is characterised by confluence of the urethra, rectum and vagina to form a common channel draining by a single opening on the perineum (see Figure 15.3). Cloacal anomalies are currently classified according to whether the common channel is less or greater than 3 cm in length, as measured on cystoscopy. In addition to the renal anomalies seen with anorectal anomalies, cloacal malformations are accompanied by a high incidence of vaginal abnormalities. Septate vagina and/or bicornuate uterus have been reported in 45% of cases, and up to 5% have an absent vagina.

The initial management of a child with a cloacal anomaly requires not only diversion of the faecal stream, usually by a colostomy, but also drainage of the urinary tract and, where necessary, decompression of hydrocolpos.

In some patients satisfactory bladder drainage can be achieved by intermittent catheterisation of the common channel, but it may be necessary to place a suprapubic catheter. Rarely, both vesicostomy and vaginostomy are required to secure adequate infection-free drainage. However, this approach is best avoided as it can complicate the definitive repair.

Cloacal malformations are now mostly corrected using the posterior sagittal approach, particularly in cases where the common channel exceeds 3 cm in length. Where the common channel is short (< 3cm) it may be feasible to use a perineal approach to relocate all three orifices on to the perineum by mobilisation of the urogenital sinus. In view of the rarity of cloacal anomalies and the complexity of their surgical correction, a case can be argued for concentrating surgical management in a small number of specialist centres.

The functional results of surgery for these children reflect the length of the common channel. In the 'low' confluence anomalies, where the common channel is less than 3 cm, 70% of children will be continent of

urine and 50% continent of faeces. In contrast, only 30% of children with a channel length greater than 3 cm will be continent of urine and faeces. The sexual outcome is not well documented, although some women are known to be sexually active and there are reports of successful pregnancy following cloacal repair.

Syndromes and associations involving the urinary tract

Abnormalities of the genitourinary tract are often seen in association with or as part of a clinical syndrome. Two of the most important associations are:

- **VACTERL association** This is comprised of vertebral, anorectal, cardiac, tracheal, oesphageal (esophageal), renal and limb anomalies. Those aspects of greatest relevance to the urologist have already been considered above.
- **CHARGE association** The components consist of coloboma of the eye, heart anomalies, choanal atresia, mental retardation, genital and ear anomalies. In one series of 32 children with CHARGE the overall incidence of genitourinary tract abnormalities was 69% (Table 15.4).

Neural tube defects

The spectrum of neural tube defects ranges from open meningomyelocoele to occult spinal dysraphism and sacral agenesis. Some degree of bladder neuropathy is almost invariably present, although, depending on the severity of the neurological impairment, this may

Table 15.4 Genitourinary malformations in the CHARGE association

	Incidence (%)
Genital anomalies	56
Hypospadias	
Micropenis	
Undescended testicle	
Vaginal and uterine atesia	
Urinary tract anomalies	42
Duplex kidney	
Vesicoureteric reflux	
Renal agenesis	
Hydronephrosis	

not always be clinically apparent. In addition to the neuropathic bladder and its consequences, notably secondary vesicoureteric reflux and upper tract dilatation, neural tube defects are also associated with an increased incidence of primary urinary tract abnormalities such as renal agenesis and hydronephrosis. The investigation and management of children with neuropathic bladder is considered in detail in Chapter 14.

Abnormal migration and fusion of the kidney

Ectopic kidney

The embryological origins of renal ectopia are considered in more detail in Chapter 1, but in essence represent the outcome of abnormalities of renal ascent or fusion. Ectopic kidneys can be divided into simple, horseshoe and crossed renal ectopia.

Simple ectopic kidney

The ectopically sited kidney may be located anywhere along the embryological path of ascent from the pelvis to the renal fossa. Pelvic kidneys are the most common of renal ectopias, accounting for 60% of all cases. In 90% the anomaly is unilateral and with a slight left-sided preponderance. In addition to its abnormal location, a pelvic kidney is frequently hypoplastic and irregular in shape (Figure 15.7). Other ectopic kidneys lie at some point between the pelvis and the normal position or, very rarely, within the thorax.

Genital and contralateral urinary abnormalities are often associated with ectopic kidneys and include absence of the vagina, retrocaval ureter, bicornuate uterus, supernumerary kidney, and ipsilateral ectopic ureter. The ectopic kidney can be a component of more complex syndromes, such as the Mayer–Rokitansky–Küster–Hauser syndrome, Fanconi's anaemia or conjoined twins.

Horseshoe kidney

Horseshoe kidneys are encountered in 1:400 and 1:1800 autopsies and the anomaly is more common in males. In 95% of cases the lower poles of the two kidneys are joined by an isthmus of renal tissue which may consist of normal parenchyma or dysplastic or

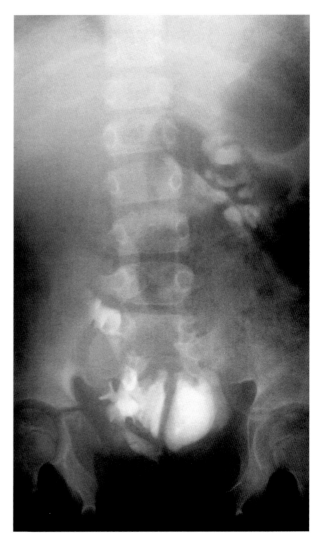

Figure 15.7 Intravenous urogram demonstrating ectopic kidney – pelvic right kidney.

fibrous tissue. In about 40% of cases the isthmus lies at the level of L4, just beneath the origin of the inferior mesenteric artery, in 20% in the pelvis (Figure 15.8), and in the remaining 40% at the level of the lower poles of normally placed kidneys. A small proportion of horseshoe kidneys are fused at their upper poles. The ureters arch anteriorly to pass over the isthmus, thus explaining the relatively high incidence of pyeloureteric anomalies (20%) associated with horseshoe kidney. Horseshoe kidney is not uncommonly found in association with other abnormalities or syndromes, notably Turner's syndrome and abnormalities of the central nervous system, the gastrointestinal tract, and the skeletal and cardiovascular systems.

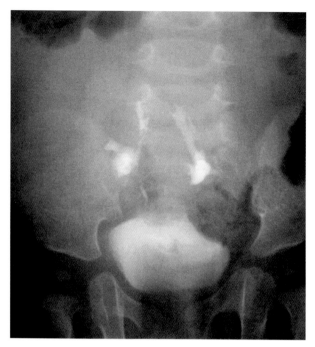

Figure 15.8 Intravenous urogram – horseshoe kidney.

Crossed renal ectopia

There are four varieties of crossed renal ectopia:

- With renal fusion (85% of cases)
- Without fusion (< 10%)
- Solitary
- Bilateral.

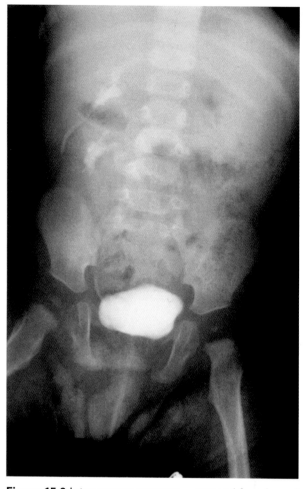

Figure 15.9 Intravenous urogram – crossed fused renal ectopia.

There is a slight male predominance, and crossing from left to right occurs more frequently than from right to left. The point of fusion is usually between the upper pole of the crossed kidney and the lower pole of the normally positioned kidney (unilateral fused type) (Figure 15.9). Associated anomalies are commonly found with renal ectopia. In addition, renal ectopia may also be a component of more complex syndromes, such as VACTERL and agenesis of the corpus callosum.

Presentation and investigation of abnormalities of ascent and fusion

Abnormalities of ascent and fusion most commonly come to light as incidental findings, typically on prenatal or postnatal ultrasound examinations. Conversely, non-dilated pelvic ectopic kidneys may be difficult to visualise on ultrasound, and absence of the kidney in

the renal fossa may be misinterpreted as renal agenesis. In such cases the presence of ectopic functioning renal tissue is best demonstrated by DMSA renography.

Crossed fused renal ectopia may sometimes present clinically as an incidentally discovered mass during the course of abdominal examination.

The occurrence of pain or symptoms associated with urinary infection generally denotes additional pathology, such as vesicoureteric reflux or pelvi-ureteric junction obstruction.

Investigation of an uncomplicated ectopic or horseshoe kidney can reasonably be limited to ultrasound and a DMSA scintigram. Additional investigations are indicated if there is hydronephrosis or a history of documented infection raising the possibility of reflux. However, it is important to stress that the majority of patients are untroubled by their abnormally placed kidney, and surgical intervention should be confined to correcting coexisting pathology, obstruction or reflux. When surgery is warranted it should be borne in mind that the anatomy may be abnormal and that the blood supply can have an aberrant course.

Further reading

Bauer S. Anomalies of the kidney and ureteropelvic junction. In: Walsh PC, Retik AB, Vaughan ED, Wein AJ (eds) *Campbell's textbook of urology*, 7th edn, Vol 2. Philadelphia: WB Saunders, 1998; 1708–1730

Boemers TM, Beek FJ, Bax NM. Guidelines for the urological screening and initial management of lower urinary tract dysfunction in children with anorectal malformations – the ARGUS protocol. *BJU Int* 1999; 83: 662–671

Kiely EM, Pena A. Anorectal malformations. In: O'Neil JA, Rowe MI, Grosfeld JL, Fonkalsrud EW, Coran AG (eds). *Pediatric surgery*, 5th edn, Vol 2 St Louis: Mosby-yearbook Inc., 1998; 1425–1448

Pena A. Anorectal malformations. *Semin Pediatr Surg* 1995; 4: 35–47

Ragan DC, Casale AJ, Rink RC, Cain MP, Weaver DD. *J Urol* 1999; 161: 622–5

Key points

- Children with anorectal anomalies have a high incidence of coexisting urinary tract abnormalities and functional urinary problems.
- It is important that management of the urological aspects of these complex malformations is not overlooked during management of the bowel.
- In addition to urinary incontinence, the bladder dysfunction in children with anorectal malformations poses a potential threat of urinary tract infection, renal damage and chronic renal failure.
- Early recognition and effective management of urological problems in children with anorectal malformations is essential to minimise these risks.
- In view of the high incidence of genitourinary tract anomalies in the CHARGE association all affected infants should be screened appropriately, initially by urinary tract ultrasound, and then with additional modalities such as renography where indicated.

Bladder exstrophy and epispadias

16

Patrick G Duffy

Introduction

Bladder exstrophy and epispadias represent a spectrum of congenital anomalies having a common underlying embryogenesis. The most frequent variant, classic bladder exstrophy (60%), occupies the middle ground as regards severity, whereas isolated epispadias (30%) represents the least severe form and cloacal exstrophy (10%) the most severe. They are rare anomalies which affect boys more commonly than girls (Table 16.1). Reconstruction, to achieve urinary continence and satisfactory sexual function, technically demanding, and especially so in the case of cloacal exstrophy, where the severity of the anomaly itself and the frequency of associated abnormalities can pose additional, ethical, dilemmas.

Embryology

Arising within the first 8 weeks of gestation, all these lesions result from some degree of abnormal mesodermal migration during development of the lower abdominal wall and of the urogenital and anorectal canals Although the aetiology is unknown, there is no linkage with parental age, birth order, identifiable chromosomal abnormalities or established teratogens.

Classic vesical exstrophy is detectable by fetal ultrasonography, the features being a permanently empty bladder, normal kidneys, a low-lying umbilicus and, in males, a short upturned penis. Cloacal exstrophy, despite being conspicuous on fetal ultrasonography, may be confused with gastroschisis.

Anatomy

Bladder exstrophy

Bladder exstrophy is characterised by the following:

- Low-lying umbilicus
- Exposed bladder plate
- Pubic symphysis diastasis
- Divarication of the rectus abdominis and pelvic floor
- Anterior ectopia of anus and vagina
- Penile epispadias.

Except for a slightly increased incidence of congenital cardiac anomalies, neonates with classic bladder

	Live-birth incidence	Male/female ratio
Isolated epispadias	1:117 000	5:1
Vesical exstrophy	1:50 000	3:1
Cloacal exstrophy	1:300 000	6:1

Table 16.1 Incidence and gender ratios of exstrophy and epispadiac anomalies

exstrophy are otherwise healthy and are typically born at term and with a birthweight within the normal range.

The umbilical cord emerges immediately above the exposed bladder plate. The latter is of variable dimensions; at one extreme the exposed bladder is of normal size or occasionally larger (Figure 16.1), whereas at the other end of the spectrum little more than the trigone is represented (Figure 16.2). At birth the mucosa is normal, but with 48 hours' exposure it becomes friable and polypoid. If it remains exposed for several decades neoplasia may supervene. The detrusor muscle, which usually has a normal autonomic innervation, is initially pliable, but with exposure becomes progressively fibrotic so that the bladder plate becomes less pliable. Musculoskeletal anomalies include divarication of the lower rectus abdominis muscles, pubic symphysis diastasis, with outward and downward rotation of the anterior pelvic ring, and splitting of the pelvic floor musculature. Perineal anomalies include anterior vaginal ectopia and a bifid clitoris in females, and anterior anal ectopia in both sexes.

Although the spine and hips are normal, patients have a slightly 'waddling' gait owing to external rotation of the acetabulae. In males the urethra is entirely deficient dorsally, with a thick urethral plate densely adherent to the underlying corpora. The corpora invariably exhibit marked dorsal chordee and are typically short but bulky, and the glans penis is similarly well developed. The prepuce is deficient dorsally. As a general rule, the greater the degree of pubic diastasis the larger the bladder plate and the less prominent the penis. The neurovascular bundles, emerging at the base of the corpora ventrolaterally, wind around to the normal dorsal disposition as they approach the glans. Vesicoureteric reflux, although almost always present following bladder closure, is usually inconsequential so long as the sphincteric mechanism remains incompetent.

Eighty per cent of boys and 15% of girls develop inguinal hernias bilaterally following bladder closure.

Epispadias

Although the bladder is normally formed, the urethra is deficient dorsally. In cases of female epispadias this deficiency is complete. In males the extent of the urethral deficiency is variable in degree, affecting only the glanular urethra in some cases (Figure 16.3), the

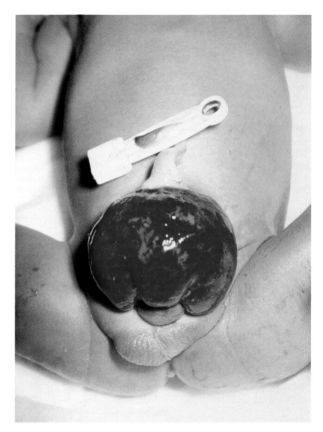

Figure 16.1 Classic bladder exstrophy with a large everted plate of exposed bladder mucosa.

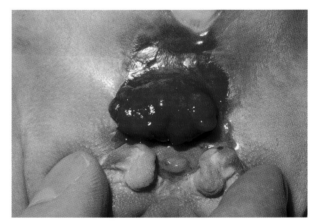

Figure 16.2 Exstrophy in a female infant. The mucosal plate comprises little more than trigone.

glans and distal penile urethra in others, and the entire urethra in a majority (60%) (Figure 16.4). Except in some cases of glanular epispadias the prepuce is deficient dorsally and, as a rule, the more severe the epispadias, the greater the associated dorsal chordee.

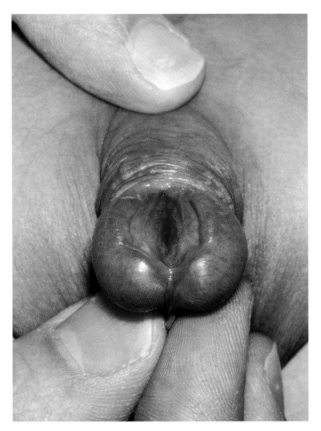

Figure 16.3 Primary epispadias: glanular.

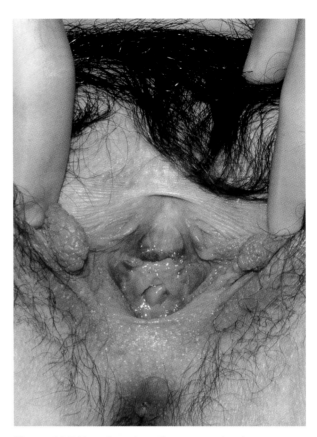

Figure 16.5 Female epispadias presenting in a postpubertal female with a history of lifelong incontinence.

Complete epispadias is associated with a bifid clitoris in females (Figure 16.5), and in both sexes with some degree of pubic diastasis and with an absent external urethral sphincter and a deficient bladder neck, so that the patient is incontinent of urine.

Cloacal exstrophy

Although several subvarieties exist, the usual configuration (Figure 16.6) is one of an exomphalos beneath which are two hemibladders separated by a midline bowel field. The bowel component has two orifices, the upper, situated at the level of the ileocaecal junction, draining the small intestine, and the lower leading to a narrow colon terminating blindly above the pelvic floor. In males the penis is typically both completely bifid and of pathologically small dimensions, and one or both testes may be absent. In contrast to epispadias and classic bladder exstrophy, other congenital anomalies are common (Table 16.2) and the situation may be further compounded by prematurity and low birthweight.

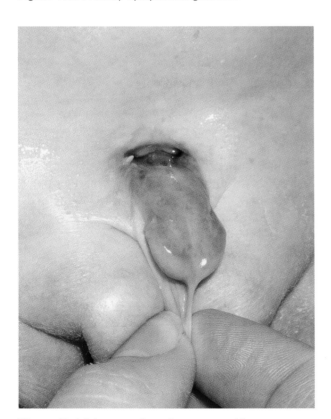

Figure 16.4 Primary epispadias: penopubic.

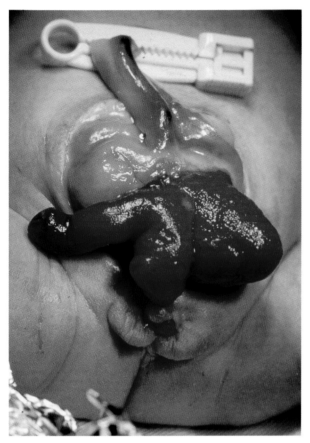

Figure 16.6 Cloacal exstrophy.

Table 16.2 Frequency of coexisting anomalies associated with cloacal exstrophy

Anomaly	Cases affected (%)
Anomalies of renal position and lesion	70
Sacral agenesis	60
Myelomeningocoele	50
Orthopaedic deformities	40
Small bowel anomalies	65
Cyanotic heart disease	<10

Clinical presentation

Although most defects are obvious at birth, glanular epispadias in males may not be apparent if the prepuce is normally formed, whereas if female epispadias is overlooked the presentation may be as primary urinary incontinence with continuous dribbling of urine.

Surgical reconstruction

Bladder exstrophy

Reconstruction is usually undertaken in stages:

- Initial anatomical repair. This consists of closure of the bladder and proximal urethra, with subsequent correction of the epispadiac deformity.
- Later functional reconstruction for continence, ideally with voiding per urethram and without the need for self-catheterisation.

Recently some centres are performing the initial anatomical repair in a single stage, and this may be combined with simultaneous functional reconstruction. For the purposes of this chapter the more traditional staged approach is described.

Anatomical repair of bladder and proximal urethra

Except when some more pressing problem exists (e.g. a congenital cardiac lesion) this is performed in the neonatal period and usually incorporates approximation of the pelvic ring anteriorly. The latter is possible without the need for pelvic osteotomies during the first 24–48 hours of life (a benefit attributed to the presence of circulating maternal relaxins). However, many centres prefer to delay closure for up to 6 weeks, finding that osteotomies permit a more reliable closure with less tense apposition of bladder and overlying soft tissues. Whichever policy is employed, the repair is identical and begins with circumcision of the bladder plate, which is then widely mobilised from the underlying recti on either side so that it may be closed in the midline anteriorly without tension (Figure 16.7a,b). In males the proximal urethral plate is mobilised and similarly closed in the midline. In females the entire urethra may be repaired at this stage or, as with males, only proximally. Although no attempt is made to achieve a competent sphincteric mechanism, it is customary to divide the pubourethral ligaments from the pelvic bones on either side and to wrap them, double-breasted, around the bladder neck, a manoeuvre which, by enhancing outlet resistance, may serve to increase bladder capacity over time (Figure 16.7c,d). Any indirect inguinal hernias are repaired extraperitoneally and the umbilicus is transposed superiorly.

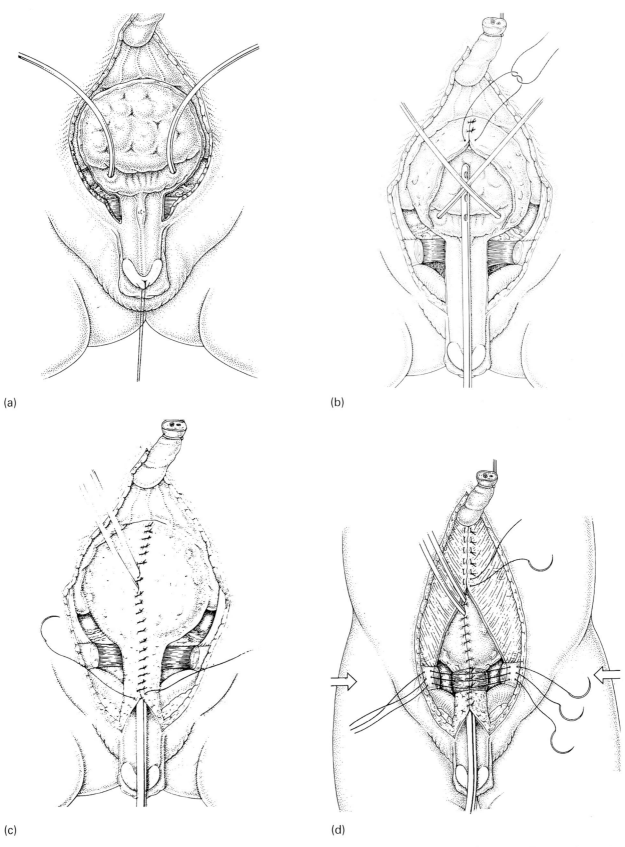

(a)

(b)

(c)

(d)

Figure 16.7 (a,b,c,d) Key steps in the primary closure of bladder exstrophy. Reproduced from *Rob Smith's Operative Surgery. Paediatric Surgery*, 5th edition published by Chapman & Hall Medical (permission applied for).

Closure of the pelvic ring anteriorly enables tension-free approximation of the lower rectus abdominis muscles and of the overlying skin.

Epispadias repair

This is usually undertaken at 1–2 years of age. The Cantwell–Ransley repair and its derivatives are the most widely used, although a number of alternatives are still employed in some centres. The Cantwell–Ransley procedure described here is based upon the premise that upward chordee is the result of inherent deformity of the corpora, rather than any deficiency of the urethral plate. The plate is incised on either side from bladder neck to glans penis and, after mobilisation from the underlying corpora, is tubularised (Figure 16.8a). The

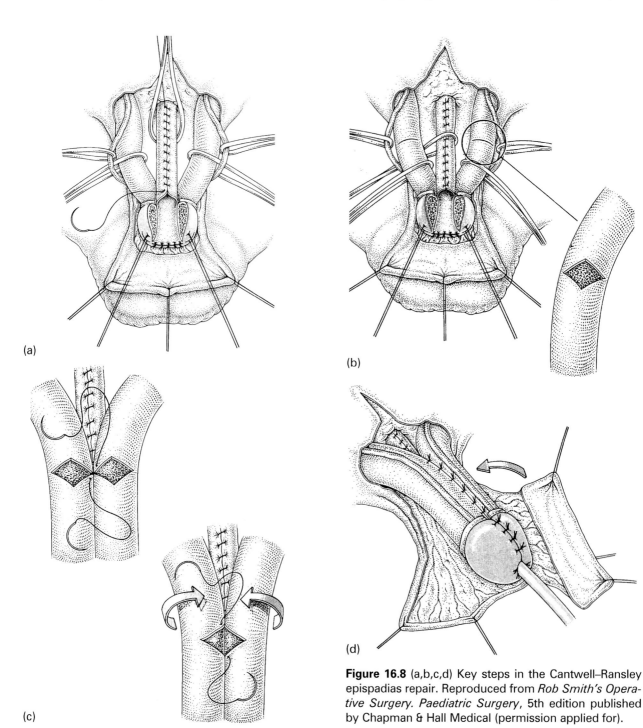

(a)

(b)

(c)

(d)

Figure 16.8 (a,b,c,d) Key steps in the Cantwell–Ransley epispadias repair. Reproduced from *Rob Smith's Operative Surgery. Paediatric Surgery*, 5th edition published by Chapman & Hall Medical (permission applied for).

glanular urethra is similarly repaired. After mobilisation of skin from the penile shaft, chordee is corrected by means of an inverting cavernocavernostomy (Figure 16.8b,c), a manoeuvre which transposes the repaired urethra ventrally. Pelvic osteotomy, if not previously undertaken, is advantageous as it renders the penis more prominent and improves the angle at which it emerges from the lower abdominal wall. Any deficiency of penile shaft skin dorsally may be rectified by transposition of a pedicled island flap raised from the redundant prepuce ventrally (Figure 16.8d).

In females in whom the epispadias has not already been fully repaired, this is also undertaken at 1–2 years of age. The repair is reinforced by fat mobilised from the prepubic area, which may also be employed to obliterate the prepubic space. On occasion this simple manoeuvre enhances urethral resistance sufficiently to secure continence. The opportunity is also taken to deal with the clitori, which are mobilised and sutured together below a reconstructed clitoral hood.

Repair of isolated epispadias lesions is undertaken by the same means, and again usually at 1–2 years of age.

Cloacal exstrophy

In cases detected by prenatal ultrasonography and where the diagnosis is beyond question, termination of the pregnancy may be offered. Prior to the era of reconstruction, beginning in 1960, no baby born with this condition survived. With more modern infant care, however, survival is possible without active surgical treatment, and for this reason reconstruction is usually advised except in cases where some other coexistent abnormality is likely to be lethal of itself or to severely compromise quality of life.

The exact form of anatomical reconstruction varies according to individual circumstances. In most cases, after repair of the exstrophy, ileum and hindgut are disconnected from the central bowel field and, following restoration of intestinal continuity, a terminal colostomy is fashioned. Occasionally it is preferable to construct a terminal ileostomy and to leave the colon in situ for later vaginal reconstruction or for augmentation cystoplasty. The central bowel field may either be left in situ, to act in effect as an 'auto-augmentation', or may be excised and the two hemibladders anastomosed together in the midline. In either case, anterior bladder reconstruction can be at this initial stage or one or 2 months later. Pelvic osteotomy is

always necessary because the pubic diastasis is exceptionally wide in these cases.

In males, gender assignment requires urgent consideration, as the penis is almost invariably severely deficient. Current practice in most cases is to advise bilateral gonadectomy and rearing as a female. However, the issues raised by gender reassignment are the subject of considerable controversy at present.

Functional reconstruction

Bladder exstrophy

Functional reconstruction should be delayed until both child and parents are well motivated, and especially so if there is any prospect that self-catheterisation will be needed. This is seldom before 5 years of age, and usually rather older than that.

In principle, the ideal of continence with spontaneous urethral voiding is achievable by bladder neck repair alone. Such repair creates a fixed outlet resistance rather than a normal dynamic sphincteric mechanism, and all of the several methods employed essentially involve tubularisation of the trigone, a procedure necessitating reimplantation of the ureters at a higher level in the bladder and which, in turn, corrects any vesicoureteric reflux. The procedure also involves loss of bladder capacity, by approximately 30 ml, and as a rule of thumb if, at 5 years of age, preoperative bladder capacity is less than 60 ml then bladder neck repair alone is most unlikely to secure continence. The success or otherwise of bladder neck repair may also depend upon detrusor function. Although this is normal in some cases, in others there is detrusor instability whereas in others there is absence of detrusor activity, so that voiding is achieved by abdominal straining. In these circumstances, bladder neck repair is unlikely to achieve continence.

Where bladder neck repair fails to achieve continence, two situations may exist:

- The bladder lacks any useful functional capacity, whether inherently, from inadequate bladder neck repair, or as a result of both factors. This may be dealt with by augmentation cystoplasty plus, when necessary, by further bladder neck repair. Because voiding is usually incomplete following augmentation cystoplasty, intermittent self-catheterisation is often required thereafter.
- The bladder neck repair is too competent, leading to a large residual urine and a small effective

bladder capacity in consequence. This is manageable by intermittent catheterisation, although augmentation cystoplasty may be necessary in the event of detrusor malfunction (instability, noncompliance) leading to secondary upper renal tract complications.

Because urethral sensation is retained, most boys and some girls are unwilling to practice urethral catheterisation and in this circumstance it is necessary to construct a Mitrofanoff channel as an additional measure. Although it enjoys the theoretical advantage of creating a variable urethral resistance, the artificial urinary sphincter has not found widespread use in patients with vesical exstrophy, mainly because of the problem of urethral erosion by the cuff. Marginal degrees of stress urinary leakage following conventional bladder neck repair may respond to α-adrenergic agonists (e.g. ephedrine) or to endoscopic submucosal injection of bulking agents. When all attempts to prevent stress urinary leakage fail, closure of the bladder neck to create, in effect, a continent diversion, represents a further resort. Lastly, there remains an occasional place for conduit urinary diversion or ureterosigmoidostomy in those children with full anal competence (the majority). Ureterosigmoidostomy has, however, fallen from favour, largely because of the appreciable long-term risk of neoplasia developing at the ureterointestinal anastomosis.

Functional reconstruction calls for regular and continued surveillance of the upper renal tracts, as bladder malfunction can result in secondary complications at any time later. The potential complications of augmentation cystoplasty are described in Chapter 14.

Epispadias

In females, as mentioned previously, a reinforced urethral repair may itself be sufficient to secure continence. With both sexes bladder neck repair gives results superior to those obtained with exstrophy because detrusor function is normal, as is bladder capacity. In males the artificial urinary sphincter also gives good results, as the cuff may be placed around virginal bladder neck. Again in males, lesser degrees of sphincteric incompetence may respond to periurethral bulking agents, although it should be noted that in this situation continence sometimes supervenes spontaneously during puberty, presumably because prostatic growth enhances urethral resistance.

Cloacal exstrophy

Functional bladder reconstruction proceeds along the same lines as those described for classic vesical exstrophy. Augmentation cystoplasty, when necessary, is usually best undertaken using the stomach, as in many of these children the small bowel is deficient in length so that sacrifice of a segment may result in 'short bowel syndrome'. Bowel management is problematical in those patients with a sacral neurological deficit due to sacral agenesis or myelomeningocoele, because pull-through procedures are almost invariably followed by faecal incontinence. A permanent terminal colostomy is preferable in this situation. For males who have undergone gender reassignment a vagina may be constructed using a short segment of bowel (small or large as appropriate) or, where there is insufficient length to spare, by means of myocutaneous flaps based on the gracilis muscle.

Outcome

Bladder exstrophy and epispadias

Anatomical reconstruction of the bladder defect is nowadays almost always achieved by the initial repair, whereas the complications of epispadias repair (principally urethral fistula) have become comparatively uncommon as a result of improved surgical techniques. The outcomes of functional bladder reconstruction, however, remain more variable and less predictable. Although some centres report continence rates exceeding 80% with bladder neck repair alone, these have not been widely replicated. In one large group of patients managed by a combination of bladder neck repair and augmentation cystoplasty, 82% were continent but at the expense of two-thirds of them needing to practice self-catheterisation. Functional reconstruction carries a risk of secondary upper renal tract complications, and in one historical series these occurred in 50% of patients. The current rate is probably lower as a result of closer surveillance and improved means of reconstruction.

Men have a normal libido and form stable partnerships with satisfactory sexual intercourse. Poor ejaculation with low quality or absent sperm usually occurs. These abnormalities result from a deformed urethra and vasal obstruction secondary to bladder neck reconstruction. Those who have undergone early urinary diversion tend to have better sperm quality. Although fertility is impaired, paternity has been reported. In females, fertility is within the normal range but uterine prolapse is a common obstetric problem.

Cloacal exstrophy

Although it is usually possible to construct a continent catheterisable urinary reservoir and thus achieve 'dryness', if not true continence, faecal continence is considerably more difficult to achieve so that most patients remain with a terminal colostomy. Although the current policy of gender reassignment avoids the catastrophe of a sexually crippled male with a minute deformed penis, it remains to be established whether patients so managed will become psychosexually adequate females any more than did their predecessors become adequate males.

Further reading

Gearhart JP, Jeffs RD. Exstrophy – epispadias complex and bladder anomalies. In: Walsh PC, Retik AB, Vaughan ED, Wein AJ (eds) *Campbell's textbook of urology*, 7th edn. Philadelphia: WB Saunders, 1998; 1939–1990

Hurwitz RS, Manzoni GM. Cloacal exstrophy. In: O'Donnell B, Koff SA (eds) *Paediatric urology*. Oxford: Butterworth–Heinemann, 1997; 514–525

Ransley PG, Duffy PG. Bladder estrophy closure and epispadias repair. In: Spitz L and Coran AG (eds) *Rob & Smiths Operative Surgery. Paediatric Surgery*, 5th ed. London: Chapman & Hall Medical, 1995; 745–759

Key points

- All forms of exstrophy and epispadias are rare and occur more commonly in males.
- Whereas vesical exstrophy and epispadias usually occur as isolated anomalies in otherwise healthy neonates, cloacal exstrophy is accompanied by a high incidence of associated abnormalities affecting both the urinary tract and other systems.
- Anatomical reconstruction of vesical exstrophy is best undertaken in the neonatal period and in conjunction with repair of the pelvic ring anteriorly; epispadias repair is usually deferred until 1–2 years of age.
- Functional reconstruction of vesical exstrophy, for continence, is nearly always deferred until at least 5 years of age, when bladder neck repair, plus or minus augmentation cystoplasty and plus or minus intermittent catheterisation, achieves continence in upwards of 80% of cases.
- Reconstruction of cloacal exstrophy, if undertaken at all, presents more formidable challenges. Although it is usually possible to construct a continent urinary reservoir, most patients remain with a terminal colostomy.
- The majority of males with a vestigial penis are nowadays usually gender reassigned to be reared as females.

Hypospadias

17

Duncan T Wilcox and Pierre DE Mouriquand

Introduction

Hypospadias can be defined as an association of three anatomical anomalies:

- An abnormal ventral opening of the urethral meatus;
- Ventral curvature (chordee) of the penis;
- A hooded foreskin, which is deficient ventrally.

Hypospadias can also be characterised as an atresia of the ventral part of the penis. The skin over the ventral surface is often poor and occasionally adherent to the urethra. The glans is deficient ventrally and the corpus spongiosum is atretic distal to the abnormal meatus; this can contribute to the penile chordee. In addition, the frenular artery is absent in patients with hypospadias.

History

One of the first descriptions of hypospadias was by Galen in the second century. He clearly describes the problem of infertility associated with a proximal meatus and penile chordee, and was the first to use the term hypospadias. Antyl described the first surgical repair during this period: his technique involved amputating the penis distal to the meatus, a method probably not acceptable today!

Following this early work little was added to our understanding of hypospadias and its treatment until the second half of the 19th century, when, between 1850 and 1900, the majority of surgical techniques employed today were first described. In the 1800s Thiersch and Duplay described tubularisation of the urethral plate; Duplay also described a technique very similar to the meatal advancement and glanuloplasty later popularised by Duckett. Bouisson, in 1860, reported the meatal-based flip-flap repair later used with great success by Mathieu. Repairs using prepuce-based pedicle tubes, later described as island flaps, were published in the 1890s. At the same time, Nove-Josserand described a two-stage repair using a preputial skin free graft. Although techniques to repair hypospadias have continued to evolve, these have been minor compared to the massive contribution made by the surgeons of the late 19th century.

Aetiology and incidence

The incidence of hypospadias has been calculated at 1 in 300 live male births and appears to be increasing in frequency. It has been suggested that this simply represents increased referral of minor forms of hypospadias for which parents would not previously have sought surgical correction. However, there is growing evidence to point to a genuine increase in incidence (possibly related to intrauterine exposure to oestrogenic environmental pollutants).

Many theories have been postulated to explain the aetiology of hypospadias; these include deficiencies in hormonal stimulation of the penis, genetic disorders, and a vascular abnormality. Hypospadias is more common in monozygotic twins and in the offspring of fathers who have hypospadias, indicating that there may be a polygenic inheritance, but as yet the aetiology is not fully understood.

Intersex and associated anomalies

Severe forms of hypospadias can present as ambiguous genitalia, especially in those with undescended testicles. In some series up to 50% of patients with hypospadias and cryptorchidism had an underlying genetic, gonadal or phenotypic sexual abnormality. It is especially important to exclude congenital adrenal hyperplasia in an apparently male baby with severe hypospadias and impalpable gonads. The abnormalities included mixed gonadal dysgenesis, gonadal agenesis, and both pseudo and true hermaphrodism (see Chapter 21). It is essential that patients with hypospadias and undescended testicles are fully investigated so that intersex anomalies can be excluded.

With the exception of an increased overall incidence of undescended testis other anomalies in patients with isolated hypospadias are rare. Abnormalities of the urinary tract are unusual, occurring in approximately 2% of patients; consequently, routine ultrasound of these children is unnecessary. The overall incidence of undescended testis is in the range 5–10%, rising to 50% in those with the severe perineal or penoscrotal forms. These severe forms are also associated with a persistent utricle in 20% of cases, which on occasions can make urethral catheterisation of the bladder difficult. However, it is rarely necessary to remove the utricle, and so routine cystography or cystoscopy to identify a utricle is not required unless the child is symptomatic.

Classification

Many authors have classified hypospadias, based on the preoperative site of the abnormal meatus (Figure 17.1). However, the position of the meatus is not always a reliable guide to the true severity of the anomaly (Figure 17.2). Some forms of proximal hypospadias may be associated with the deceptive presence of a flimsy ('paper-thin') penile urethra which must be fully excised before correction can be under-

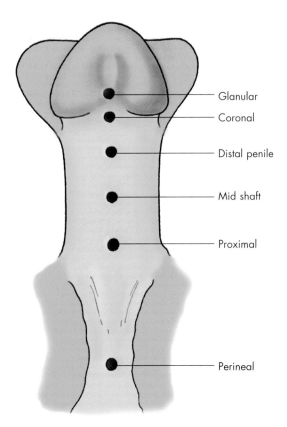

Figure 17.1 Standard classification of hypospadias.

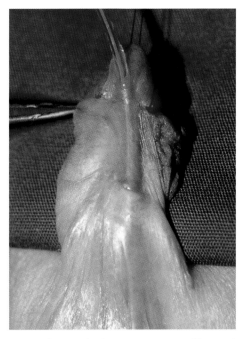

Figure 17.2 Deceptively severe case illustrating the potential pitfalls of classification based on the position of the urethral meatus. The urethra terminates with an opening on the glans but the entire urethra is 'paper thin', and this case is in effect a proximal form of hypospadias with chordee.

taken. In other cases the abnormal meatus can become significantly more proximal once the chordee tissue has been fully excised.

General surgical principles

Magnification

The precise nature of this delicate surgery means that most surgeons use some form of optical magnification. Operating microscopes have almost unlimited magnification power, but they are cumbersome and often too powerful for most cases of hypospadias. Most surgeons therefore use standard operating loupes which are easy to use and provide magnification in the range 2.5–4×. The important thing is that the surgeon should feel comfortable using the optical magnification.

Sutures

The suture material used needs to be fine, absorbable and easy to use. Traditionally chromic catgut was the most commonly used suture, but with developments in suture technology others are now available. We prefer 7-0 or 6-0 polydioxanone (PDS): these fine absorbable monofilament sutures provide excellent strength and disappear before suture tracts are formed.

Haemostasis

As in all operations haemostasis is essential; however, the vascularity of the glans can make this difficult. Three techniques are currently used:

- A **tourniquet** at the base of the penis provides an excellent bloodless operating field, but care must be taken not to leave it on too long, as there is the theoretical problem of reperfusion injury. In addition, a compressive dressing is required to prevent postoperative haemorrhage.
- **Adrenaline 1:100 000** can also be used, up to a maximum dose of 10 mg/kg. In theory this might compromise the the vascularity of skin flaps, although Duckett did not report this complication.
- **Diathermy** Bipolar diathermy is generally preferred, but the safe use of monopolar diathermy has been described. Diathermy may be inadequate to control bleeding from the glans.

It is currently our policy to use a tourniquet followed by a compressive dressing at the end of the operation.

Urinary drainage

The indications for urinary diversion depend upon the type of reconstruction. Some forms of distal hypospadias repair may not require any form of urethral catheter drainage. We use transurethral catheter drainage for all but the most minor repairs in general a 6–8 Fr dripping stent. A standard indwelling urinary catheter may cause some concern in that once the balloon is deflated it can catch on the anastomosis as it is withdrawn. Some surgeons use a suprapubic catheter: we do not feel that this is necessary, except perhaps after complex or 'salvage' redo surgery.

Dressing

The dressing serves many purposes, which ideally include providing gentle compression of the penis to reduce haemorrhage and oedema, and immobilising it to reduce postoperative pain. Many dressings are available and and are subject to preference of the surgeon. These include silastic foam, a clean bandage, and bio-occlusive dressings (Tegaderm). The dressings stay in place for between 2 and 7 days, depending on the complexity of the repair.

Specific surgical principles

There are three specific parts to the surgical correction of hypospadias:

- Correction of the penile chordee
- Reconstruction of the urethra (urethroplasty)
- Covering the penis.

Correction of penile chordee

Penile chordee can result from a number of factors, including:

- Abnormal tethering of the penile shaft skin on to the underlying structures;
- Tethering of the urethral plate to the corpora cavernosa;
- Atretic corpora spongiosum tissue extending from the abnormal meatus to the glans;
- Abnormal flexion of the corpora cavernosa (Figure 17.3).

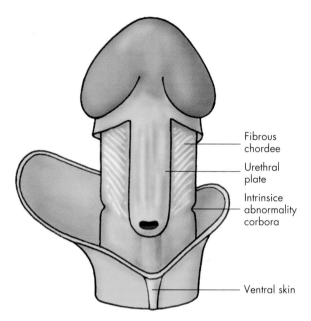

Fibrous chordee

Urethral plate

Intrinsice abnormality corbora

Ventral skin

Figure 17.3 Causes of penile curvature associated with hypospadias.

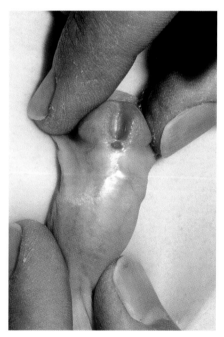

Figure 17.4 Anterior hypospadias – well suited to a meatal advancement and glanuloplasty (MAGPI) repair.

Correction of penile chordee can involve a number of steps, which should be addressed in the following order:

1. **Degloving of the penis**. In the majority of patients this is all that is required to correct the chordee.

2. **Excision of the atretic and fibrous corpora spongiosum** proximally and distally to the abnormal meatus.

3. **Dissection of the urethral plate**, which is carefully elevated off the corpora cavernosa. In some patients after these steps the penis still has ventral curvature, in which case it is necessary to plicate the dorsal aspect of the tunica albuginea (Nesbit procedure).

The correction of penile chordee is controversial, with some surgeons preferring to plicate the tunica albuginea if chordee persists once the penis has been degloved. We prefer to avoid plication, as the long-term results are unknown and the manoeuvre may affect penile growth, leading to secondary deformities.

When correction of the penile chordee is completed and confirmed with an artificial saline erection test, it is necessary to reconstruct the urethra.

Urethroplasty

Reconstruction of the urethra can be performed in one stage or in two stages as described by Cloutier. Although some surgeons prefer a two-stage repair most paediatric urologists now prefer a one-stage procedure. The current techniques for a urethroplasty are described below.

Urethral repositioning

MAGPI procedure (Figure 17.5)

Meatal advancement and glanuloplasty was originally described by Duckett. It is more accurately described as a refashioning of the glans penis, with only minor meatal advancement, and can only be used if the urethra is mobile (Figure 15.4). This can be confirmed if simple traction can move the meatus to the tip of the glans. A vertical incision between the tip of the glans and the meatus is created (Figure 17.5a,b) and then closed transversely, thereby advancing the meatus. A circumferential incision is made in the skin below the corona and the meatus. The glanuloplasty is then performed in two layers (Figure 17.5c), and finally the penis is circumcised and the skin closed. It is not normally necessary to leave a urinary catheter in for this procedure (Figure 17.5d).

Urethral advancement

Many authors have described techniques in which the urethra is mobilised and repositioned at the tip of the glans. Urethral mobilisation was reported over 100

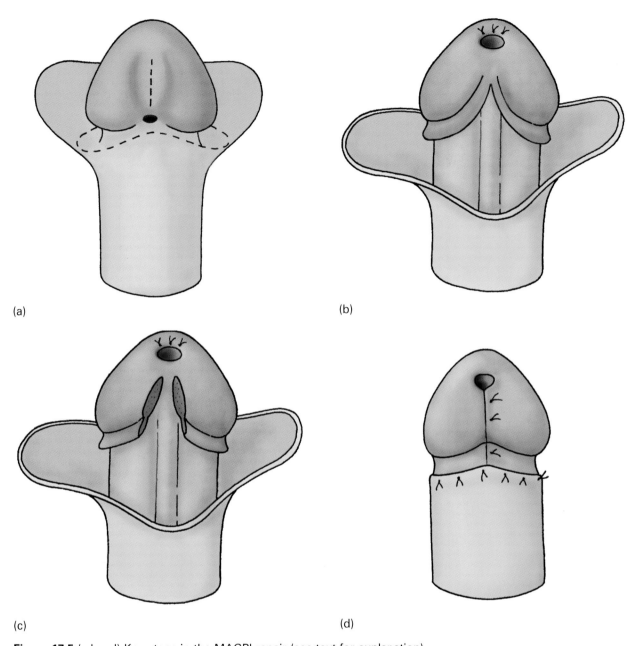

(a)

(b)

(c)

(d)

Figure 17.5 (a,b,c,d) Key steps in the MAGPI repair (see text for explanation).

years ago, but has recently been repopularised by Koff and colleagues. The technique requires mobilisation of the urethra to the scrotum and has not gained widespread acceptance.

Tubularising the urethral plate (Figure 17.6)

The urethral plate was originally used in the late 19th century to form the neourethra, but the procedure fell out of favour. Ransley redescribed the urethral plate and used it in his modified Cantwell epispadias repair.

This was later adapted for hypospadias repair by both Duckett and Mollard, and is rapidly becoming an adaptable and widely used technique.

If the urethral plate is wide enough to be tubularised over an 8 Fr catheter, it can be rolled into a tube (Duplay procedure). If it is too narrow the plate can be incised vertically, as described by Snodgrass; this enables it to be tubularised. In this procedure the urethral plate is marked and then incised (Figure 17.6a); its width is then assessed. If it is wide enough tubularisation is performed; if not,

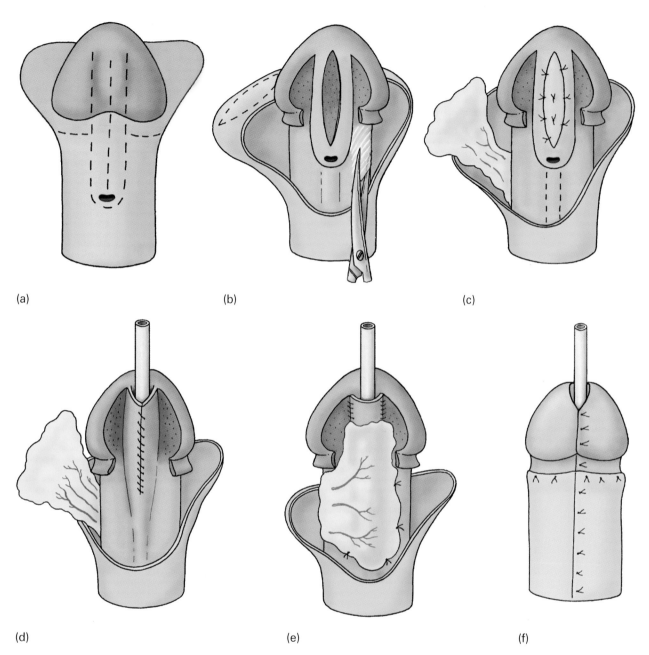

Figure 17.6 (a,b,c,d,e,f) Key steps in a tubularised incised plate (Snodgrass) repair (see text for explanation).

the urethral plate is incised and then rolled once any chordee has been corrected (Figure 17.5b). In a modification described by Hayes a free graft of preputial skin is inlaid into an incision in the urethral plate to reduce the risk of contraction and stenosis of the neourethra (Figure 17.5b,c). The urethral plate is then rolled or 'tubularised' over a size 8 Fr tube (Figure 17.6d). Once the neourethra is formed a vascularised de-epithelialised pedicle of tissue is placed over the anastomosis to reduce fistula formation (Figure 17.6e).

The glanuloplasty is performed by reapproximating the glans wings in two layers. The skin is closed, ensuring that there is adequate coverage on the ventral surface so that penile chordee does not recur (Figure 17.6f). A dripping stent or urethral catheter is usually left draining for 7 days.

Pedicle flaps

Two types of pedicle flap are commonly used: these are the meatal-based and the preputial flap. Both of these procedures are skin flaps, using the urethral plate as a mooring for the flap.

Meatal-based flap (Mathieu procedure) (Figure 17.7)

The urethral plate is incised (Figure 17.7a) and the glans flaps developed. A flap of proximal penile skin is created using the meatus as the base (Figure 17.7b).

The flap is then placed on to the urethral plate and both lateral edges are sutured. Adjacent subcutaneous tissue is used to cover ('waterproof') the suture line (Figure 17.7c). Once the neourethra is created the glanuloplasty is performed. A urinary catheter is left in for 4–7 days, although some authors have reported that no drainage is necessary. The maximum length of this flap is three times the base; as a rule this technique cannot be used to cover more than 1.5 cm.

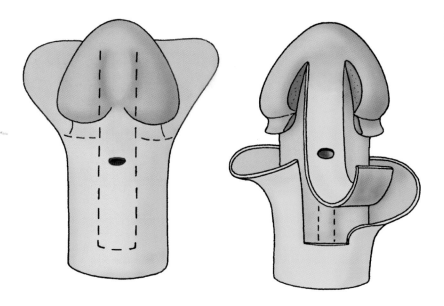

(a) (b)

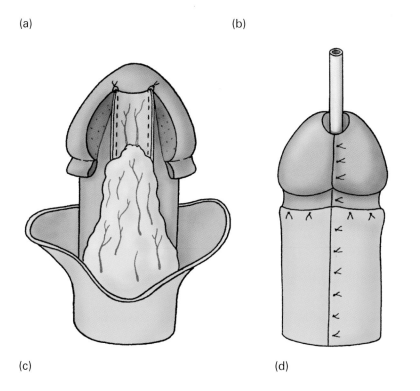

(c) (d)

Figure 17.7 (a,b,c,d) Key steps in a perimeatal-based flap (Mathieu) repair (see text for explanation).

Preputial flap (onlay island flap procedure) (Figure 17.8)

The urethral plate is incised vertically using two parallel incisions. The penis is then degloved back to its base using a circumferential subcoronal incision. Once this is complete, the penile chordee, if present, is corrected. The glans flaps are then created and the proximal thin urethra is cut back until normal urethral tissue is found.

A pedicle flap is then created out of the inner prepuce, as shown in Figure 17.8a,b. The preputial flap is wrapped around the side of the penis and anastomosed to the urethral plate (Figure 17.8c).

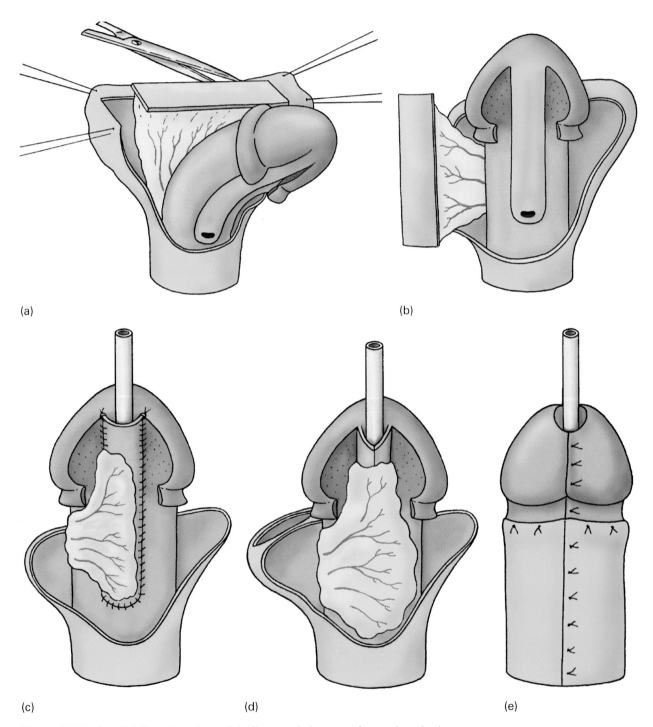

(a)   (b)   (c)   (d)   (e)

Figure 17.8 (a,b,c,d,e) Key steps in pedicle flap repair (see text for explanation).

Once the flap is sutured the pedicle is sutured to the tunica albuginea lateral to the urethral anastomosis (Figure 17.8d). This covers the anastomosis and acts to reduce the ventral bulkiness. Occasionally it is necessary to divide the urethral plate in order to correct the chordee. In these rare cases the preputial flap can be tubularised, thereby creating the neourethra alone.

The lateral glans wings are then approximated in two layers to recreate the glans, and the skin is closed (Figure 17.8e).

Free flaps

The techniques described above are all one-stage repairs: they have the theoretical advantage of only one operation and hospital stay, and consequently are the most widely used. Some surgeons, however, prefer a two-stage repair, arguing that it can be used for all forms of hypospadias, is technically easy, and provides a superior cosmetic result. We do not routinely use the two-stage repair, but reserve its use for patients with hypospadias and severe chordee, and those unfortunate individuals who have undergone multiple procedures and who in the past were labelled 'hypospadias cripples'.

The first stage of the operation involves correcting the chordee (described above), preparing the glans and taking the free flap. Once the chordee has been corrected a midline ventral incision is made from the most dorsal part of the new meatus on the glans to the current meatus. Glans wings are created so that the glans opens like a book. When haemostasis has been achieved the free flap can be placed into the glans.

The ideal material for the flap should be easy to harvest, without leaving a long-standing cosmetic defect. It should be supple and non-hair bearing. The most commonly used material is inner preputial skin; postauricular Wolfe skin grafts can also be used. Buccal skin and bladder mucosa are less frequently used for standard two-stage repairs, but do have a role in 'salvage' hypospadias. When the donor graft has been taken all the fat and subepithelial tissue is removed to enhance graft revascularisation. The graft is then placed into the glans and tacked with absorbable sutures; 'windows' are made in the graft to allow haematomas to escape, and a few midline quilting sutures are placed to prevent the graft shearing on its base. A firm dressing is applied, with a catheter, which holds the graft in place and minimises haematoma formation. After 1 week the dressing and catheter are removed.

The second stage of the repair is usually performed after 6 months. This step involves tubularisation of the graft into the neourethra and then placing a second vascularised layer over the anastomosis. Once this is completed the glans is recreated and the penile skin closed. This second stage is very similar to one-stage tubularisation of the urethral plate already described.

Covering the penis

When the urethra has been reconstructed it is necessary to recreate the meatus and glans. Glanuloplasty is performed by bringing the two wings of the glans around to cover the urethra; the glans is then closed in two layers. The distal end of the neourethra is sutured to the new meatus, thereby creating a slit-like meatus. Once this is complete, mucosa is brought around the ventral side of the penis to produce a mucosal collar surrounding the glans. Skin cover is provided by moving the excess skin from the dorsal side to the ventral side: this gives a good cosmetic result that is superior to the Byars flaps previously used.

'Salvage' or 'redo' surgery often calls for ingenuity and familiarity with a number of different techniques. Where the neourethra is largely intact and the surrounding skin is healthy, a procedure using locally available skin may suffice, but where there is extensive scarring, and particularly in the presence of residual chordee it is usually preferable to abandon the unhealthy existing neourethra and perform a substitution procedure with an onlay or tubularised free graft. Postauricular skin is suitable, but buccal skin, harvested from the lower lip (Figure 17.9) or cheek, is also widely used for this purpose.

Common variants include:

- **Chordee without hypospadias** (Figure 17.10) Most cases do in fact represent a form of hypospadias in which the distal penile urethra is flimsy, despite the presence of a glanular meatus and circumferential prepuce. It may be possible to achieve good correction by degloving the shaft and excising chordee tissue while preserving an intact urethra. At the time of operation, however, it may prove necessary to excise the abnormal urethra back to healthy spongiosum-supported urethra and proceed to urethroplasty as if it were the corresponding degree of true hypospadias.

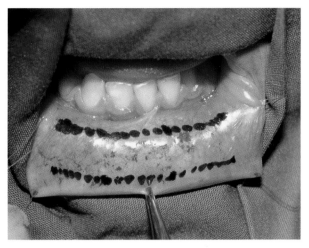

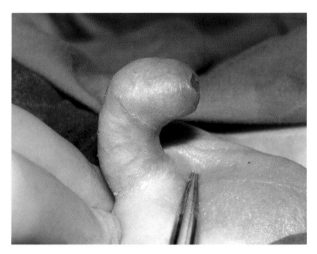

Figure 17.9 Donor site on buccal aspect of the lower lip marked out prior to harvesting of buccal skin for free graft salvage repair.

Figure 17.10 Chordee without hypospadias.

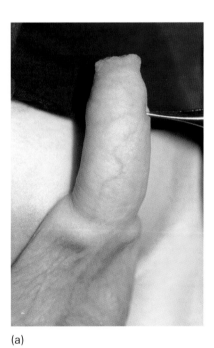

(a)

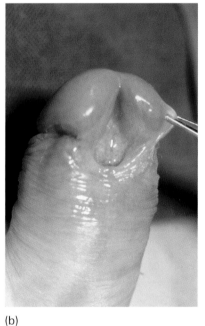

(b)

Figure 17.11 Megameatus intact prepuce variant. (a) Normal external appearances before the prepuce is retracted. (b) Glanular anomaly revealed by retraction of the prepuce. Deep glans groove with 'fishmouth' megameatus.

- **Mega meatus intact prepuce** (Figure 17.11) Because there is no external clue to the presence of this variant it sometimes comes to light for the first time in a boy who is about to undergo circumcision. In this situation the planned circumcision should be abandoned, the child returned to the ward and the findings discussed with the parents. If the parents opt for surgical correction of the glanular defect referral to a specialist is advisable. A suitable technique has been described by Duckett, who also specifically cautioned against the use of

the MAGPI repair in view of its high failure rate when used for the attempted repair of this variant.

Over 300 different techniques have been described to repair hypospadias. This chapter describes the most widely used methods and principles. Most surgeons today use a one-stage repair unless the severity of the defect requires a two-stage approach. In order to perform hypospadias surgery adequately most of the techniques described above need to be mastered so that all patients can be treated appropriately.

Outcome

The results of hypospadias repair are dependent on the original defect, and consequently on the type of operation performed.

Urethral advancement

Duckett has reported his experience with the MAGPI procedure: in his series of over 1000 patients only 1.2% required a secondary procedure. Partial meatal regression is, however, a common problem with this procedure and leads to a poor cosmetic result. The technique is still used to repair glanular hypospadias.

Tubularisation of the urethral plate

Tubularisation of the urethral plate, as originally described by Duplay, has a secondary operation rate of around 10%. The reoperations were mainly required for urethral fistulae. This technique does have the advantage of creating a slit-like meatus, which is more cosmetically appealing. Snodgrass' modification of Duplay's procedure appears to have a slightly better success rate, with only 7% developing a complication.

Pedicle flaps
Meatal based

In the Mathieu repair distal strictures are rare (1%) and fistulae occur in approximately 4% of cases. However, the meatus is often crescentic in appearance, giving a poor cosmetic result. Wide glans mobilisation and a midline dorsal incision of the urethral plate may reduce this problem.

Preputial flaps

This method of repair is often reserved for the more complex cases of hypospadias: consequently the rate of complications is higher. There is wide variability in the published fistula rate, from 4% to 69%. Duckett, who popularised this repair, reported a complication rate of under 10%, with urethral fistulae being the commonest problem.

Free flaps

Bracka has reported a series of 600 patients who underwent a two-stage procedure, the majority of which were free preputial skin grafts. In these patients the fistula rate was 6%, but he also reported a high stricture rate of 7%, which occurred mainly in the complex redo cases. This technique does, however, give an excellent cosmetic result.

Psychosexual outcome

Sexual function following successful hypospadias correction should be normal. Erections should be obtainable and fertility should not be affected unless the patient had associated undescended testicles. There has been considerable concern about the psychosocial and sexual outcome of these men. A recent psychosocial study appears to refute this concern, showing that men operated on for hypospadias had a similar outcome to those age-matched controls who underwent inguinal herniotomy.

Complications
Early

Operations to correct hypospadias are susceptible to all general surgical complications, which can severely affect the outcome of the procedure. Because of the hypervascularity of the penis haemorrhage can often be a concern. Intraoperatively bleeding can usually be controlled by one of the methods previously discussed. Postoperatively most surgeons prevent delayed haemorrhage with a compressive bandage; this also acts to reduce the postoperative oedema that occurs following most hypospadias repairs. It is essential to minimise haematoma formation, as this can act as a focus for infection and subsequent fistula formation. Care needs to be taken to avoid wound infections. Apart from controlling haematoma formation, meticulous skin preparation is necessary: some surgeons use prophylactic antibiotics, although Duckett did not feel they were necessary. Infections, haematoma formation and ischaemic tissue flaps can all lead to poor wound healing, resulting in fistulae and/or complete breakdown of the repair. Complete dehiscence of the repair is fortunately rare, but when it does occur the secondary repair of the hypospadias 'cripple' is a daunting task.

Late

The long-term complications of hypospadias surgery are well known and, sadly, all too common. The rate depends on the initial severity of the hypospadias, making the right choice of operation, the type of operation and, of course, the skill and experience of the surgeon.

Fistulae

These are the most common complications following hypospadias surgery, and can occur in up to 30% of patients. A fistula can present acutely immediately after the catheter is removed, or many years after the repair. If the fistula appears acutely many surgeons would replace the catheter for 14 further days to allow it to close spontaneously. Using this method some fistula will close, but many will persist and require further treatment. The location of the fistula varies, but it is often just proximal to the glans and lateral. Occasionally large or multiple fistulae occur, usually indicating that the original urethroplasty was unsatisfactory and needs to be repeated. Before attempting to repair the fistula it is imperative to exclude meatal and/or distal urethral strictures, as these predispose to further fistulae formation. In addition, fistulae can be associated with urethral diverticula, which need to be excised at the time of the fistula repair.

Repair of fistulae should not be undertaken lightly: in some series there has been a 50% recurrence rate. The timing of the closure is important: although initially the closure was performed soon after diagnosis, most surgeons have discovered that unless the original surgery has completely healed then recurrence rates are very high. Now it is recommended to wait at least 6 months after the hypospadias repair before attempting fistula closure. Many techniques have been described: simple closure, by freshening and then closing the fistula edges and the overlying skin, is associated with a high recurrence rate and is therefore not recommended. A flap-based repair has also been described, in which the fistula is dissected down to the urethra and the urethral defect closed by inserting absorbable sutures. A flap of skin is then formed from which a vascularised subcutaneous layer is created and placed over the urethral repair. Once the urethra is covered the skin flap is advanced to close the skin defect. This technique has been more successful, with Duckett reporting a 90% cure rate. In some cases the fistula is very large and represents a failure of the original urethroplasty, and in these patients a repeat of the original operation is required. In patients who have unsuccessful fistula repairs a subsequent repair appears to have the same chance of success.

The use of a urinary catheter following repair is much debated: the success rate in those diverted or left undiverted seems very similar in most series. Therefore, unless there is some doubt about postoperative micturition it is possible to perform a fistula repair without draining the bladder.

Meatal stenosis

Meatal stenosis results from either ischaemic glans flaps or an inadequately mobilised glans wrap. It can present with difficulty in micturatition, a fine spray stream, and in some patients urinary tract infections can occur as a result of poor bladder emptying.

Meatal stenosis can be treated initially with gentle dilatation of the meatus; in minor cases this can be an outpatient procedure using a fine-tipped catheter. Some patients require intraoperative dilatation. In more severe or recurrent cases of meatal stenosis a formal meatotomy is required. In most patients this simple procedure is successful.

Urethral stenosis

Urethral stenosis is a rare problem with modern procedures, which avoid a circular anastomosis. Although strictures can occur at any point along the urethroplasty they most commonly occur at the distal and proximal ends of the neourethra. Distal stenosis is often associated with a fistula and can usually be treated with regular dilatation; in severe cases a formal surgical repair is necessary. Proximal stenosis is a serious complication which, if severe, often requires complete reconstruction of the urethra.

Persistent chordee

The persistence of penile chordee after hypospadias repair is usually due to inadequate correction at the time of the original repair; however, in rare cases it may be due to postoperative fibrosis. The best treatment is to avoid the complication by a good repair and confirmation of correction by an intraoperative artificial erection test. When persistent chordee does occur it is necessary to deglove the penis completely to ensure that the cause of the problem is not skin tethering. If chordee still persist then dorsal plication of the tunica albuginea is usually sufficient to correct it.

Balanitis xerotica obliterans

This is a rare complication caused by chronic inflammation and fibrosis of the glans and meatus, which results in scarring and meatal stenosis. Topical steroids help in some patients, but the majority require a formal meatoplasty to correct the stenosis.

Hairy urethra

A hairy urethra forms when hair-bearing skin is used for the urethroplasty, but with modern techniques this should no longer occur. The main problem is that the hair acts as a focus for urethral stone formation. If a hairy urethra becomes symptomatic the patient requires a new, non-hair bearing urethroplasty.

Urethrocoele

A urethrocoele may result from distal obstruction, with proximal dilatation of the neourethra. It may also be secondary to an absent corpus spongiosum, when the lack of supporting tissue for the urethra results in urethrocoele formation. A urethrocoele can present with a poor urinary stream and postmicturition dribbling, urinary tract infections, and urethral calculi secondary to stasis. Surgical treatment requires excision of the redundant urethral tissue and treatment of the distal stenosis as necessary.

Key points

- Despite advances in technique, instrumentation and aftercare, the correction of hypospadias remains one of the most technically challenging aspects of paediatric urology.
- There is no place for the 'occasional' hypospadias surgeon, even in the correction of so-called 'minor' hypospadias. Surgeons should have a detailed understanding of the various concepts and surgical techniques and maintain a clinical workload that is sufficient to obtain consistently good results.
- Preservation of the urethral plate is the keystone of modern single-stage procedures.
- With improving functional results the challenge is now to obtain the optimal cosmetic result to provide patients with a penis of normal appearance regardless of the severity of the original abnormality.

Further reading

Bracka A. Hypospadias repair: the two-stage alternative. *Br J Urol* 1995; 76 (Suppl 3): 31–41

Mouriquand PDE, Persad R, Sharma S. Hypospadias repair: current principles and procedures. *Br J Urol* 1995; 76 (Suppl 3): 9–22

Mureau MA, Slijper M, Slob AK, Verhulst FC. Psychosocial functioning of children, adolescents, and adults following hypospadias surgery: a comparative study. *J Pediatr Psychol* 1997; 22: 371–87

Rajfer J, Walsh PC. The incidence of intersexuality in patients with hypospadias and cryptorchidism. *J Urol* 1976; 116: 769–770

Redman JF. Results of undiverted simple closure of 51 urethrocutaneous fistulae in boys. *Urology* 1993; 41: 369–371

Smith ED. The history of hypospadias. *Pediatr Surg Int* 1997; 12: 81–85

The prepuce

18

AMK Rickwood

Topics covered
Development of the prepuce
Preputial function

Preputial disease and abnormalities
Circumcision
Alternatives to circumcision

Introduction

Although the practice of circumcision dates back at least 5000 years, for most of this time the operation was undertaken principally as an item of religious protocol. Only during the last 150 years have other indications come to the fore, namely procedures as prophylaxis against putative future ailments ('routine circumcision') and procedures for some immediate medical problem. During the 1930s, upwards of a third of English boys underwent 'routine' circumcision in infancy. Although this practice has subsequently dwindled to negligible proportions, there can be little doubt that its legacy has lingered on in the form of an excessive number of procedures undertaken for supposed medical reasons. An understanding of the true medical indications for circumcision (and for alternative procedures) calls for a knowledge both of preputial development before and after birth, and of preputial pathology.

Development of the prepuce

Prenatally

First appearing at 8 weeks' gestation as a ridge of thickened epithelium, the prepuce grows forward over the developing glans so that preputial construction is complete by 16 weeks' gestation. At this stage, however, the epithelia lining the prepuce and covering the glans are contiguous, with no plane of separation between them, so that 'preputial adhesions' represent a feature of normal development, not a pathological process. Spontaneous separation, commencing late in gestation and usually proceeding proximally, occurs

by desquamation, with areas of cell nests degenerating to form a series of spaces which ultimately enlarge and coalesce to furnish a continuous preputial sac.

Postnatally

Preputial separation after birth proceeds at a rate that varies from one individual to another and is uninfluenced by environmental or genetic factors: even at 5 years of age some degree of preputial adherence persists in upwards of 70% of boys. Separation may be accompanied by mild inflammatory episodes, possibly owing to infection of retained smegma, and which can mimic true balanoposthitis. At birth the prepuce is almost always unretractable, and attempted retraction results in the appearance of a blanched and apparently constricting ring of skin *proximal* to the preputial meatus (Figure 18.1). Viewed end-on, the preputial

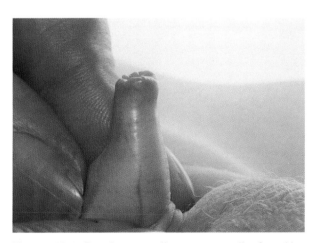

Figure 18.1 Developmentally non-retractile foreskin: attempted retraction reveals an apparent constriction ring a few millimetres proximal to the preputial meatus.

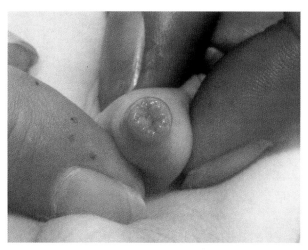

Figure 18.2 Developmentally non-retractile foreskin: on attempted retraction, the preputial orifice opens as a flower (same patient as in Figure 18.1).

orifice is supple and unscarred, opening as a flower as the foreskin is pulled back (Figure 18.2). In some infants still in nappies the margins of the orifice are adherent owing to a film of fibrinous exudate, which must be gently broken down to demonstrate the flowering: this state accounts for almost all referrals with 'pinhole' meatus.

Developmental non-retractability of the foreskin is often termed 'phimosis' (Greek Ψιμοσις, 'muzzling'), although this description is misleading as it implies the existence of pathology when in reality there is none. 'Non-retractile foreskin' or 'physiological phimosis' are thus more appropriate terms.

In younger boys the natural history of non-retractile foreskin and of preputial adhesions was classically described by Gairdner in 1949, and that in older boys

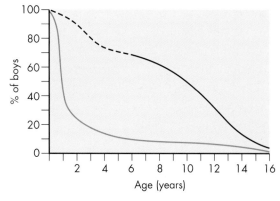

Figure 18.3 Natural history of non-retractile foreskin (red) and of preputial adhesions (black) (from Gairdner (1949) and Øster (1968)).

by Øster in 1968. Their findings are summarised in Figure 18.3, from which it is clear that, if left alone, the foreskin becomes fully and easily retractable by physical maturity in all but a tiny minority of boys – 1% at most. At a time when the foreskin remains non-retractile, but after substantial preputial separation has taken place, there is frequently 'ballooning' during micturition. This phenomenon, typically occurring between 2 and 4 years of age, does not signify urinary obstruction and resolves as the foreskin becomes more easily retractable.

Preputial function

Although it is self-evident that the prepuce serves no physiologically essential function, it is not wholly without purpose. In the first instance, the foreskin typically remains unretractable prior to toilet training, and so – perhaps coincidentally, perhaps not – protects the glans penis and its meatus from ammoniacal inflammation and hence the risk of meatal ulceration and subsequent stenosis. By analogy, the prepuce is to the glans as the eyelid is to the eye.

The second consideration is that of sexual function. In contrast to the glans, which is innervated principally by free nerve endings subserving poorly localised sensations, the prepuce has a rich somatosensory innervation forming an important component of the normal complement of penile erogenous tissue. Amputation neuromas may follow circumcision. Moreover, this procedure removes some 30% of the penile skin plus the greater part of the muscular component of the dartos layer, while the surface of the glans undergoes keratinisation. However, because of the highly subjective nature of sexual pleasure it impossible to draw meaningful comparisons between the circumcised and the uncircumcised state, except on an anecdotal basis.

Preputial diseases and abnormalities

Pathological phimosis

This is characterised unambiguously by cicatrisation of the preputial orifice (Figures 18.4, 18.5) and, except for a few examples of non-specific dermal fibrosis, the histological appearances are those of **balanitis xerotica obliterans (BXO)**. Apart from a few cases thought to occur following forcible retraction of the foreskin, the aetiology of BXO is

unused

ignore

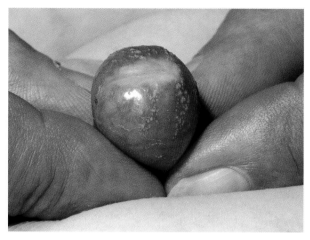
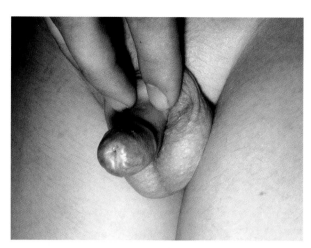

Figure captions:

Figure 18.4 Pathological phimosis due to balanitis xerotica obliterans. Characteristic pallor, scarring and stenosis of the prepuce.

Figure 18.5 Balanitis xerotica obliterans.

unknown. Although histologically identical to lichen sclerosus et atrophicus, the extragenital features of this disorder, notably anal involvement, are very rarely encountered in boys with pathological phimosis. Similarly, although the histological appearances of BXO resemble some of the generalised collagen disorders, it has none of the systemic associations of these conditions. There is no familial predisposition, nor is there any identifiable causative bacterial or viral agent. Contrary to widespread belief, BXO does not result from recurrent balanoposthitis. There is no association with puberty, although the age distribution is conspicuous for the rarity of the condition in those under 5 years of age (Figure 18.6). BXO is

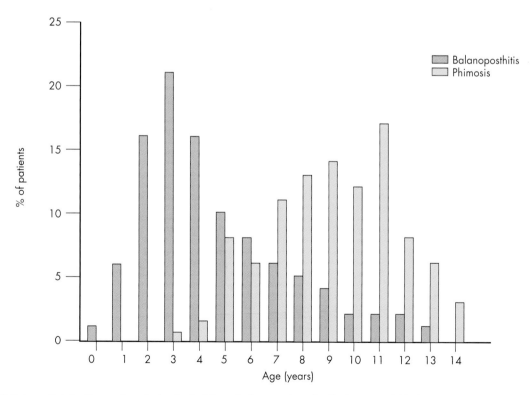

Figure 18.6 Age distributions of pathological phimosis (orange) and of balanoposthitis (purple) (Urology Department, Alder Hey Children's Hospital, 1984–99).

end

done

z

The prepuce — 183

estimated to affect 0.6% of boys in the age range up to 15 years.

In 20% of cases the glans is involved at the time of presentation, although the meatus is affected in only a small proportion. What proportion go on to develop secondary glanular or urethral involvement in adult life is unknown, although this is probably only a minority.

The **presentation** includes secondary non-retractability of the foreskin, irritation, bleeding and dysuria. Although 'ballooning' is an uncommon complaint, BXO may cause a poor urinary stream or, less often, acute or chronic urinary retention. Long-standing obstruction may be associated with ultrasound findings of a thick-walled bladder and upper tract dilatation.

Treatment

Although a few cases respond to topical application of high-potency steroids, BXO represents the one absolute indication for circumcision. Preputioplasty is not an option, as the continuing inflammatory process results in recurrent stenosis of the preputial orifice. Glanular involvement may persist following circumcision and may necessitate treatment with a topical steroid. Follow-up is advisable in view of the risk of subsequent meatal stenosis, which is reported to occur in up to 25% of cases and may require meatotomy or meatoplasty. Although more extensive involvement of the anterior urethra leading to stricture formation has been reported in adults, this complication is not encountered in children.

Acute balanoposthitis

This term describes acute pyogenic infection of the prepuce and the **presenting symptoms** comprise erythema and oedema of the foreskin and a purulent discharge from the preputial orifice. In some cases the oedema spreads to involve the entire penile shaft. Bleeding from the prepuce is rare, but dysuria is a common complaint. In the absence of preputial discharge, urinary infection is the principal differential diagnosis. In a sizeable proportion of boys referred as having balanoposthitis there is no history of preputial discharge, and in such cases, if oedema and erythema have been strictly limited to the preputial orifice, the inflammation resulting from spontaneous lysis of adhesions represents a possible cause. Young boys are apt to 'fiddle' with their foreskin, and the resulting inflammation represents a further source of diagnostic difficulty.

If diagnosis is confined to those experiencing preputial discharge, the **incidence** of balanoposthitis is of the order of 3% of boys, of whom less than a third experience multiple episodes. The **age distribution** (Figure 18.6), as would be expected, indicates that the complaint is most apt to occur at a time of life when the foreskin is commonly wholly or partially non-retractable. However, it is comparatively infrequent prior to toilet training, perhaps because ammonia inhibits the growth of pathogens. Common causative organisms are *Staphylococcus aureus*, *Escherichia coli* and *Proteus* spp., although in a third of cases the preputial discharge is sterile on culture. Balanoposthitis occasionally occurs when the prepuce is fully and easily retractable, and in older boys may be the presenting feature of diabetes mellitus.

Treatment comprises antibiotic therapy for acute episodes, where indicated, and attention to hygiene. Surgical intervention is best limited to those suffering multiply recurrent episodes. Because the complaint is typically associated with complete or partial non-retractability of the foreskin, preputioplasty or preputiolysis – whichever is more appropriate in any individual case – constitute alternatives to circumcision.

Paraphimosis

This condition, which is rare in boys, represents preputial abuse, not disease, and cannot occur in the presence of physiological or pathological phimosis. Reduction under general anaesthesia is almost always possible without the need for a dorsal slit, and circumcision is indicated only for exceptional cases troubled by recurrence.

Preputial cysts

Most boys so referred, with one or more lumps on the penis, prove to have nothing more sinister than smegma entrapped by preputial adhesions. As the latter lyse spontaneously so the smegma is released, and no active treatment is needed. Occasional examples are seen of true retention cysts of the prepuce (Figure 18.7). Localised retention cysts can be enucleated, but more diffuse lesions call for circumcision.

Megaprepuce

This deformity, only recently recognised and almost certainly congenital, is characterised by an enormously

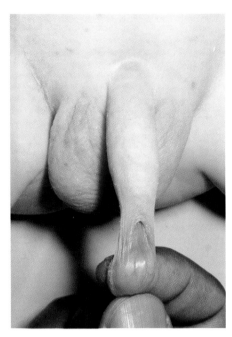

Figure 18.7 Preputial retention cyst.

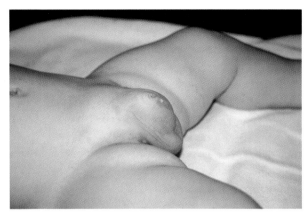

Figure 18.8 Congenital megaprepuce. The penile shaft is no longer visible, being surrounded by urine collecting within a dilated subcutaneous preputial sac.

capacious preputial sac which becomes hugely distended during micturition (Figure 18.8). The severity of the 'ballooning' is gross and cannot be mistaken for the minor degree associated with physiological phimosis. Affected boys typically present within the first year of life. Various reconstructive procedures have been described.

Circumcision

Religious circumcision

Here the principal concern for surgeons is ethical, as scarcely any boys undergoing the procedure are in a position to give informed consent. The present position in the United Kingdom varies in different regions but, in essence, surgeons may decide for themselves whether or not to undertake religious circumcisions. Some health authorities with sizeable ethnic populations have established a circumcision service for their local communities.

'Routine' circumcision

This practice has declined to negligible proportions in the UK, although circumcision remains culturally entrenched in the USA. Arguments previously advanced in justification include a reduced risk of venereal disease or carcinoma of the penis for the patient, or of carcinoma of the cervix in a prospective spouse. These arguments have largely been discounted, although the possible role of the prepuce in the transmission of HIV infection remains unclear as the evidence is contradictory. Currently only one consideration deserves attention, namely the risk of urinary infection.

It has long been recognised that during the first year of life urinary infections occur more frequently in boys than in girls. Moreover, the risk of urinary infection is six to ten times higher in uncircumcised than in circumcised boys. Nevertheless, the absolute incidence of urinary infection is low, and it it has been calculated that 180 boys would be required to undergo circumcision to prevent one urinary infection. Routine neonatal circumcision is clearly not justified as a routine prophylactic measure on this basis. However, there is more persuasive anecdotal evidence that circumcision is beneficial in reducing the risk of urinary infection in male infants with predisposing urinary tract pathology, such as vesicoureteric reflux or urinary tract dilatation resulting from congenital urethral obstruction. However, as yet the perceived benefit of circumcision in boys who are predisposed to urinary infection remains unproven, as this has never been subjected to a controlled trial.

Circumcision for medical indications

In the UK 'phimosis' and balanoposthitis are the most commonly cited medical indications for circumcision. Given the incidence of pathological phimosis and of recurrent balanoposthitis, it would be expected that 2% of boys, at most, would be circumcised for medical reasons – the figure pertaining in the Scandinavian countries. In the UK, however, the 'medical' circumcision rate has consistently been considerably higher, and although the number of circumcisions performed annually is declining there is no doubt that a large number of unnecessary procedures are still being performed. The principal area of poor practice relates to circumcisions performed for 'phimosis' on boys under 5 years of age (i.e. at a time of life when pathological phimosis is scarcely ever encountered).

Surgical aspects

The techniques employed for neonatal circumcision will not be considered here. Circumcision performed for genuine medical indications should be undertaken as a formal surgical procedure under general anaesthesia, with additional local anaesthesia (caudal or penile block) to provide postoperative analgesia. The details of technique are a matter of individual surgical preference, but the following general points should be observed:

- Care should be taken to ensure that the prepuce is completely separated from the underlying glans and coronal sulcus prior to circumcision. Failure to do so may result in the formation of persistent skin bridges between the glans and the penile skin.
- The outer and inner layers of preputial skin should be excised separately and trimmed further if necessary to ensure the best cosmetic result. For this purpose some surgeons delineate the planned incisions with a marking pen. Failure to excise sufficient of the outer layer may leave redundant penile skin, resulting in an unsatisfactory cosmetic outcome (incomplete circumcision) and a requirement for secondary surgical revision.
- Conversely, the removal of too much skin may leave insufficient to cover the penile shaft. This risk is greatest in boys with so-called 'buried penis', in whom even a standard circumcision may result in a denuded penile shaft and a requirement for skin grafting. A modified technique is required in such cases, to redistribute rather than remove preputial skin.
- Careful attention to haemostasis is important to minimise the risk of postoperative haemorrhage. Bipolar diathermy is more effective than ligation of individual vessels.

The choice of postoperative dressing (if any) is also a matter of individual preference. Many surgeons avoid dressings because of the distress caused by their removal.

Complications of circumcision

Parents should be alerted to the fact that there is an appreciable incidence of postoperative distress and morbidity following circumcision. Early complications include urinary retention and haemorrhage. The former can be prevented by adequate analgesia or intraoperative local block with bupivacaine. Haemorrhage of sufficient severity to require early reoperation is reported to occur in 2–5% of boys. The most common postoperative problem is encrustation, scabbing and infection of the exposed glans. The authors of a prospective study undertaken in a British paediatric surgical unit found that 26% of boys could not wear underpants for more than a week, and that in 23% of cases healing was delayed for more than 14 days. Serious complications such as urethral injury and partial amputation of the glans or penile shaft are virtually confined to religious circumcisions performed in the community (Figure 18.9).

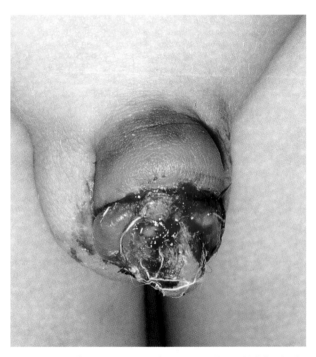

Figure 18.9 Complication of circumcision. Child admitted to hospital following religious circumcision. Excoriation and infection of the glans.

Alternatives to circumcision

These are designed not to treat phimosis but rather to render a normal foreskin fully retractable at an earlier age than would otherwise have been the case. Although intervention may be legitimate for boys experiencing balanoposthitis, it is more dubious when performed in response to pressure from parents who are concerned by non-retractability of the foreskin or 'ballooning'.

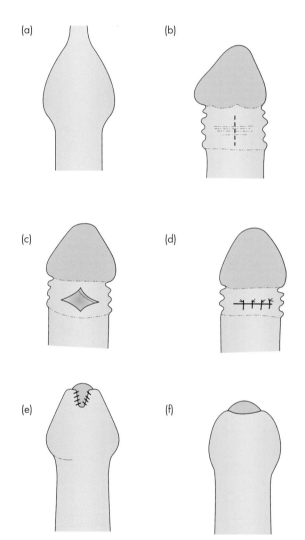

Figure 18.10 Technique of preputioplasty. (a) Adhesions divided, prepuce retracted. (b) Constricting ring incised and (c, d) incision closed transversely. (e) 'Dorsal slit' appearance on completion of the procedure evolves into normal retractile prepuce (f) if retraction is undertaken regularly in the ensuing weeks.

Low-potency steroids

There is evidence that topical application of such agents (e.g. Betnovate) speeds up lysis of preputial adhesions and, possibly, the process of retractability generally.

Preputioplasty

This consists of incising the 'constriction ring' that is seen when the prepuce is retracted under anaesthesia and closing the incision transversely with interrupted sutures. When the prepuce is drawn over the glans again the incision assumes the appearance of a limited dorsal slit, but with regular retraction of the prepuce in the weeks following the procedure the cosmetic appearances evolve into those of a normal retractile foreskin. The regimen of regular retraction, which is important to prevent contraction of the preputial orifice, is commenced as soon as the initial postoperative discomfort has settled. Preputioplasty is contraindicated in the presence of BXO. It is a good alternative to circumcision when used selectively – ideally in older boys who are willing to cooperate with the postoperative regimen of regular retraction (Figure 18.10).

Preputiolysis

Surgical release of preputial adhesions enjoys a very limited role in the management of recurrent balanoposthitis: the foreskin must be fully and often retracted postoperatively to prevent adhesions reforming.

Further reading

Cold CJ, Taylor JR. The prepuce. *BJU Int* 1999; 83 (Suppl 1): 34–44

Cuckow PM. Circumcision. In: Stringer MD, Oldham KT, Mouriquand PDE, Howard ER (eds) *Paediatric surgery and urology: longterm outcomes.* London: WB Saunders, 1998; 616–624

Dunsmuir WD, Gordon EM. The history of circumcision. *BJU Int* 1999; 83 (Suppl 1): 1–12

Gairdner D. The fate of the foreskin. A study in circumcision. *BMJ* 1949; 2: 1433–1437

Øster J. The further fate of the foreskin. *Arch Dis Child* 1968; 43: 200–203

Rickwood AMK, Hemalatha V, Batcup G, Spitz L. Phimosis in boys. *Br J Urol* 1980; 52: 147–150

Key points

- Although the foreskin is almost always unretractable at birth, it spontaneously becomes fully and easily retractable in 99% of boys by 16 years of age.
- Pathological phimosis, due to balanitis xerotica obliterans, affects only 0.6% of boys and scarcely ever occurs in those under 5 years of age.
- Balanoposthitis principally troubles younger boys at a time when their prepuce remains wholly or partially non-retractable. Consequently, it is usually a self-limiting complaint.
- Pathological phimosis (usually the result of balanitis xerotica obliterans) is the one absolute indication for circumcision.
- Surgical intervention for balanoposthitis can reasonably be considered for boys troubled by recurrent episodes, and may take the form of preputioplasty and/or preputiolysis rather than circumcision.

Testis, hydrocoele and varicocoele 19

Nicholas P Madden

Topics covered
Undescended testis
    Epidemiology
    Impalpable testis, retractile testis
    Fertility, malignancy

Hydrocoele
Varicocoele

Introduction

Orchidopexy and operations for hydrocoele (so-called 'groin surgery') are among the commonest elective surgical procedures of childhood, and the management of varicocoele is increasingly entering the sphere of paediatric surgical practice. Despite the frequency of these conditions, several important aspects of the long-term functional outcome of orchidopexy and the treatment of varicocoele remain unresolved. The reasons lie partly in the lengthy interval between intervention and outcome (plus the difficulty of devising reliable prospective studies) and partly in the problems inherent in measuring fertility. The embryological basis of cryptorchidism and hydrocoele, the normal mechanism of testicular descent and the role of the processus vaginalis are described in Chapter 1.

Incidence

The incidence of cryptorchidism appears to be increasing. An authoritative study in the 1950s put the figure at 0.8% at 1 year of age, whereas subsequent work in the 1980s based on similar criteria documented an incidence of 1.55%. The rate of orchidopexy in England and Wales is considerably higher than either figure, with approximately 3% of boys undergoing orchidopexy. This discrepancy may be due partly to inappropriate procedures on retractile testes, and perhaps partly to the now well-described phenomenon of secondary testicular ascent. A recent report indicates that in 10–20% of boys undergoing orchidopexy in

Table 19.1 Incidence of undescended testis in low birthweight premature infants

Birthweight (g)	Incidence of undescended testes (%)	
	At birth	At 3 months
< 2000	45.4	7.7
2000–2499	13.4	2.5
> 2500	3.8	1.4

later childhood the testis had previously been noted to be present in the scrotum.

In boys born at term the testis should be in the scrotum, and where it is not spontaneous descent thereafter is comparatively unusual. By contrast, premature infants have a significantly higher incidence of undescended testes, and here spontaneous testicular descent frequently occurs during the first 3 months of life (Table 19.1).

Pathology

Undescended testes develop progressive histological changes during the first few years of life, with hypoplasia of Leydig cells and defective transformation of gonocytes. These changes are most apparent from 2 years of age onwards. In gonads not brought into the scrotum, this histological picture progresses to one of atrophy and aspermia, and eventually carcinoma in situ may supervene, being present in up to 25% of testes retained in an intra-abdominal position into adult life. The histological changes observed in cryptorchidism probably represent the outcome of a combination of temperature-related damage, pituitary–gonadal dysfunction and underlying dysplasia. Undescended testes are also associated with an appreciable incidence of coexisting congenital abnormalities of the epididymis and vas which, in their own right, may further contribute to impaired fertility in later life.

It should be noted that congenitally maldescended testes are almost always associated with a completely patent processus vaginalis or, occasionally, a frank complete inguinal hernia. However, genuinely ectopic testes represent an exception to this rule, as these gonads have descended fully but to the wrong site.

Classification

Because of the implications for clinical management, the most practical distinction lies between the **palpable** and the **impalpable** testis.

The anatomical classification of undescended testis can be further subdivided into maldescended testes, lying somewhere along the normal line of descent, and ectopic testes lying outside that line. Ectopic gonads are most commonly encountered in the perineum, lateral to the scrotum (Figure 19.1), occasionally in the thigh, and exceptionally, as crossed ectopia, in the contralateral hemiscrotum. Although undescended testes are often to be found within the 'superficial inguinal pouch', this location is no longer considered to be 'ectopic'.

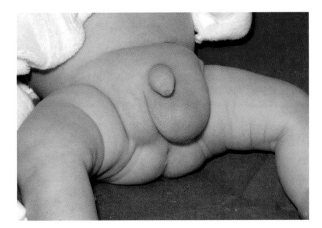

Figure 19.1 Right ectopic testis. Empty right hemiscrotum, and a visible swelling (ectopic testis) in the perineum lateral to the scrotum.

Presentation

In the United Kingdom, undescended testes are most frequently diagnosed during the course of the examination routinely performed in all newborns. If at this stage the testis is not in the scrotum, its position should be reassessed at 3 months of age (or 52 weeks postconceptual age in premature infants). It should be noted that at birth, and for the first 3 months of life, the cremasteric reflex is absent, so that the true location of the gonad is easier to assess than at other times in infancy and childhood. Testicular maldescent is also sometimes identified for the first time during routine developmental assessments at 6–8 months of age, or during school medical examinations.

The right testis is more commonly undescended than the left, and in approximately 25% of cases of cryptorchidism the condition is bilateral.

Older boys referred with 'undescended testis' more commonly prove to have a retractile or ascending gonad. The term 'retractile testis' should be confined to those where the testis, wherever sited initially, can nevertheless be brought fully to the floor of the scrotum without tension on the spermatic cord. It is important to note that a cremasteric reflex can sometimes also be elicited in congenitally maldescended testes, and hence the distinction between maldescent and retractility is not always so clear-cut as was once believed.

History

This is straightforward when referral is made directly from a maternity unit. When boys are referred at any later stage the information recorded in the neonatal notes regarding the location of the testes at birth can prove instructive, if it is available. However, it should be borne in mind that these findings are not always reliable. In most instances, however, this information is lacking, and here the history assumes importance. Occasionally transient testicular descent has been observed, typically during the course of a warm bath, and in this circumstance the diagnosis is almost certainly one of retractile testis. In the absence of such a history the parents should be asked whether the possibility of testicular maldescent was mentioned at birth, at subsequent routine checks during infancy or, in older boys, at any school medical examination. If the answer to these questions is 'no', there is strong presumptive evidence that the testis was, at some stage, fully descended.

Examination

This begins with scrotal inspection. Not infrequently, both gonads are to be seen at the base of the scrotum, in which case the diagnosis is evidently one of retractile testis. Sometimes there is obvious asymmetry of the scrotum, whereas in other instances, where bilateral maldescent is suspected, the scrotum appears to be 'small'. However, because the scrotal skin is highly sensitive to external temperature, a 'small' scrotum, or one exhibiting asymmetry, can not be taken as reliable evidence of true testicular maldescent. The examiner's hands must not be cold and examination should be conducted in a relaxed, warm environment. Palpation may be facilitated by the application of talcum powder to minimise friction between the examiner's hands and the patient's skin. Starting lateral to the internal ring, the left hand moves down the inguinal canal, 'milking' the testis towards the scrotum. Once the left hand reaches the pubic tubercle, the right hand is employed to locate the testis and to draw it downwards towards the scrotum.

A testis which can be readily manipulated from the groin to the floor of the scrotum, and which remains

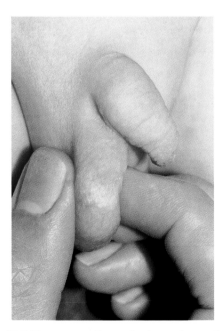

Figure 19.2 True retractile testis, brought easily to the floor of the scrotum without undue traction.

there, is evidently 'retractile' and, as such, normal (Figure 19.2). In other instances, although the testis can be brought to the base of the scrotum, this is only with some difficulty and is followed by immediate ascent once the manipulation has been concluded, a situation commonly termed 'high retractile testis'.

Thickening of the spermatic cord may be indicative of a persistent processus vaginalis, and very occasionally – usually in infants – there is a frank inguinal hernia. Care should be taken not to overlook ectopic gonads, which are most often to be found in the perineum immediately lateral to the scrotum. Where one testis is impalpable, hypertrophy of the contralateral testis suggests that the impalpable gonad is absent, although this finding is not sufficiently reliable to avoid the need for laparoscopy.

Management

Hormonal treatment

This may consist of a 3-week course of intranasal luteinising hormone-releasing hormone administered four to six times daily, or of human chorionic gonadotrophin given by intramuscular injection once or twice weekly for the same period. Success rates in excess of 50% have been reported in uncontrolled studies, although the findings of a double-blind placebo cross-over trial demonstrated conclusively that hormone therapy is ineffective in treating congenitally undescended testes. None the less, hormonal manipulation does have its uses, sometimes when administered preoperatively to facilitate a potentially difficult orchidopexy, and otherwise to distinguish between true maldescent and 'high retractile testis'.

Surgery

Palpable undescended testis

Standard single-stage orchidopexy is usually undertaken as a day-case procedure, ideally before the boy's second birthday. In experienced hands, the incidence of testicular atrophy following orchidopexy before 2 years of age is no greater than when the procedure is undertaken at a later stage. However, for surgeons unused to operating on the very young a measure of compromise is reasonable, with the procedure being deferred until the patient is 3 or 4 years of age.

Impalpable testis

Some 10–20% of undescended testes are impalpable. Before embarking upon definitive surgery, it is necessary to establish whether the testis is absent (anorchia), is intra-abdominal, or is represented by an atrophic nubbin of tissue within the inguinal canal. In approximately 40% of cases of 'impalpable testis' the gonad lies intra-abdominally; in 30% it has 'vanished', with vas and vessels ending blindly deep to the internal inguinal ring; in 20% similarly but with vas and vessels ending blindly within the inguinal canal; and in 10% the testis is normal but concealed within the inguinal canal.

Ultrasound is unreliable in distinguishing between anorchia and intra-abdominal testis, giving both false positive and false negative findings, but it is sometimes helpful in visualising a testis within the inguinal canal. Magnetic resonance imaging (MRI) is also unhelpful alone although more reliable when combined with angiography, but this requires a general anaesthetic.

Consequently, laparoscopy remains the investigation of first choice in cases of impalpable testis, being both highly reliable and providing positive guidance for further management. In this regard, there are five possible laparoscopic findings:

- Vas and vessels ending blindly together at or above the internal ring. Such 'vanished' testes presumably result from intrauterine torsion and no further exploration is required.
- Vas and vessels seen entering the inguinal canal. Here it is impossible to be certain whether the canal contains a normal testis or an 'atrophic nubbin' of testicular tissue. Inguinal exploration is indicated.
- Testis lying adjacent to the internal inguinal ring. Such gonads are usually amenable to a single-stage orchidopexy using a conventional or a preperitoneal approach. An experienced laparoscopist may be able to manipulate the testis towards the inguinal canal so as to assess the feasibility of a single-stage procedure.
- Testis located on the posterior abdominal wall or ectopically within the pelvis (Figure 19.3). This calls for a decision as to whether to remove the gonad (either laparoscopically or as an open procedure), or whether to embark upon orchidopexy. Here the options lie between open or laparoscopically assisted orchidopexy, as either a single or a staged procedure.
- Failure to visualise blind-ending vessels or testis. In this rare situation, a limited laparotomy is indicated in view of the high risk of subsequent malignancy associated with an undetected intra-abdominal testes left in situ.

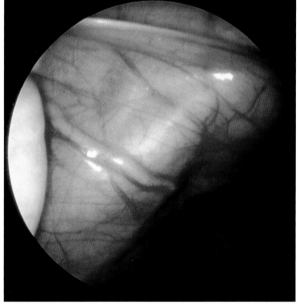
(a)

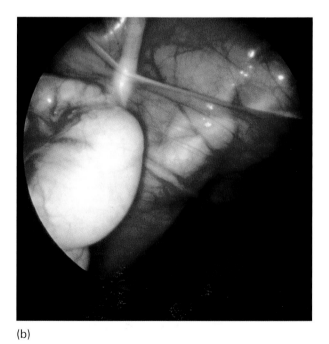
(b)

Figure 19.3 (a,b) Intra-abdominal testis and vas viewed laparoscopically.

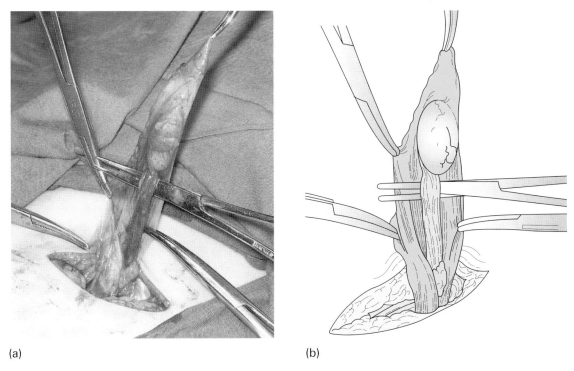

(a)   (b)

Figure 19.4 Conventional inguinal orchidopexy. (a) Intraoperative photograph. (b) Diagrammatic representation illustrating mobilisation of cord structures from the processus vaginalis.

Bilateral impalpable testes

Determination of karyotype is always worthwhile in this situation, looking for sex chromosome mosaicism or for chromosomal aberrations such as the Prader–Willi syndrome. A human chorionic gonadotrophin stimulation test may be undertaken to determine the presence or otherwise of functioning testicular tissue. However, although a positive result is encouraging for the parents, a negative result does not obviate the need for laparoscopy.

Orchidopexy: surgical considerations

For a detailed account of standard orchidopexy for a palpable testis, the reader is referred to one of the textbooks of operative paediatric surgery or urology listed under Further reading. In cases of true congenital maldescent the crucial step is clean separation of the patent processus vaginalis from the cord structures so as to facilitate full mobilisation of the testicular vessels, extended retroperitoneally if necessary (Figure 19.4). In the absence of a patent processus vaginalis orchidopexy is usually straightforward, with the gonad coming readily to the scrotum following separation of the cremasteric coverings from the cord structures.

More specialised techniques are required for testes lying high within the inguinal canal or within the abdomen. The options comprise:

- **Preperitoneal approach (Jones)** A skin incision at or slightly higher than for a standard inguinal approach is employed and the oblique abdominal muscles are split to gain access to the preperitoneal space above the inguinal canal. Thereafter, the testis is mobilised extraperitoneally or transperitoneally and is passed to the scrotum through the inguinal canal or, if necessary, more directly through the posterior wall of the canal medial to the inferior epigastric vessels.
- **Fowler–Stephens procedure** (Figure 19.5) With intra-abdominal testis, failure to mobilise the gonad to the scrotum is usually the result of inadequate length of the testicular vessels rather than of the vas deferens. The existence of a collateral blood supply to the testis via the artery to the vas represents the rationale for this procedure, and the results are better when it is conducted in two stages. At the first stage, undertaken either via an open approach or laparoscopically, the testicular vessels are isolated and divided close to the testis, taking care not to disturb

(a)

(b)

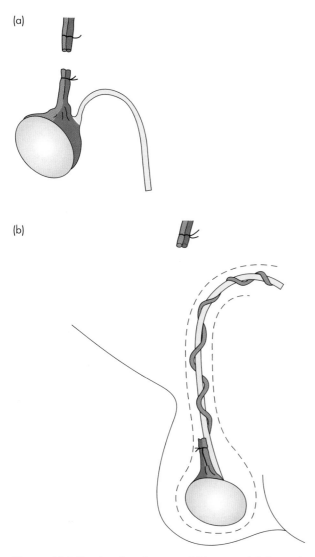

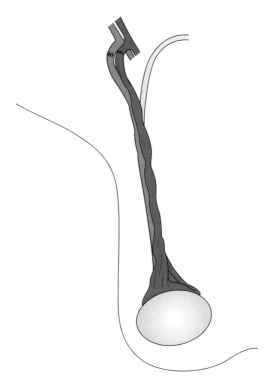

Figure 19.6 Microvascular orchidopexy. Testicular artery and single vein anastomosed to inferior epigastric vessels (or branches).

Figure 19.5 Fowler–Stephens orchidopexy. (a) Stage I, testicular vessels ligated or clipped in continuity. (b) Stage II, collateral vascularisation of the testis via the artery to the vas. After 6 months the testis is mobilised on the vas and a strip of surrounding peritoneum and brought to the scrotum by the most direct route.

the vas and its all important collateral vessels. The second stage is undertaken 6 months later, when this collateral supply has become more robust following ligation of the testicular vessels proper. Testis and vas are mobilised, along with a broad strip of overlying peritoneum, and brought transinguinally to the scrotum. This may be undertaken as an entirely open procedure or with laparoscopic assistance.

● **Microvascular orchidopexy** is appropriate for intra-abdominal testes, especially if the vas is too short for a Fowler–Stephens procedure or, rarely, if

the vas is absent. The testicular vessels are mobilised and divided as high as possible, following which testis and vas are brought to the scrotum and the testicular vessels anastomosed to the inferior epigastric vessels in the inguinal canal (Figure 19.6).

● **Laparoscopically assisted orchidopexy** (Figure 19.7) The intraperitoneal pedicle of testicular vessels is extensively mobilised laparoscopically, and when sufficient length has been obtained the testis is placed in the scrotum by either an open inguinal approach or an entirely laparoscopic procedure.

Even an experienced surgeon may occasionally operate for what is thought to be a palpable testis only to find, having opened the inguinal canal, that it is empty. This situation should be managed not by exploring retroperitoneally but by incising the peritoneum in the posterior wall of the canal. Intra-abdominal or intra-canalicular testes and their vessels are typically enclosed within a mobile pedicle of peritoneum and can be brought down more easily into the inguinal canal by opening the peritoneum of the empty proccessus vaginalis.

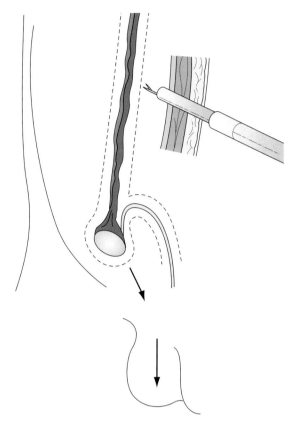

Figure 19.7 Laparoscopic or laparoscopically assisted orchidopexy. Extensive intraperitoneal mobilisation of testicular vessels enables the testis to be brought down to the scrotum with its vascular pedicle intact.

Management of retractile testis

In clear-cut cases parents may be reassured that retractile testes are common, particularly between the ages of 3 and 7 years, and that surgical intervention is rarely required. Moreover, one study has shown that men with bilateral retractile testes during childhood subsequently have normal testicular volume and fertility.

It is not possible to be so confident where the diagnosis lies between 'high retractile testis' and true congenital maldescent. In these circumstances the history may be more informative than the examination. Where any doubt exists, regular reassessment at 6–12-monthly intervals should be undertaken, and the parents should be advised that the need for surgery cannot be discounted.

If, during follow-up, it becomes apparent that a 'high retractile testis' is assuming an increasingly abnormal position, hormonal manipulation may be employed as both a diagnostic and a therapeutic trial. Where orchidopexy proves necessary, either following

unsuccessful endocrine treatment or as the procedure of first choice, this may be undertaken via a scrotal approach. Mobilisation of the cord structures and complete separation from the overlying cremasteric coverings is usually sufficient to allow a retractile testis to be positioned in a satisfactory scrotal position without tension on the spermatic cord.

During recent years the distinction between 'high retractile testis' and 'secondary testicular ascent' has become increasingly debated. The aetiology of the latter condition is unknown, although obliteration of a patent processus vaginalis with contraction of the remnant has been advanced as a possible cause. In almost all series of 'secondary testicular ascent' orchidopexy was undertaken prior to puberty, so that it is impossible to be sure whether or not spontaneous descent would ultimately have occurred.

Complications of orchidopexy

The principal complications are postoperative testicular atrophy, injury to the vas and reascent of the testis. Among a total of 8425 procedures in 64 published studies, the failure rate, including atrophy, was 8% when the testis lay beyond the external inguinal ring, 13% when the testis was within the inguinal canal, and in the case of intra-abdominal testes 16% for microvascular procedures and 27% for two-stage Fowler–Stephens procedures. A 5% incidence of testicular atrophy following inguinal orchidopexy reported from one specialist paediatric surgical centre in the United Kingdom is probably representative of current practice.

The incidence of injury to the vas is more difficult to determine, and although a figure of 1–2% is sometimes cited the true incidence is probably higher, as direct injury may go unnoticed or unreported. Post ischaemic obliteration of the vas resulting from intraoperative damage to the delicate blood supply is likely to remain unrecognised except in individuals who undergo exploration or vasography in later life.

Long-term follow-up studies following prepubertal orchidopexy indicate that testicular volume is ultimately influenced by the initial position of the gonad, but not by the age at which the surgery was performed.

Long-term outcomes of orchidopexy
Fertility

Assessment of fertility is inexact, as almost all long-term studies have been retrospective, with the limitations inherent in such studies. In addition, the ability to father children does not consistently correlate with parameters of semen quality.

Among men previously undergoing bilateral orchidopexy during childhood, approximately 25% have normal semen analysis, 50% are azospermic and 25% have oligospermia. As for men who had previously undergone a unilateral procedure, 57% have normal semen analysis.

Paternity rates, by contrast, are somewhat more encouraging. Approximately 50% of men who had undergone bilateral orchidopexy achieve paternity, and for those who underwent a unilateral procedure the overall paternity rate is 80%, which is only marginally less than normal. However, men with a history of unilateral cryptorchidisim do demonstrate some degree of subfertility, as evidenced by the fact that 11% of those attempting paternity fail to achieve conception within 12 months, compared to only 5% of controls.

Figures for both semen analysis and paternity are based upon men who underwent orchidopexy comparatively late in childhood. It seems reasonable to anticipate an improvement in fertility as a consequence of the recent trend toward earlier orchidopexy before the age of 2 years. Some evidence is emerging to this effect, but it will be some time before the presumed benefit of earlier orchidopexy can be confirmed by reliable long-term data.

Malignancy

Men with a history of cryptorchidism are undoubtedly at increased risk of testicular malignancy. A recent large case–control study in the United Kingdom put the relative risk at 3.8 times greater than normal when orchidopexy had been performed after 9 years of age. However, the relative risk was not found to be significantly increased if the procedure was undertaken before that age. Other studies based on recent figures for the incidence of testicular cancer and cryptorchidism have generally placed the increased relative risk at between 5 and 10 times greater than that for the normal population. The lifetime risk of developing cancer in an undescended testis has been calculated to lie in the order of 1 in 100, compared with 1 in 500 in the population at large. However, this risk is somewhat less if maldescent is unilateral, and correspondingly somewhat greater if bilateral.

In adults the incidence of carcinoma in situ, a precursor of invasive malignancy, is strongly linked to the anatomical position of the testis, being found in 25% of gonads retained intra-abdominally into adult life. This and other evidence suggests that the original position of the testis may be a factor influencing the long-term risk of malignancy. During the first year of life undescended testes develop Leydig cell hypoplasia and delayed disappearance of gonocytes. There is some evidence that these gonocytes may degenerate into carcinoma in situ cells, thus providing further justification for the trend towards earlier orchidopexy in the belief that this will be accompanied by a reduction in the risk of malignancy.

Regardless of the age at which orchidopexy has been performed, men who have undergone the procedure should be encouraged to practise testicular self-examination.

Testicular microcalcification

This disorder, which is characterised by the presence of multiple small echogenic foci of calcification (Figure 19.8), has come to light as a result of the introduction of testicular ultrasound as a screening tool in adult urology. Although it may occur as a sporadic finding in the absence of other testicular pathology, testicular microcalcification has been identified as a potential marker of carcinoma in situ and gonadal dysgenesis. Testicular ultrasound is performed far less frequently in children and adolescents but, nevertheless, cases of testicular microcalcification are being identified. At present the risk of malignancy posed by this finding in young people is uncertain, but until further information becomes

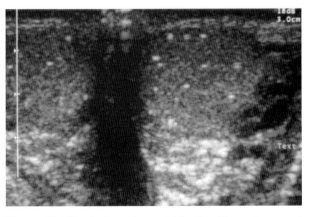

Figure 19.8 Testicular microcalcification. Two ultrasound images demonstrating characteristic appearances.

available affected individuals should certainly be advised to undertake regular testicular self-examination from puberty onwards. In the light of current knowledge regular ultrasound surveillance is justifiable, but testicular biopsy is not indicated in this age group.

Hydrocoele

With few exceptions, hydrocoeles in boys share a common underlying aetiology with indirect inguinal hernias, namely, failure of closure of the patent processus vaginalis following descent of the testis (see Chapter 1). The difference between the two conditions lies in the diameter of the processus, which in communicating hydrocoeles is narrow and allows no more than the passage of intraperitonal fluid. Non-communicating hydrocoeles are very rare in boys and occur principally around or after the time of puberty (Figure 19.9).

Communicating hydrocoeles are common in newborn males, with an incidence of 2–5%. Upwards of 90% of these congenital lesions resolve during the first year of life as a result of spontaneous closure of the processus. For reasons that are unclear, a processus occluded at birth can sometimes recanalise and result in the appearance of a hydrocoele at some time later during childhood, although usually before the age of 5 years.

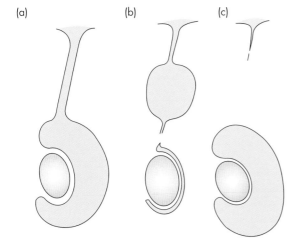

(a)　　　(b)　　　(c)

Figure 19.9 Anatomical classification of hydrocoele. (a) Communicating hydrocoele. (b) Hydrocoele of the cord ('encysted hydrocoele'). (c) Non-communicating hydrocoele.

Presentation

Most hydrocoeles present as a painless scrotal swelling which may vary in size throughout the day, being comparatively small first thing in the morning and enlarging during the course of the day. Sometimes hydrocoeles develop following the insertion of a ventriculoperitoneal shunt for hydrocephalus, whereas others present acutely, and sometimes painfully, usually during the course of a viral illness causing an increased production of intraperitoneal fluid. Although rare, it should always be remembered that hydrocoeles may be a secondary phenomenon associated with testicular tumours.

Encysted hydrocoeles of the cord typically present as a painless swelling in the groin and, being 'irreducible', are apt to be confused with an incarcerated inguinal hernia.

Examination

The principal differential diagnosis is one of a complete inguinal hernia, the latter being reducible whereas hydrocoeles are not. Transillumination, the classic physical sign of a hydrocoele, is not reliably diagnostic as a scrotal hernia in infancy will also transilluminate in bright light. A hydrocoele of the cord is distinguished from an incomplete and irreducible inguinal hernia in that downward traction on the testis causes a corresponding movement in the hydrocoele.

Although investigation is usually unnecessary, ultrasonography is helpful whenever there is any suspicion of testicular tumour.

Management

Congenital hydrocoeles should be managed conservatively, as almost all will resolve spontaneously during the first 12 months of life. The only indication for surgical treatment during this time is a scrotal swelling so large as to cause discomfort.

Surgical intervention is indicated for the occasional congenital hydrocoele that persists beyond 1 year of age, and for those appearing for the first time in later childhood. Hydrocoeles of the cord are rarely present at birth and usually treated surgically, especially where there is any doubt about the diagnosis.

Operative technique

With communicating hydrocoeles the operative technique closely resembles that employed for indirect inguinal hernia. Through a short skin-crease incision in the groin the spermatic cord is delivered, with or without opening the inguinal canal according to the surgeon's preference. The patent processus vaginalis is isolated from the testicular vessels and vas, traced back to its junction with the peritoneal cavity, and trans-fixed, ligated and divided at this point. The hydrocoele sac is then drained by incising the distal portion of the processus, or by percutaneous needle aspiration of the sac.

Recurrence is most unusual, occurring in less than 1% of cases. Most recurrences result from a failure to identify or deal adequately with the patent processus at the original procedure. Less often, recurrence is owed to the fact that the underlying pathology was of a non-communicating hydrocoele, a situation that may be rectified by a Jaboulay or a Lord's procedure.

Varicocoele

Although the significance of varicocoeles lies princi-pally in their association with subfertility, there is considerable variation in both the clinical characteris-tics of these lesions and their impact, if any, upon fertility. Opinion therefore remains divided on the indications for surgical intervention in childhood or adolescence. There is also debate as to the preferred surgical technique.

Incidence

Varicocoeles can be demonstrated in 6% of 10-year-old boys and 15% of 13-year-olds, the latter figure being comparable to the prevalence among adult males generally. Among the male partners of infertile couples the incidence of varicocoele is 30%.

Aetiology

The tortuosity and dilatation of the veins of the pampiniform plexus is the result of incompetence of the valvular mechanism that normally protects the spermatic veins from the pressure of venous blood transmitted from the great veins. The fact that more than 90% of varicocoeles are left-sided reflects differ-ences in venous anatomy, with the left testicular vein draining into the renal vein, whereas the right testicu-lar vein drains into the vena cava. Several patterns of abnormal venous anatomy predisposing to varicocoele formation have been described:

- Absence of valves within an otherwise normal single testicular vein;
- Anomalous venous drainage, for example between testicular and retroperitoneal veins;
- Bifurcation of the left renal vein, with an abnormal point of entry of the spermatic veins.

Although renal tumours account for less than 1% of varicocoeles during childhood, this possibility should never be overlooked.

Pathology

The application of heat-sensitive strips to the scrotal skin confirms that the presence of a varicocoele elevates the temperature of the scrotal contents, leading to loss of the normal temperature differential necessary for spermatogenesis. The role, if any, of venous pressure-related damage to the testis is more difficult to assess. Testicular biopsies in the presence of a varicocoele show reduced spermatogonia, seminiferous tubal atrophy, endothelial cell proliferation and Leydig cell abnormal-ities. When found in patients under 18 years of age the Leydig cell changes are potentially reversible, but the more extensive histological changes found in older men are not – an observation that argues in favour of treat-ing varicocoeles during adolescence rather than later.

Classification

The classification devised by Hudson is widely employed:

- **Subclinical**: neither palpable nor visible, but demonstrable by Doppler ultrasound
- **Grade I:** palpable only on Valsalva manoeuvre
- **Grade II:** palpable at rest but not visible
- **Grade III:** visible and palpable at rest.

Presentation

Varicocoeles may be detected during the course of some routine medical examination or may present symptomatically, either as a scrotal swelling, classically likened to a 'bag of worms', or by a dragging sensa-tion within the scrotum, which is often worse during hot weather (Figure 19.10).

Diagnosis and investigation

The patient should be examined both lying and, more importantly, standing, the latter both with and without

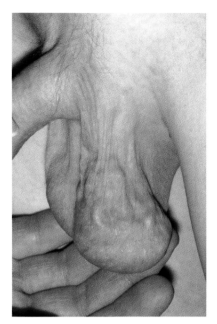

Figure 19.10 Grade III varicocoele. Visibly distended cremasteric veins ('bag of worms').

a Valsalva manoeuvre. Testicular size and volume should be assessed. The traditional method using a Prader orchiometer or callipers is prone to considerable observer variation. Ultrasound assessment of testicular volume is more reliable and can be combined with abdominal examination to exclude a renal tumour.

Treatment

Indications

The existence of symptoms is generally accepted as an indication for surgical intervention, as is impairment of testicular growth. Among adolescent boys with asymptomatic lesions, however, the issue of 'prophylactic' intervention is altogether more controversial. The arguments in favour can be summarised as follows:

- Persistence of an untreated varicocoele into adult life leads to a demonstrable reduction in testicular volume, and there is evidence that surgical correction may partly reverse this process, leading to some degree of subsequent 'catch-up growth'.
- The incidence of varicocoele among men investigated for infertility is higher than in the male population at large.
- Some studies have found an improvement in semen quality and pregnancy rates following treatment of varicocoele in subfertile men.

Arguments against prophylactic intervention in adolescence are that:

- varicocoeles exist in some 15% of adult males, most of whom, as judged by paternity, have normal fertility.
- although a link exists between varicocoele and infertility or subfertility, there is no consistent correlation between the presence or size of the lesion and semen quality or fertility.

Although only time will ultimately resolve this controversy, the present tendency is to advise 'prophylactic' intervention in the case of the larger, grade III, lesions.

Surgical treatment (Figure 19.11)

Embolisation

This may be carried out under sedation, although a general anaesthetic is usually used for prepubertal boys. A catheter introduced via the right femoral or

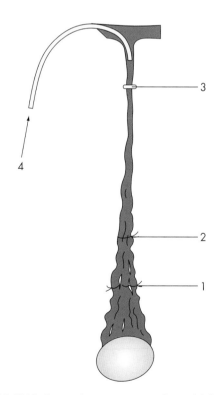

Figure 19.11 Varicocoele treatment options. (1) Surgical ligation of individual veins, inguinal approach. (2) Surgical ligation of veins and artery, high approach. (3) Laparoscopic clipping, all vessels or selective 'artery sparing'. (4) Embolisation.

internal jugular vein is screened into the left renal vein and thence into the spermatic vein. Venography is performed to identify collaterals. Embolisation is undertaken using coils inserted into the testicular vein or, less often, by the injection of a sclerosant.

Surgical ligation

Using the **inguinal approach** (Ivanissevich), the internal inguinal ring is exposed via the inguinal canal; the spermatic vein is exposed deep to the transversalis fascia and divided at this level.

Using the **high approach** (Palomo), a short transverse incision is performed lateral to the internal inguinal ring. The testicular vessels are identified extraperitoneally above the divergence of the vas deferens. In Palomo's description, the testicular artery, vein and lymphatics are all ligated and divided but many surgeons ligate only the veins

Microvascular procedures are nowadays sometimes performed for local ligation of varicoceles. Although usually undertaken beyond the external inguinal ring, in prepubertal boys, the dissection is better performed within the inguinal canal. Magnification of 6–25 times is employed and papaverine and introperative ultrasound are helpful in identifying and preserving the arteries. Care is taken to preserve the testicular and cremasteric arteries, the vas deferens and its artery, and also the lymphatics as preservation of the lymphatics is believed to minimise the incidence of postoperative hydrocoele.

Other direct approaches to the dilated veins distal to the internal ring carry an unacceptably high risk of testicular atrophy and should be avoided.

With **laparoscopic ligation** three ports are placed and the testicular vessels identified. The veins can either be dissected and divided alone or clipped and ligated *en masse*, along with the artery, as in the Palomo technique. This approach also allows easy identification and division of any abnormal veins associated with the vas deferens, and is also especially applicable to the rare case of bilateral varicocoele. As with open techniques, lymphatic vessels should be preserved as far as possible.

Complications and outcome

That fact that several surgical techniques continue to be employed for treating varicocoeles argues that no single technique gives consistently satisfactory results.

The failure rate for all procedures is up to 20%, although this figure appears to be rather lower when the testicular artery, as well as the veins, is occluded. The incidence of complications, notably hydrocoele and testicular atrophy, is in the region of 5%. Almost all published results relate principally to adult men, and there is insufficient information relating specifically to boys and adolescents from which to draw meaningful conclusions about the best form of treatment in this age group.

Improved fertility has been documented in subfertile men following varicocoele ligation, although these represent only a minority of all men with varicocoeles. Whether prophylactic treatment of asymptomatic varicocoeles in adolescents is beneficial for fertility has yet to be ascertained.

Key points

- The optimal age for orchidopexy remains uncertain. Paediatric urologists and paediatric surgeons favour the second year of life. For non-specialist surgeons it may be reasonable to defer orchidopexy until 3–4 years of age.
- The risk of testicular atrophy should be specifically discussed with parents when obtaining consent for orchidopexy.
- Laparoscopy is the investigation of choice for impalpable testes.
- In infants a clear diagnostic distinction must be made between an inguinal hernia (which requires prompt surgical intervention in this age group) and a communicating hydrocoele (which generally resolves as a result of spontaneous closure of the patent processus vaginalis in the first year of life).
- The available evidence suggests that treatment of varicocoeles in adolescence should be limited to boys with grade III varicocoeles and evidence of impaired testicular growth.

Further reading

Ashcraft KW, Holder TM (eds) *Paediatric surgery*, 2nd edn. Philadelphia: WB Saunders, 1993
Barthold JS Redman JF. Congenital anomalies of the testis and scrotum. In: Whitfield HN, Hendry WF, Kirby RS,

Duckett JW (eds) *Textbook of genitourinary surgery.* Oxford: Blackwell, 1998; 254–260

Genitourinary surgery. In: *Rob & Smith's Operative Surgery, Paediatric Surgery.* 5th edn. Oxford: Butterworth–Heinemann, 1993; 601–605 and 745–751

Hendry WF. Testicular, epididymal and vasal injuries. *B J Urol Int* 2000; 86: 344–348

Stringer MD, Oldham KT, Mouriquand PDE, Howard ER (eds) *Paediatric surgery and urology: long term outcomes.* London: WB Saunders, 1998

The acute scrotum

20

David FM Thomas

Topics covered
Epidemiology
Diagnostic features, symptoms and signs
Torsion of the testis

Torsion of testicular appendage
Epididymo-orchitis
Idiopathic scrotal oedema
Other acute scrotal pathology

Introduction

Management of the acutely painful or swollen scrotum is one of the few real surgical emergencies in paediatric urology. Testicular torsion accounts for 80–90% of cases of 'acute scrotum' in teenage boys. In this age group the high probability of torsion justifies immediate surgical exploration unless there is compelling evidence of an alternative diagnosis. In prepubertal boys the differential diagnosis is more varied, but it is important to recognise that testicular torsion figures prominently as a cause of acute scrotal pathology across the entire paediatric age range.

Surgical intervention can sometimes be avoided if a reliable alternative diagnosis, such as torsion of a testicular appendage, can be established rapidly, but it is generally wiser to observe the time-honoured adage: Whenever doubt exists, it is safer to explore.

Epidemiology

The relative frequency of the various causes of acute scrotum in the different age groups is illustrated in Figure 20.1. Between the ages of 13 and 21 years, testicular torsion accounts for nearly 90% of acutely

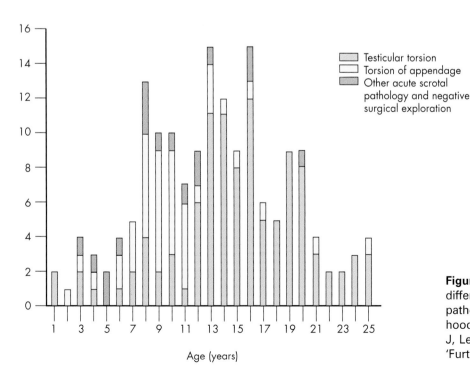

Age (years)

Figure 20.1 The relative frequency of different causes of acute scrotal pathology at different ages in childhood and early adult life (Ben-Chaim J, Leibovitch I, Ramon J et al – see 'Further reading').

presenting scrotal symptoms. However, in prepubertal boys torsion of a testicular appendage (hydatid of Morgagni) is the most frequent acute scrotal condition, accounting for 45–50% of cases, testicular torsion accounts for approximately 35% of acutely presenting scrotal symptoms, and epididymo-orchitis, ideopathic scrotal oedema, acute hydrocoele and Henoch–Schönlein vasculitis comprise the remaining 15–20%.

Diagnosis

Clinical features

The differential diagnosis of the acute scrotum and the relative importance of the different pathologies in pre- and postpubertal boys in one sizeable series are detailed in Table 20.1. Establishing a clinical diagnosis may be straightforward in the presence of a characteristic history and distinctive physical findings, but in many cases the history is not specific and examination simply reveals a swollen, reddened tender scrotum. In other instances the history or initial findings may be frankly misleading.

- Contrary to textbook descriptions pain is not always a prominent feature of testicular torsion. In infants and young children pain may be virtually absent until changes secondary to established testicular infarction are apparent.
- Pain arising from a right-sided testicular torsion may radiate to the right iliac fossa, mimicking appendicitis.
- Oedema and erythema of the scrotal skin are not

apparent in the first few hours of testicular torsion. Absence of these physical signs should not be allowed to delay surgical exploration.

- The pathognomic 'blue dot sign' associated with torsion of a testicular appendage (hydatid of Morgagni) is present in fewer than 20% of cases.
- Urinary symptoms (frequency, dysuria), which can sometimes feature in the clinical picture of testicular torsion, may be wrongly attributed to urinary infection and epididymo-orchitis.

Diagnostic imaging

Colour Doppler ultrasound provides simultaneous real-time anatomical imaging of the scrotal contents together with colour-encoded characteristics of blood flow. Perfusion of the testis is absent or dramatically reduced in testicular torsion. Drawbacks include operator dependency, limited out-of-hours availability, and falsely reassuring findings in early or intermittent torsion.

Radionuclide testicular scanning (RTS) Sodium pertechnetate labelled with ^{99m}Tc is injected intravenously. Testicular torsion is characterised by a central 'cold' area of poor isotope uptake corresponding to the ischaemic testis surrounded by a halo of vascular activity in hyperaemic scrotal tissue. The limited availability and time-consuming and invasive nature effectively precludes its use in everyday clinical practice.

The role of diagnostic imaging, notably colour Doppler ultrasound, is largely confined to prepubertal boys in whom testicular torsion is thought to have been excluded on clinical grounds but where further confirmation is sought.

Table 20.1 Relative frequency of different causes of 'acute scrotum' in 154 cases

Diagnosis	0–12 years		13–21 years	
	n	%	n	%
Torsion of testis	24	34	72	86
Torsion of appendix	33	47	8	9
Negative exploration	8	11	4	5
Epididymitis	3	4		
Acute scrotal oedema	1	2		
Acute haematocoele	1	2		
Total	70	100	84	100

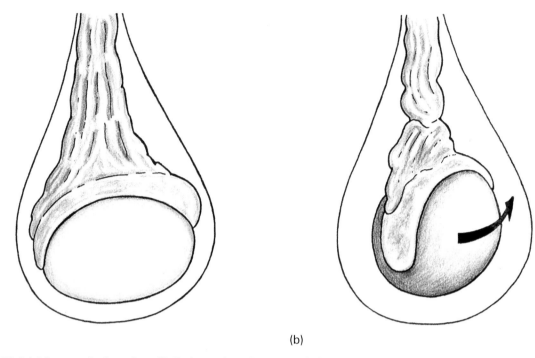

(a)   (b)

Figure 20.2 (a) Intravaginal torsion. 'Bell-clapper' testis suspended on an abnormally long leash of vessels (mesorchium) within the tunica vaginalis. (b) Undue mobility of the testis predisposes to torsion around the axis of the spermatic cord.

Testicular torsion

Although the peak incidence lies between the ages of 14 and 16 years (see Figure 20.1), torsion can occur at any age from the neonatal period through to late adult life. The annual incidence has been estimated at 1 in 4000 males below the age of 25 years. The left testis is affected more commonly than the right. Predisposing factors may include cold weather (precipitating activity of the cremasteric muscle) and testicular trauma. Maldescended testes account for approximately 5% of cases.

Aetiology

Neonatal or intrauterine testicular torsion is of the **extravaginal** pattern, in which the testis and coverings twist in their entirety within the scrotum. In contrast, testicular torsion in all other age groups is generally **intravaginal**, i.e. the testis twists within the confines of the tunica vaginalis. It is generally accepted that an anatomical variant termed the 'bell clapper' testis, with a long mesentery-like leash of vessels (mesorchium), predisposes to torsion by permitting an abnormally mobile testis to twist around the axis of the spermatic cord (Figure 20.2). Although a rotational twist of

360–720° is commonly encountered at the time of surgical exploration, the degree of rotation required to produce testicular ischaemia is poorly documented. Experimental studies, coupled with the findings of a limited number of clinical follow-up studies, indicate that a viable testis can only be salvaged if the blood supply is restored within 4–6 hours of the onset of ischaemia. Varying degrees of atrophy ensue when surgical exploration is delayed by 6–8 hours after the onset of symptoms. When the history exceeds 8–10 hours ischaemic necrosis and atrophy are virtually inevitable.

Presentation

Unilateral scrotal pain and swelling of acute onset are the pathognomic features of testicular torsion, but the clinical picture is variable and fewer than 50% of cases present with a classic 'full house' of history and clinical findings. Pain is often referred to the groin or lower abdomen, and vomiting is a feature of approximately 40% of cases. The potentially misleading painless form of presentation is encountered more frequently in younger children (Figure 20.3) but may also give rise to diagnostic confusion in the postpubertal age group.

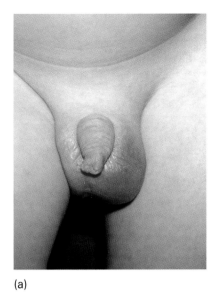

(a)

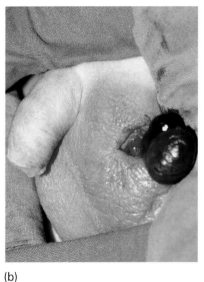

(b)

Figure 20.3 (a) Deceptively painless presentation of testicular torsion in an infant with a 3-day history of minimal symptoms. Discoloration of the scrotum prompted his parents to seek medical advice. (b) Prompt surgical exploration nevertheless revealed a necrotic testis.

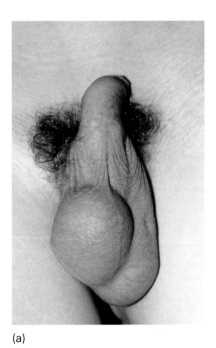

(a)

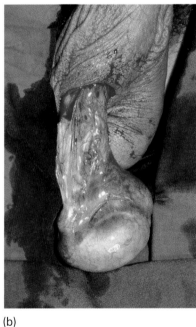

(b)

Figure 20.4 (a) Characteristic appearances of early torsion (3-hour history). The right testis is tender, mildly swollen, and lies in an elevated position within the scrotum. (b) This testis was judged to be viable in view of the short history and operative findings indicating good return of perfusion following detorsion.

Management

External non-operative detorsion in the emergency room has been advocated, but although this may have a place in young adults it is not generally feasible in children.

Urgent **surgical exploration** is the keystone of management. Following exposure of the testis via a scrotal incision, the spermatic cord is untwisted and testicular viability assessed. Factors influencing the decision to conserve or remove the testis include the duration of the history, the appearance of the testis,

and arterial bleeding on incising the tunica albuginea (Figure 20.4). Unless the testis is clearly viable it is generally best to err in favour of orchidectomy (assuming the contralateral testis is healthy). Fixation of the contralateral testis is mandatory in view of the bilateral nature of the anatomy predisposing to torsion. Via a scrotal incision the tunica vaginalis is opened and the healthy testis anchored to the scrotal wall using two or three non-absorbable sutures, e.g. 4/0 or 5/0 Prolene. (Cases of further torsion despite fixation have been reported following the use of catgut sutures.) Implantation of a testicular prosthesis is an option available to young men following unilateral orchidectomy or testicular atrophy, but because of the risk of infection this should be a subsequent elective procedure via an inguinal incision, rather than at the time of acute surgical exploration.

Prognosis

Fertility

Follow-up studies in adults have revealed that semen quality is significantly reduced following unilateral torsion in adolescence. In one such study semen quality was reduced in 50% of men, and in another study of 36 patients only 16% had normal parameters of semen quality on follow-up. The mechanism is unclear, but possibilities include antisperm antibodies and pre-existing abnormalities of the spermatogenic tissue in the 'healthy' contralateral testis.

Very little information exists on the prognosis for fertility following torsion in prepubertal boys, but the limited clinical data and some experimental evidence suggest that it may not have the same potential impact on fertility as torsion in adolescents and young adults.

Endocrine function

In contrast to the impaired spermatogenesis, endocrine function is unaffected and uniformly normal plasma levels of testosterone have been documented following unilateral torsion (regardless of the outcome for the twisted testis). FSH levels may be elevated, reflecting impaired spermatogenesis in these patients.

Neonatal torsion

More strictly this should be termed intrauterine or 'perinatal' torsion, as with rare exceptions the event dates from the late stages of intrauterine life and cases of testicular torsion have been diagnosed on prenatal ultrasound. Typically, the surgeon is called to the postnatal ward to see an infant with scrotal discoloration and an indurated testis. In these circumstances the prospects of salvaging a viable testis are effectively zero. Reviewing the outcome of torsion in 30 neonates presenting over a 20-year period, Burge did not encounter a single viable testis. The almost invariably disappointing findings at surgical exploration, coupled with the belief that extravaginal

torsion does carry the same risk to the contralateral testis, have prompted a shift in policy. In many centres neonatal torsion is now managed conservatively, with regular ultrasound follow-up to monitor the process of testicular atrophy. The main risk associated with non-operative management lies in the remote possibility of failing to recognise a congenital testicular tumour masquerading as 'neonatal' testicular torsion. If the ultrasound appearances are in any way suspicious, or the indurated testis fails to involute, surgical exploration and orchidectomy should be performed.

Torsion of testicular appendage (hydatid of Morgagni)

Children of any age can be affected, although the peak incidence is between 10 and 12 years. In prepubertal boys torsion of a testicular appendage occurs more frequently than torsion of the testis itself (Table 20.1).

Presentation

Although pain is the usual presenting symptom it is typically less severe and more gradual in onset than that of testicular torsion. However, the two conditions cannot always be distinguished reliably on clinical grounds, particularly in younger children. Haemorrhagic infarction of the hydatid of Morgagni, visible as a localised area of discoloration at the upper pole of the testis ('blue dot sign'), is pathognomic of the condition but is only present in a minority of cases. Similarly, although examination may reveal tenderness confined to an indurated nodule, more generalised tenderness is often present and accompanied by oedema and erythema of the hemiscrotum.

Diagnosis

The clinical features may be sufficiently distinctive to enable an experienced clinician to make a firm diagnosis. Colour Doppler ultrasound can provide additional confirmation.

Management

Surgical intervention is indicated when testicular torsion cannot be excluded or when discomfort is severe. Treatment consists of simple excision of the infarcted hydatid of Morgagni. Prophylactic excision of the contralateral testicular appendage is unnecessary. When a firm clinical diagnosis has been established, and where pain is mild or resolving, conservative management is appropriate.

Epididymo-orchitis

Aetiology

Bacterial infection of the epididymis progressing to involve the testis occurs as a result of retrograde bacterial colonisation via the ejaculatory ducts and vas deferens. Vasal reflux of infected urine is usually present. Epididymo-orchitis (particularly when recurrent) may be linked to an underlying urological condition such as neuropathic bladder, persistent müllerian remnant or ectopic ureter. However, it also occurs in infants with urinary infection associated with low-grade vesicoureteric reflux, or urinary infection for which there is no identifiable predisposing cause.

Presentation

Scrotal pain may be accompanied by evidence of urinary infection, e.g. dysuria or offensive urine. Examination typically reveals marked scrotal erythema and tenderness, and induration of the testis, often accompanied by fever and systemic upset.

Diagnosis

In boys of all ages testicular torsion is considerably more common than epididymo-orchitis, and this diagnosis should be viewed with suspicion. Moreover, epididymo-orchitis cannot be reliably distinguished from testicular torsion on clinical grounds alone. For these reasons surgical exploration should be performed, unless the child is known to have a predisposing urological abnormality and the clinical features point strongly to epidiymo-orchitis. Confirmatory investigations include:

- Urine microscopy – pyuria, bacteriuria and positive urine culture
- Doppler ultrasound – hyperaemia and increased vascularity.

Management

Surgical

Surgical intervention is indicated:

- To exclude the diagnosis of testicular torsion
- To drain a scrotal or testicular abscess.

In cases of recurrent symptomatic epididymo-orchitis it may be necessary to consider vasectomy if the underlying urological abnormality is not amenable to surgical correction.

Medical

Non-operative management comprises **analgesia** (epididymo-orchitis is an acutely painful condition) and an **intravenous antibiotic**, e.g. gentamicin or ciprofloxacin, pending the result of urine culture. Antibiotic treatment should be instituted postoperatively when the condition is discovered at exploration.

Prognosis

The fate of the testis cannot be reliably assessed until all the induration has resolved, and this is generally a matter of several months. Following an isolated and promptly treated episode in a child without underlying urological abnormalities, the prognosis is generally good. However, after recurrent attacks of epididymo-orchitis varying degrees of testicular atrophy supervene.

Idiopathic scrotal oedema

This condition is virtually confined to the prepubertal age group, with a peak incidence between the ages of 5 and 6 years.

Aetiology

Although the condition is genuinely idiopathic the association with anal pathology and the occasional finding of erythema extending from the perineum has been interpreted as evidence of reactive oedema secondary to localised lymphangitis.

Presentation

The clinical picture is characterised by marked oedema of the scrotum, which is usually unilateral in

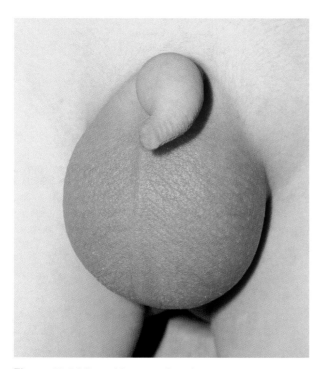

Figure 20.5 Idiopathic scrotal oedema.

distribution but which may occur bilaterally and may also extend upwards to involve the subcutaneous tissues of the inguinal region (Figure 20.5). Pain is minimal or absent. The diagnosis presents few problems to those acquainted with the condition.

Management

The condition settles spontaneously, usually within 24–48 hours. Antihistamines or antibiotics are sometimes prescribed but there is no evidence of benefit, and in general no specific treatment is required.

Other acute scrotal conditions

Incarcerated hernia

In infancy, scrotal swelling may be the most striking visible manifestation of an inguinoscrotal hernia. Palpation will distinguish between an inguinoscrotal hernia (which extends from the inguinal region to the scrotum) and true intrascrotal pathology.

Acute hydrocoele

A tense, rapidly developing hydrocoele can give rise to diagnostic uncertainty. However, acute hydrocoeles

are rarely painful (unless associated with underlying pathology of the testis). Transillumination confirms the diagnosis.

Henoch–Schönlein vasculitis

Involvement of the testis, giving rise to tenderness, swelling and scrotal discoloration, is a well documented complication of Henoch–Schönlein vasculitis. The presence of a purpuric rash should give the clue to the diagnosis and thus avert unnecessary surgical intervention.

Key points

- Torsion of the testis accounts for 90% of acutely presenting scrotal symptoms in postpubertal boys and adolescents. **Urgent surgical exploration is mandatory unless there is compelling evidence of an alternative diagnosis.**
- Most cases of so-called 'neonatal' torsion have actually occurred in utero and the affected testis is almost invariably non-viable.
- Torsion of a testicular appendage (hydatid of Morgagni) in a prepubertal boy can be managed conservatively provided a confident diagnosis has been made by an experienced clinician.
- Epididymo-orchitis is uncommon in childhood and always merits investigation of the urinary tract.

Further reading

Bartsch G, Frank S, Marbeger J, Mikuz G. Testicular torsion: late results with special regard to fertility and endocrine function. *J Urol* 1980; 124: 375–378

Ben-Chaim, J, Leibovitch, I, Ramon, J et al. Etiology of acute scrotum at surgical exploration in children, adolescents and adults. *Eur Urol* 1992; 21: 45–47

Ben-Chaim J, Pinthus JH. Testicular torsion. *European Board of Urology Update Series* 1998; 7: 39–44

Burge DM. Neonatal testicular torsion and infarction: aetiology and management. *Br J Urol* 1987; 59: 70–73

Nour S, MacKinnon AE. Acute scrotal swelling in children. *J Roy Coll Surg Edin* 1991; 36: 392–394

Puri P, Barton D, O'Donnell B. Prepubertal testicular torsion: subsequent fertility. *J Pediatr Surg* 1985; 20: 598–601

Schutte N, Becker H, Vydra G. Exocrine and endocrine testicular function following unilateral torsion – a retrospective clinical study of 36 patients. *Urologe Ausgabe A* 1986; 25: 142–146

Intersex and paediatric gynaecology

21

Henri Lottman

Introduction

The newborn infant with ambiguous genitalia represents a rare and potentially urgent diagnostic problem. Congenital adrenal hyperplasia (CAH), the most important intersex condition, is associated with disorders of adrenal metabolism which may pose a threat to the survival of the affected infant. Even when the underlying condition does not carry this risk, it is important to investigate every infant with ambiguous genitalia without delay. This is best achieved by involving a specialised multidisciplinary team comprising a paediatric endocrinologist, urologist, radiologist, biologist and geneticist. Transfer to a specialist centre may be required if the relevant specialist expertise is not available locally. Parents should be advised against registering the birth of a child with ambiguous genitalia until the diagnosis has been established and agreement reached on the assignment of gender.

Although the overall incidence of intersex disorders is low it is subject to geographical variation, for example there is a relatively high incidence of true hermaphroditism in South Africa and of 5α-reductase deficiency in the Dominican Republic.

Normal sexual differentiation

A knowledge of the embryological development of the internal and external genital tracts is essential in understanding intersex states. The embryology of the genital tracts has already been considered in Chapter 1 but to facilitate understanding of this chapter the key elements are summarised again:

1. The precursors of the gonads, genital ducts and external genitalia are present in an identical undifferentiated state in both 46XX and 46XY embryos until around the 6th week of gestation.
2. The genital tract of the embryo and fetus is genetically programmed to develop by a process of passive differentiation down a female phenotypic pathway, unless positively switched into a pattern of male phenotypic differentiation by the influence of certain genetic and endocrine factors.
3. With the exception of true hermaphrodites (individuals with both testicular and ovarian gonadal tissue) intersex abnormalities fall into two broad categories:
   - Inappropriate virilisation of a 46XX fetus owing to intrauterine exposure to virilising agents (female pseudohermaphroditism);
   - Incomplete virilisation of a 46XY fetus (male pseudohermaphroditism).

Differentiation of the male genital tract

Testis

Differentiation of the testis commences at around 6 weeks, when the gonadal primordium situated at the anterior aspect of the mesonephros is colonised by extraembryonic primordial germ cells. The process of differentiation is initiated during the 7th week, when the pre-Sertoli cells aggregate to form the seminiferous tubules secreting the glycoprotein hormone müllerian inhibitory substance. Leydig cells appear at around 8–9 weeks, increasing until 12–14 weeks, when their number remains stable until 24 weeks before declining. At birth the tesis contains relatively few Leydig cells, a state that persists until puberty, when there is proliferation of Leydig cells within the pubertal testis.

Internal genitalia

In the undifferentiated state the genital ducts of both XX and XY embryos comprise the mesonephric (wolffian) and paramesonephric (müllerian) ducts. Regression of the müllerian ducts in the male begins at 8 weeks in response to müllerian inhibitory substance, and is complete by 10–12 weeks. Under the influence of androgens secreted by the fetal testis each mesonephric duct develops into epididymis, vas deferens and seminal vesicle. The prostatic bud develops around the distal end of the mesonephric ducts at approximately 11–13 weeks. The prostatic utricule forms at the junction of the paired mesonephric ducts and the urogenital sinus (Figure 21.1).

External genitalia

The undifferentiated state of the external genitalia in both XX and XY embryos comprises a genital tubercle, and a urogenital groove surrounded by urethral folds and labioscrotal swellings. Without exposure to androgenic stimulation the external genitalia of a XY fetus are destined to retain these features and hence develop into the external genitalia of a female phenotype. Conversely, in the presence of circulating androgens the genital tubercle elongates and the urethral folds fuse over the urethral groove to create the penile urethra surrounded by the corpus spongiosus; meanwhile, the genital swellings fuse posteriorly to form the scrotum. Male anatomical differentiation is essentially complete by the 13th week of gestation, except for testicular descent (see Chapter 1) and further penile growth and development, which continues from 20 weeks to term.

Differentiation of the female genital tract

Ovary

Differentiation is triggered around the 6th week of gestation by the interaction of the primordial germ cells and the mesenchymal tissue of the genital ridge. Oögonia enter the meiotic phase at 12–13 weeks, and all the germ cells have entered the meiotic prophase by 7 months. The oöcytes then remain in a state of arrested division until the onset of puberty. From the 12th week of gestation the fetal granulosa cells produce oestrogens.

(a)

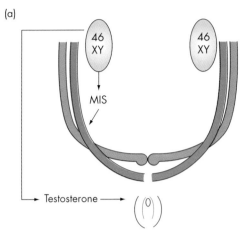

(b)

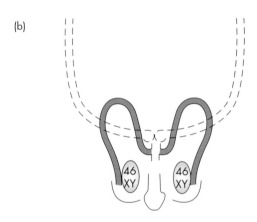

Figure 21.1 Normal male development. (a) Undifferentiated state. (b) Regression of paramesonephric ducts (red) under the influence of MIS, and persistence of mesonephric ducts (blue) in response to localised testosterone secretion by the fetal testis. Virilisation of external genitalia by circulating androgens.

Internal genitalia

The mesonephric ducts undergo spontaneous degeneration at around 10 weeks, while the paramesonephric ducts develop into the fallopian tubes, the uterus and the upper vagina. The lower vagina is derived from urogenital sinus. Separation of the urethra and vagina results from downgrowth towards the perineum of the junction of the paired paramesonephric ducts and urogenital sinus at the level of the sinuvaginal bulb (Figure 21.2).

External genitalia

Differentiation of the genitalia to the female phenotype occurs without any known requirement for

(a)

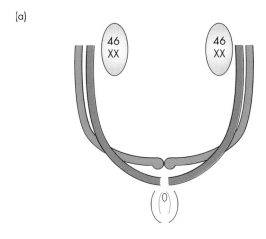

(b)

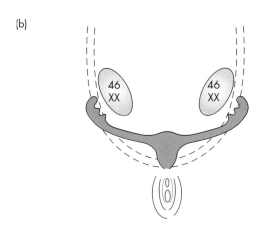

Figure 21.2 Normal female development. (a) Undifferentiated state. (b) Persistence of paramesonephric duct derivatives (no exposure to MIS). Spontaneous regression of meonephric ducts. Passive differention of external genitalia to female phenotype.

endocrine stimulation, and begins with the formation of a dorsal commissure between the labioscrotal swellings. The genital tubercle persists as the clitoris, and the urethral folds become the labia minora and the labioscrotal swellings the labia majora.

The role of sex-determining genes

Determination of sexual differentiation in mammalian species is governed primarily by the presence of genes located on the Y chromosome. Of these, by far the most important is the testis-determining gene, which is located at the distal part of the short arm of the Y chromosome and has been named *SRY* (sex-determining region Y). Although the *SRY* gene is ultimately responsible for intiating testicular differentiation, many

downstream genes located on the sex chromosomes and autosomes are also involved in the complex sequence of subsequent events contributing to the embryological development of the genital tracts.

It has been thought that in the absence of the Y chromosome the gonad adopts a default pattern of differentiation to form an ovary. Evidence is emerging, however, indicating that this is not an entirely passive process and that normal ovarian differentiation is dependent on the presence of the paired X chromosomes. In particular, survival of the germ cells requires the presence of two X chromosomes. In 45XO female patients (Turner's syndrome) the ovaries degenerate into fibrous streaks containing no surviving germ cells.

Phenotypic sex differentiation

Experimental studies conducted by Jost and Josso in animals such as the rabbit and rat have provided a detailed picture of the endocrine factors implicated in male sex differentiation. As already indicated, müllerian inhibitory substance and androgens play key roles which can be summarised as follows:

- **Müllerian inhibitory substance (MIS)** Produced within the testis by the Sertoli cells, MIS, a glycopeptide, induces resorption of the müllerian (paramesonephric) ducts, stimulates the Leydig cells, and is implicated in the initial phase of testicular descent. The genes coding for MIS and its receptor have been mapped on chomosomes 19 and 12, respectively.
- **Testosterone and dihydrotestosterone** Testosterone, secreted by the Leydig cells of the embryonic testis, is responsible for maintenance of the mesonephric ducts and virilisation of the urogenital sinus and external genitalia. The production of testosterone by the fetal testis is detectable at 9 weeks, with a peak around 15–18 weeks and then a sharp fall. Testosterone is released into the bloodstream, enters target cells and is converted to dihydrotestosterone (DHT) by the enzyme 5α-reductase. DHT binds to androgen receptors with a greater affinity than does testosterone. The androgen receptors are coded by genes located on the X chromosome. A local source of androgen is essential for mesonephric duct development, which does not occur if testosterone is supplied only via the peripheral circulation (as in female pseudohermaphroditism due to adrenal hyperplasia). The

fetus is exposed to high levels of maternal and intrinsic **gonadotrophins**, and also to **oestrogens** of fetal and maternal origin. Their role in sexual differentiation is ill understood.

Classification of intersex states

Intersex disorders are generally the outcome of hormonal dysfunction, which may result from a variety of underlying causes, including:

● Chromosomal abnormalities or gene mutations;
● Endocrine abnormalities due to exposure to excessive or inadequate hormone levels;

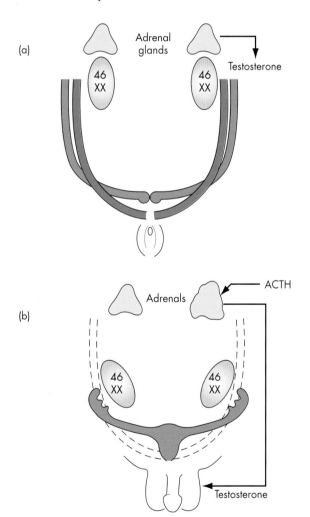

Figure 21.3 Congenital adrenal hyperplasia. (a) Undifferentiated state. (b) Persistence of paramesonephric duct derivatives (no exposure to MIS). Regression of mesonephric ducts (no localised secretion of testosterone by the gonad–ovary). Virilisation of external genitalia caused by circulating adrenal-derived testosterone.

● Insensitivity of target tissues to hormones, as either a receptor deficiency or an intracellular defect.

Occasionally the cause cannot be established, such cases presumably representing a defective component of sexual differentiation which has yet to be identified.

The intersex disorders are conventionally classified as follows:

● **Female pseudohermaphroditism** – virilisation of a 46XX female;
● **Male pseudohermaphroditism** – inadequate virilisation of a 46XY male;
● **Gonadal dysgenesis** – a spectrum of gonadal and genital abnormalities associated with absence of one of the pair of sex chromosomes, e.g. 45XO, 45XO/46XY, and often present in mosaic form (see Chapter 1);
● **True hermaphroditism** – 46XX/46XY – i.e. ovarian and testicular tissue present in the same individual and with a variable phenotype.

Female pseudohermaphroditism

This group of intersex abnormalities consists almost entirely of 46XX females whose external genitalia have been virilised by intrauterine exposure to androgens at a critical phase in differentiation (Figure 21.3). Affected individuals have ambiguous external genitalia but normal ovaries and internal genitalia (fallopian tubes, uterus, upper vagina).

Virilisation by androgens of fetal origin
Congenital adrenal hyperplasia (CAH)

CAH is not only the most common cause of female pseudohermaphroditism but also accounts for approximately 85% of all infants with ambigouous genitalia. The disorder can arise as a result of one of three enzymatic defects occurring at different points on the biosynthetic pathways for the production of cortisol and aldosterone in the adrenal gland. All three result in ACTH-stimulated overproduction of androgenic precursors (Figure 21.4).

● **21-Hydroxylase deficiency** is the most common form of CAH (estimated incidence 1:15 000 births) and is an autosomal recessive disorder associated with a mutation of a gene located on chromosome 6. The diagnostic feature is elevation

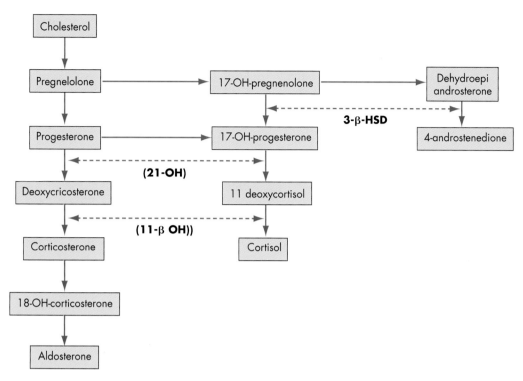

Figure 21.4 Congenital adrenal hyperplasia. Sites of enzyme block in metabolic pathway.

of plasma 17α-hydroxy progesterone. Prenatal diagnosis is possible and treatment has been described using dexamethasone to supress the fetal pituitary–adrenal axis from the 9th to the 17th weeks of gestation.

Fifty per cent of cases are complicated by a salt-losing statem which may represent a potentially life-threatening neonatal emergency. Management comprises gluco- and mineralocorticoid replacement therapy, female gender assignment and feminising genitoplasty. **11β-Hydroxylase deficiency** is a rare cause of CAH associated with severe virilisation, salt retention and potassium loss with, in some instances, hypoglycaemia and impaired stress response. The diagnosis is based on the elevation of plasma levels of 11-desoxy-cortisol.

Prenatal diagnosis is feasible in the siblings and the offspring of affected individuals. Sex determination and a range of genetic studies with gene probes for CAH can be performed on fetal cells obtained by chorionic villus sampling or amniocentesis. In addition, the external genitalia of a 46XX fetus can be assessed with ultrasound for evidence

of virilisation. Prenatal treatment has been reported, consisting of the administration of dexamethasone to the mother with the aim of suppressing the fetal pituitary–adrenal axis.

3β-Hydroxysteroid dehydrogenase deficiency is the rarest form. Virilisation is moderately severe, but salt loss and hyponatraemia are severe. Plasma dehydroepiandrosterone 17OH pregnenolone and ACTH (adrenocorticotrophic hormone) are both elevated. The management is similar to that for 21-hydroxylase deficiency.

- **Aromatase deficiency** This oestrogen synthetase enzyme is present in particularly high concentrations in the placenta and is involved in the synthesis of oestrogens from androgenic precursors. Deficiency of this enzyme results in an accumulation of androgens and consequent fetal virilisation.

Virilisation by androgens of maternal origin

This is a rare cause of female pseudohermaphroditism, possible factors being **androgen-secreting tumours of the adrenal or ovary,** and **maternal treatment with progestational agents.**

Other virilising anomalies of the external genitalia in 46XX females

These rare anomalies have a teratogenic rather than an endocrine aetiology. Examples include isolated clitoral hypertrophy, or abnormalities associated with urogenital sinus and cloacal anomalies.

Male pseudohermaphroditism

In this group of disorders 46XY male infants exhibit varying degrees of inadequate virilisation which can be ascribed either to defects in androgen production or metabolism or to abnormalities of receptor sensitivity in the target tissues.

Defects of testosterone production

These may be the outcome of rare testicular abnormalities such as testicular dysgenesis or Leydig cell aplasia. Alternatively, the testes may be morphologically normal but the production of testosterone is impaired by an enzymatic block in the biosynthetic pathway.

Defects of testosterone metabolism

The enzyme 5α-reductase is responsible for converting testosterone to the more potent androgen dihydrotestosterone. 5α-Reductase deficiency is responsible for a particular pattern of virilisation defects found in inbred communities in the Dominican Republic, and, rarely, in certain other parts of the world.

Defects of receptor sensitivity

Failure of virilisation can occur despite the presence of normal levels of testosterone and/or dihydrotestosterone if the target tissues are resistant to androgens.

Androgen insensitivity syndrome is inherited as an X-linked recessive disorder associated with a mutation on the long arm of the X chromosome. In the complete form (previously termed testicular feminisation syndrome) the external genitalia are phenotypically female. In contrast, the internal genitalia have differentiated normally down a male pathway in response to MIS secreted by the fetal testis. Typically the condition is discovered during the investigation of primary amenorrhoea, or following the discovery of a testis during hernia surgery in a girl. Partial androgen insensitivity has a broad phenotypic spectrum.

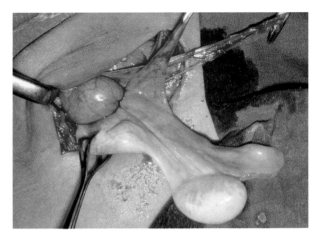

Figure 21.5 Laparotomy findings in a case of MIS deficiency. Intra-abdominal testes, persistence of paramesonephric duct structures – vestigal fallopian tubes and uterus.

Abnormalities of MIS activity

Deficiency of MIS or insensitivity of MIS receptors result in an externally masculinised 46XY male with internal genitalia derived from persistent müllerian structures (uterus, tubes, upper vagina) (Figure 21.5). The condition usually comes to light during a surgical procedure for cryptorchidism or inguinal hernia. The diagnosis is confirmed by measuring circulating MIS: the level is low in case of MIS gene mutation and high in cases where there is a mutation of the gene encoding for the MIS receptor.

Idiopathic male pseudohermaphroditism

In up to 50% of cases no genetic or hormonal abnormality is identifiable. In such instances the malformation of the genitalia may be attributed to teratogenic factors, to mutations in yet unknown genes, or to genes acting downstream of androgen or MIS receptors.

Gonadal dysgenesis

Dysgenesis is a term applied to a fundamental abnormality of gonadal development in which the degenerate testis or ovary persist as a non-functioning 'streak' gonad. In a 46XY fetus the failure of the dysgenetic testes to produce testosterone and müllerian inhibiting substance results in an entirely female phenotype. Partial gonadal dysgenesis may be unilateral or bilateral, and so gives rise to varying degrees of sexual ambiguity.

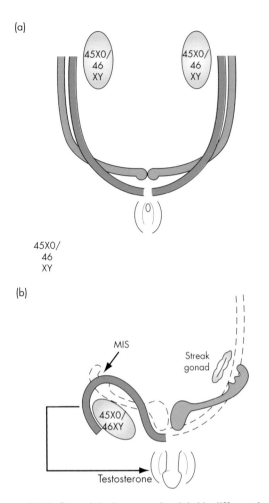

(a)

45XO/
46
XY

45XO/
46
XY

45XO/
46
XY

(b)

MIS

Streak
gonad

45XO/
46XY

Testosterone

Figure 21.6 Gonadal dysgenesis. (a) Undifferentiated state. (b) Varying embryological patterns and phenotypes. For example, non-functional streak gonad with persistence of paramesonephric structures (left). Mosaicism, right gonad, with male internal genital tract owing to presence of Y chromosome and MIS and testosterone production. Incomplete external virilisation.

Mixed gonadal dysgenesis is most commonly the result of 45XO/46XY mosaicism. A mixed phenotype ensues, for example an inguinal testis (with limited endocrine function) on one side accompanied by a contralateral dysgenetic streak gonad with persistent müllerian derivatives. Affected individuals are characterised by virilisation defects of varying severity (Figure 21.6). Ovarian dysgenesis (Turner's syndrome, 45XO or 45XO/46XX mosaicism) does not result in sexual ambiguity. Streak or dysgenetic gonads carry a significantly increased risk of malignant change.

True hermaphroditism

True hermaphroditism is a variant of gonadal dysgenesis in which the individual possesses both testicular and ovarian tissue, either in separate gonads or coexisting in the same gonad as an ovotestis.

The genitalia are invariably ambiguous. Several karyotypes have been documented, including 46XX/46XY, 46XX and 46XY. The diagnosis is suggested by exclusion of other causes of intersex and is confirmed by macroscopic and microscopic examination of the gonads. The choice of sex of rearing may raise difficulties. In case of female rearing, spontaneous puberty may occur and even pregnancy; in case of male rearing, pubertal development may require sex hormone therapy and there is a significant risk of gonadal malignancy.

Investigation of an intersex case

In the newborn period the aims are twofold:

- To recognise any life-threatening underlying metabolic disorder (notably congenital adrenal hyperplasia);
- To establish a precise diagnosis so as to permit an informed decision on gender assignment. Legal registration of the birth should not be performed until such investigation is complete.

Clinical evaluation

History should include an enquiry about siblings and other family members and details of the pregnancy.

Examination of the newborn should focus on:

- Appearances of the external genitalia, assessment of the degree of virilisation and the presence of pigmentation (favouring a diagnosis of CAH) (Figure 21.7);
- The presence or absence of palpable gonads;
- Associated extragenital abnormalities (as indicative of a probable teratogenic aetiology).

Laboratory investigations

In addition to routine initial investigations (karyotype, 17OH progesterone and plasma electrolytes) more detailed evaluation may include plasma testosterone (basal and post-hCG (human

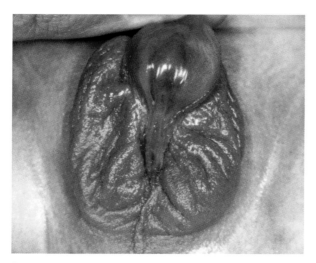

Figure 21.7 Ambiguous genitalia in a newborn infant. Empty scrotum and severe hypospadias.

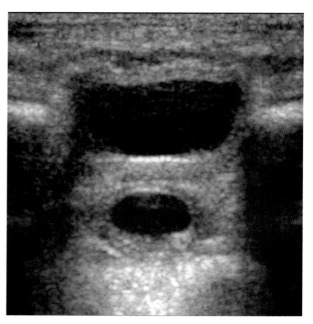

Figure 21.8 Pelvic ultrasound. Transverse view illustrating the bladder (top) and dilated müllerian structure lying posteriorly.

chorionic gonadotrophin) stimulation), steroid assay, e.g. 11-deoxycortisol, MIS levels, DNA analysis to look for specific gene mutations, and studies of binding capacity and androgen receptor activity in genital skin fibroblasts.

Diagnostic imaging

Ultrasound is aimed at identifying gonads and/or a uterus within the pelvis. An enlarged müllerian remnant can often be visualised in the undervirilised male (Figure 21.8).

Genitogram Also termed a 'sinogram', this contrast study is performed via a catheter introduced into the urethra, vagina or the opening of a common urogenital sinus. It demonstrates the anatomy of the urogenital sinus and the junction of the vagina/müllerian structure and lower urinary tract (Figure 21.9). This information is of value when planning the surgical approach to genital reconstruction. In addition, it may be possible to visualise the uterine cervix, uterine canal, fallopian tube(s) or vas deferens.

Surgical investigations

In addition to the information yielded by non-invasive investigations, diagnostic surgical intervention is often required:

- Endoscopy of the lower urinary and genital tracts;
- Laparoscopy to identify internal structures (uterus, tubes, gonads); and eventually
- Pelvic laparotomy and biopsy of the gonads.

Diagnostic features of intersex disorders

Where the abnormal physical findings are confined to ambiguous genitalia with no palpable gonads the diagnosis is most likely to be **congenital adrenal hyperplasia**. An elevated plasma level of 17OH progesterone associated with positive visualisation of a uterus and ovaries on ultrasound is confirmatory. Although an emergency buccal smear for sex chromatin determination (positive in case of CAH) can also be performed, modern techniques of karyotyping are preferable and will provide rapid authoritative confirmation of an XX genotype within 48–72 hours. A contrast genitogram will define the level of confluence of the vagina with the urogenital sinus.

The finding of palpable gonads in conjunction with an abnormal sex chromosome karyotype (typically 45XO/46XY) points to a diagnosis of **mixed gonadal dysgenesis** or some form of **true hermaphroditism** (e.g. 46XX/46XY), whereas a normal male 46XY karyotype suggests **partial androgen insensitivity**. The presence or absence of müllerian structures (uterus, fallopian tubes) indicates a lack of müllerian inhibiting substance consistent with a diagnosis of **gonadal dysgenesis** or **true hermaphroditism**. The absence of müllerian structures (reflecting the activity

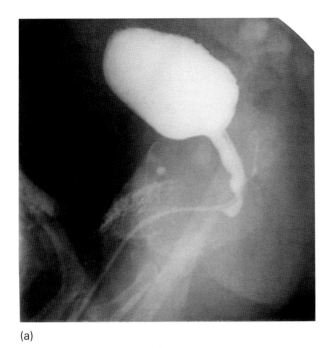

(a)

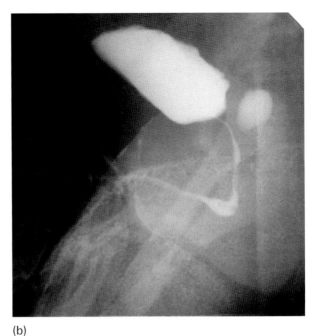

(b)

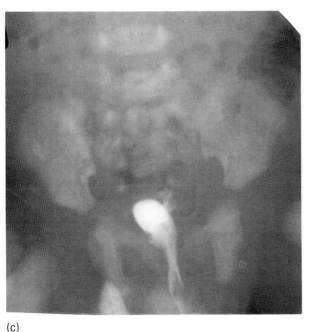

(c)

Figure 21.9 Contrast sinogram (genitogram). (a) Injection of contrast through a catheter positioned too low in the urethra/urogenital sinus may fail to fill the müllerian structure. (b,c) Visualisation of müllerian structure in relation to the lower urinary tract.

of MIS) indicates a diagnosis of **male pseudohermaphroditism** due to **androgen insensitivity** or, rarely, a block in testosterone synthesis.

Gender assignment

This is the defining step in management of an intersex case. **The decision on the sex of rearing should be delayed until a precise diagnosis has been established and the functional potential of the genitalia adequately assessed.** This may take some time, particularly when it is necessary to await the outcome of hCG tests or assessment of the potential for penile development in response to androgen stimulation.

Advice on gender should be carefully considered before it is communicated sympathetically to the parents by the key members of the multidisciplinary team. At that time, the plan of further management should be detailed as precisely as possible. Once a decision on gender has been agreed it is vital that no uncertainty should persist about the sex of rearing of the child (e.g. ambiguous first names should be avoided).

Although management may have to be individualised according to the particular features of each case, the following broad generalisations apply to the more common categories of intersex anomalies:

- **Female pseudohermaphroditism** (mostly virilised females with CAH). These individuals have normal female internal genitalia, normal ovaries and a normal expectation for fertility. Female sex of rearing is invariably advised, and only in the most exceptional circumstances (e.g. late presentation with established male identity) would it be appropriate to consider male gender assignment.
- **Male pseudohermaphroditism** Female gender assignment is generally advised where the external genitalia are predominantly female and there is no realistic prospect of constructing a functional phallus. The presence of androgen insensitivity strengthens the case for female sex of rearing. By contrast, where there is a significantly male phenotype and where a positive stimulation test indicates responsiveness to androgens, male gender assignment is preferable. Typically the phenotype in such cases is characterised by severe hypospadias and bilateral cryptorchidism.
- **Mixed gonadal dysgenesis and true hermaphroditism** In both conditions the sex of rearing depends on the phenotype (notably the size of the phallus) and upon the potential for androgen production as revealed by stimulation tests. In practice, female assignment is usually judged the better option, but a male sex of rearing may be considered appropriate if the phallus is amenable to reconstruction and functioning gonadal tissue is predominantly testicular.
- **Isolated deficiency of müllerian inhibitory substance** With the exception of bilateral cryptorchidism and the persistence of some internal müllerian remnants, the phenotype is male. Affected individuals are reared as males.

Cultural considerations may impinge upon the decision regarding sex of rearing. For example, in some situations parents and their medical advisers may believe it is better for a highly virilised female pseudohermaphrodite to be raised as a male. Conversely, in some communities an affected individual may find it easier to lead an independent adult life as an undervirilised male than as a sterile female.

Surgical management

Once the sex of rearing has been determined with the parents, appropriate surgical correction of the genital abnormalities should be planned, with the timing being dependant on the nature and severity of the genital abnormality and the preference of the surgeon. As a rule, feminising genitoplasty should be undertaken during the first 6 months of life, and masculinising genitoplasty completed between the ages of 6 and 18 months.

The steps in **masculinising genitoplasty** comprise:

- **Hormonal treatment** with testosterone preparations to stimulate phallic enlargement;
- **Excision of müllerian structures**;
- **Phalloplasty** Surgical reconstruction of the severe hypospadias combines correction of chordee to achieve a straight penis and urethroplasty to create an orthotopic meatus. In addition, transposition of scrotal skin may be required to overcome the 'buried' phallus and to improve the overall cosmetic appearances of the genitalia;
- **Orchidopexy** is frequently required (see below).

The key steps involved in **feminising genitoplasty** include:

- **Clitoroplasty** to reduce the size of the glans and shaft. This is achieved by combining excision of corporal erectile tissue with preservation of the neurovascular bundles so as to maintain normal sensation of the glans (Figure 21.10).
- **Vaginoplasty and labioplasty** Surgery consists of separating the vagina and urethra from the common urogenital sinus to create two separate perineal orifices (Figure 21.11). The introitus and vagina should be adequate to permit normal menstruation and intercourse in adult life. Flaps of 'scrotalised' skin are fashioned so as to create as far as possible normal labial appearances (Figures 21.12, 21.13). Vaginoplasty may be technically challenging in cases when the vagina opens high in the urogenital sinus. A number of surgical techniques have been advocated to overcome this problem, including perineal, abdominal or anterior sagittal transanorectal approaches (ASTRA).

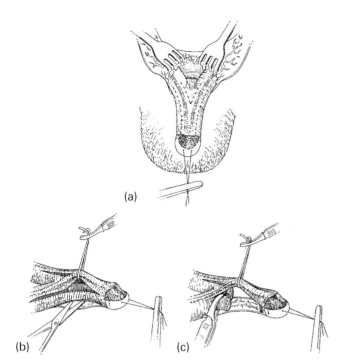

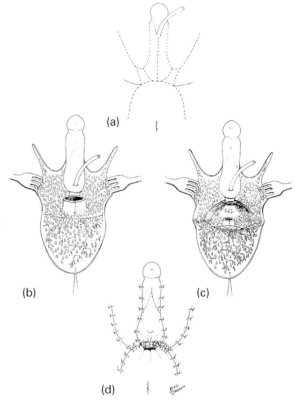

Figure 21.10 Feminising genitoplasty: clitoroplasty. (a) Exposure of the corpora and neurovascular bundles. (b) Mobilisation of the neurovascular bundles. (c) Resection of erectile tissue (the corporal bodies).

Figure 21.11 Feminising genitoplasty: vaginoplasty. (a) Lines of incision. (b) Exposure of low-lying vagina. (c) Exposure of high vagina. (d) Completed vaginoplasty and labioplasty.

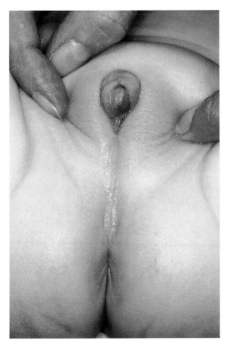

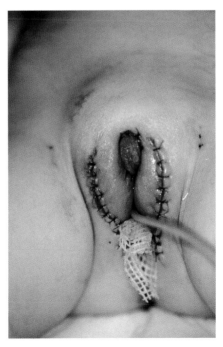

Figure 21.12 Feminising genitoplasty for congenital adrenal hyperplasia: preoperative appearances.

Figure 21.13 Following completion of the procedure in the patient in Figure 21.13.

Alternatively, as the vagina serves no functional role in a prepubertal girl surgical correction of the 'high vagina' may be deferred until after puberty. Genital skin is more robust and amenable to flap formation at that age, and the relative anatomy of the vagina and perineum may be more favourable than in infancy.

CAH is the most common indication for feminising genitoplasty. In conditions not associated with external virilisation and where the vagina is a absent or grossly atretic, it is generally agreed that vaginoplasty should be deferred until after puberty.

Gonadal management

- **Female pseudohermaphrodites** The ovaries are normal and no specific treatment is required.
- **Male pseudohermaphrodites** Where female gender is assigned (as in complete androgen insensitivity) the testes should be removed, although the timing of orchidectomy is subject to debate. Where it is decided to rear an affected individual as a male, orchidopexy is performed to bring the testes to the scrotum.
- In **mixed gonadal dysgenesis** and **true hermaphroditism** gonadal biopsy may be required to define the nature and distribution of the different gonadal tissues. Streak (dysgenetic) gonads are excised, whereas gonadal tissue concordant with the sex of rearing is conserved. Sex hormone replacement therapy may be needed at and after puberty.

In view of the high risk of malignancy after puberty any retained testicular tissue should be placed surgically within the scrotum to facilitate careful monitoring. This is particularly important in cases of gonadal dysgenesis or true hermaphroditism. Lifelong follow-up is required, involving autopalpation, ultrasound and, eventually, postpubertal testicular biopsy for evidence of carcinoma in situ.

Long-term outcome

This is considered in Chapter 23.

Gynaecological disorders of childhood

Symptoms relating to the external genitalia of prepubertal girls are common and often generate considerable parental anxiety. A balanced approach is required to avoid causing unnecessary distress by overinvesti-

gating healthy children while recognising those clinical features that may denote more significant pathology.

'Vulvovaginitis'

Strictly speaking the term vulvitis is more accurate in most cases, as true vaginitis is rare in childhood whereas non-specific inflammation of the non-oestrogenised prepubertal skin of the intoitus and vulva is very common. Irritation and itching are the dominant symptoms, accompanied by localised dysuria and slight discharge.

Many parents interpret the symptoms of vulvitis as evidence of 'cystitis' or of urinary infection. It is therefore important to enquire specifically about those aspects of the history, such as frequency, fever, suprapubic or loin pain, which help to distinguish genuine urinary infection from localised vulvitis (although the two diagnoses may sometimes coexist).

Hyperaemia of the vulval skin may be apparent if there is florid active inflammation, but examination generally reveals normal external genitalia.

Treatment is aimed at correcting any identifiable predisposing causes, such as poor perineal hygiene, tight-fitting clothes and threadworm infestation. Antibiotic treatment is sometimes effective and may be justified on an occasional short-term basis where symptoms are severe (although culture swabs generally reveal a mixed growth of perineal commensal flora).

Longer-term antibiotic usage should be avoided. Similarly, the use of antimicrobial pessaries is inappropriate in children. Unfortunately, some girls continue to experience troublesome episodes of symptomatic non-specific vulvitis despite a range of simple preventative measures. Reassurance and an explanation of the aetiology and self-limiting nature of the condition is often helpful in allaying parental anxiety.

Labial adhesions

These are inflammatory in aetiology and are a consequence of vulvitis. The condition presents most commonly between the ages of 2 and 6 years. Gentle separation of the labia majora reveals flimsy midline fusion of the labia minora occluding part or most of the introitus.

In time, labial adhesions always resolve spontaneously. However, active measures to separate the adhesions may be indicated if anxious parents seek positive reassurance that their daughter's genitalia are normal. Active intervention is also justified if occlusion of the introitus by labial adhesions results in dribbling of urine which has pooled in the vagina.

The simplest **treatment** comprises a 7–10 day course of an oestrogen or topical steroid cream applied to the area of adhesions. Alternatively, where it is thought justifiable to intervene surgically, the adherent labia are separated with a probe or pair of artery forceps under general anaesthesia. Parents should be warned that recurrent adhesions are not uncommon.

Vaginal discharge

A copious or purulent vaginal discharge is uncommon and should be investigated. Possible causes include a vaginal foreign body, specific bacterial infections and perineal ectopic ureter. Although vaginal **rhabdomyosarcoma** typically presents with a bloody discharge, this is not always the case. Depending upon the clinical picture, initial investigation generally includes ultrasound imaging of the pelvis and urinary tract and examination under anaesthesia. The possibility of **sexual abuse** and **sexually transmitted infection** should be considered and the relevant bacteriological examinations performed (i.e. for *Neisseria gonorrhoeae*) at the time of the examination under anaesthesia.

Vaginal bleeding

Although inflammation of the vulval region may occasionally be associated with slight spotting of blood on the underclothes, the passage of frank blood or a bloodstained vaginal discharge is potentially an ominous sign demanding prompt investigation at a specialist centre.

Rhabdomyosarcoma of the vagina (sarcoma botryoides) is a tumour of infancy and early childhood, whereas uterine rhabdomyosarcomas occur from the teens onward. Other causes of vaginal bleeding include **trauma**, **foreign body**, **vascular malformations** and **precocious puberty**.

Congenital anomalies of the vagina

In girls with **imperforate hymen** the vagina is obstructed but otherwise embryologically normal. Accumulation of secretions within the obstructed vagina and/or uterus (hydocolpos or hydrometrocolpos) characteristically presents clinically as a bulging introital mass in the newborn period, or as primary amenorrhoea (or occasionally urinary retention) in pubertal or postpubertal girls. Nowadays the distended vaginal and/or uterine mass may be detected on prenatal ultrasound. Treatment comprises incision of the hymenal membrane.

Vaginal agenesis (Mayer–Rokitansky syndrome) occurs as an isolated anomaly or, more often, as part of a spectrum of congenital abnormalities resulting from abnormalities of paramesonephric and mesonephric duct development. Depending upon the extent of the vaginal agenesis the external genitalia may appear normal or the vaginal opening may be represented as a dimple. Mayer–Rokitansky syndrome is the most common cause of primary amenorrhoea.

Ovarian pathology

Streak gonads and ovarian dysgenesis are considered above. Unilateral ovarian agenesis may be associated with unilateral renal agenesis as an isolated anomaly, or as part of a more complex manifestation of the Mayer–Rokitansky syndrome.

Ovarian cysts in infants and young girls are generally benign follicular cysts. Small to medium-sized cysts (5 cm in diameter) detected incidentally on pre- or postnatal ultrasound can be managed expectantly and monitored with ultrasound. The management of larger, asymptomatic cysts is controversial, with the rationale for surgery hinging on diagnostic uncertainty and the risk of torsion.

The classification of ovarian tumours in children is beyond the scope of this book. Benign teratoma is the most common pathology, although malignancy can arise in any of the cell lines of which the teratoma is comprised. Some present acutely with torsion of the bulky ovarian mass (Figure 21.14).

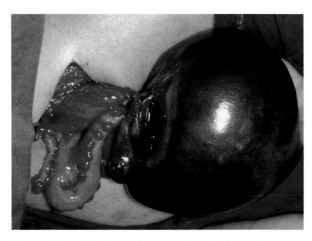

Figure 21.14 Torsion of a large (benign) ovarian cyst. Laparotomy findings.

Key points

- The management of intersex should be concentrated in the hands of specialised multidisciplinary teams working in collaboration with local paediatricians and primary care physicians.
- Errors in diagnosis or early management can have disastrous and lifelong consequences for affected individuals and their families. Gender should not be assigned until a firm diagnosis has been established and a clear plan of management defined.
- Congenital adrenal hyperplasia (CAH), causing virilisation of a 46XX fetus, is the most common form of ambiguous genitalia in western Europe, accounting for approximately 80–85% of cases. Affected individuals are almost invariably reared as females.
- Fifty per cent of newborns with CAH have the salt-losing form of the condition which, if unrecognised, is potentially life-threatening.
- Gonadal dysgenesis (associated with differing patterns of sex chromosome abnormalities) represents the second largest group. Sex of rearing and surgical management are individualised according to the phenotype and the potential for sexual function.
- Mild inflammatory vulvitis and labial adhesions are common in young girls. Simple measures are generally helpful but there is no uniformly effective treatment. Other gynaecological symptoms in this age group are uncommon and merit specialist referral for further investigation.

Further reading

Aaronson, IA. Sexual differentiation and intersexuality. In: Kelalis P, King L, Belman B (eds) *Clinical Pediatric Urology*. Philadelphia: Saunders, 1992; 977–1014

Gonzales ET. Gynaecological disorders in children. In: O'Donnell B, Koff SA (eds) *Pediatric urology*. Oxford: Butterworth–Heinemann, 1997; 834–844

Rappaport R, Forest MG. Disorders of sexual differentiation. In: Bertrand J, Rappaport R, Sizonenko PC (eds) *Pediatric Endocrinology*. Baltimore: Williams and Wilkins, 1993; 305–332

Rink RC, Adams MC. Feminising genoplasty: state of the art. *World J Urol* 1998: 16; 218–219

Schober JM. Feminizing genitoplasty for intersex. In: Stringer MD, Oldham KT, Mouriquand PDE, Howard ER (eds) *Pediatric surgery and urology: long-term outcomes*. London: WB Saunders, 1998; 549–558

Genitourinary malignancies 22

Patrick G Duffy

Topics covered
Wilms' tumour (nephroblastoma)

Rhabdomyosarcoma
Testicular tumours

Wilms' tumour (nephroblastoma)

Introduction

Nephroblastoma, with an incidence of 7 per 1 000 000 children per annum, accounts for 6–7% of all childhood cancers, and approximately 80–90 cases occur in the UK each year. Although Jessop performed the first nephrectomy in 1877, the tumour is named after Max Wilms, who described a group of children with this malignancy in 1889. Radiation treatment was originally described in 1915, however, the prognosis was much improved following Farber's introduction, in 1956, of actinomycin as a chemotherapeutic agent. The current 5-year survival rate, exceeding 90%, has been achieved by the judicious use of surgery, chemotherapy and radiotherapy. Such progress is a result of collaborative national and international clinical trials, including the National Wilms' Tumour Studies in the United States, the United Kingdom Wilms' Tumour Study and the International Society of Paediatric Oncology Trial.

Epidemiology/aetiology

Wilms' tumour is by far the most common renal neoplasm of childhood, although other forms do occur (Table 22.1). Clear cell sarcoma and rhabdoid tumour were once considered as part of the Wilms' tumour spectrum, but are now thought to be distinct entities. With the exception of clear cell sarcoma, which is commoner in boys, the sexes are equally affected.

The prevalence of Wilms' tumour is 50% higher among Afro-Caribbean children than those of other races. Cases usually arise sporadically, but some occur with 'predisposition' syndromes (Table 22.2), and

Table 22.1 Classification of childhood renal tumours

Benign	Malignant
Mesoblastic nephroma (< 1 year of age)	Wilms' tumour
Cystic nephroma	Clear cell sarcoma (bone secondaries)
Angiomyolipoma	Rhabdoid tumour (bone/brain secondaries)
Haemangioma/lymphangioma	Neuroblastoma (usually retroperitoneal)

Table 22.2 Syndromes predisposing to Wilms' tumour

Denys–Drash	Renal disease (glomerulosclerosis/male pseudohermaphrodite)
WAGR	Wilms' Andiridia Genitourinary malformation, mental Retardation
Beckwith–Weidemann	Macroglossia, omphalocoele, visceromegaly

others are associated with aniridia, hemihypertrophy, cryptorchidism and hypospadias as isolated anomalies.

At least three genes are associated with Wilms' tumour. Located on chromosomes 11p13, 11p15 and 16q, they are found mainly in children with the predisposition syndromes. Specific gene mutations are found in only some 10% of the sporadic Wilms' tumours that account for over 90% of cases. The peak age of presentation of sporadic Wilms' tumour is 3–4 years, but children with bilateral disease (5%) or a predisposition syndrome usually present earlier. Mesoblastic nephroma is a tumour that occurs only in those under 1 year of age.

Presentation

Nephroblastoma is the most common solid abdominal tumour of childhood and typically presents as a painless abdominal mass in an otherwise well child (Table 22.3). Pain is uncommon and usually results from bleeding into the tumour. Haematuria occurs in 10–15% of cases. Tumour rupture may result from minor trauma and so lead to presentation with an acute abdomen. A left varicocoele sometimes occurs in association with unusually large tumours. Hypertension is more often seen in mesoblastic nephroma.

Symptoms of metastatic spread are rare. Ultrasound alone can confirm the diagnosis of Wilms' tumour in most instances, although occasionally the appearances are mimicked by xanthogranulomatous pyelonephritis, a chronic inflammatory reaction within the kidney usually associated with renal calculi. This latter condition also presents with a large renal mass, but typically with a long-standing history of listlessness and with a finding of anaemia (see Chapter 12).

Investigations

The routine tests for malignancy are performed (Table 22.4). Specific features to be assessed by ultrasound are extension of the tumour into the renal vein or inferior vena cava, and the blood lakes characteristic of bleeding into the tumour. CT scanning clearly demonstrates the renal origin of the tumour, as well as the anatomy of the opposite kidney, and contributes to assessment of tumour within the inferior vena cava which, if detected, should be treated by chemotherapy prior to surgery. Proteinuria may be indicative of the Denys–Drash syndrome, with a concomitant increased risk of bilateral disease. Wilms' tumour may occasionally manufacture an anti-von Willebrand factor leading to a bleeding disorder. The presence of elevated VMA (vanylmandelic acid) in the urine raises suspicion of neuroblastoma, a retroperitoneal tumour usually of non-renal origin.

Histopathology

Wilms' tumour histology falls into two categories:

* Favourable: triphasic nephroblastoma;
* Unfavourable: rhabdoid, clear cell and anaplastic lesions.

Table 22.3 Differential diagnosis – childhood abdominal mass

Benign	Malignant
Xanthogranulomatous pyelonephritis	Nephroblastoma
Large hydronephrosis	Neuroblastoma
Renal cysts	Hepatic tumour
Splenomegaly	Soft tissue sarcoma
Bowel duplication	

Table 22.4 Investigations for suspected Wilms' tumour

Abdominal ultrasound	– to include renal vein and inferior vena cava
Chest X-ray	– AP and lateral
CT scan	– abdomen and lungs
Urinalysis	– protein, vanylmandelic acid
Brain/bone scan	– clear cell sarcoma and rhabdoid tumours only
Blood count	– to include partial thromboplastin time

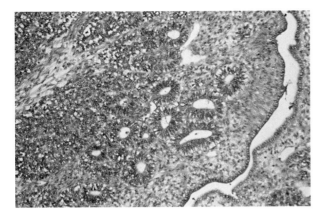

Figure 22.1 Triphasic nephroblastoma – 'favourable' histology.

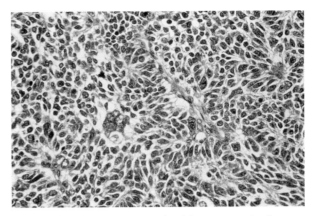

Figure 22.2 Anaplastic nephroblastoma – 'unfavourable' histology.

Classic Wilms' tumour, a triphasic nephroblastoma, comprises three elements, blastema, tubular cells and stroma (Figure 22.1), which is described as 'favourable histology' as it carries a generally good prognosis. Unfavourable histology, accounting for only 10% of tumours but 60% of deaths, has rhabdoid, clear cell or anaplastic features. The anaplastic group (Figure 22.2) takes two forms, diffuse and focal, with the focal variety having a relatively good prognosis. Nephroblastomatosis is a curious tumour-like condition consisting of small groups of mesoblastic cells with no pseudocapsule. These are assumed to be precursor lesions and are noted in all cases of bilateral Wilms' disease. They are also present in 28% of tumour specimens removed for unilateral Wilms' tumour.

Treatment

- Surgery
- Chemotherapy/radiotherapy.

Treatment is determined by tumour staging, which is based on histopathology, lymph node involvement and the completeness of surgical excision (Figures 22.3, 22.4). Management consists of surgery combined with

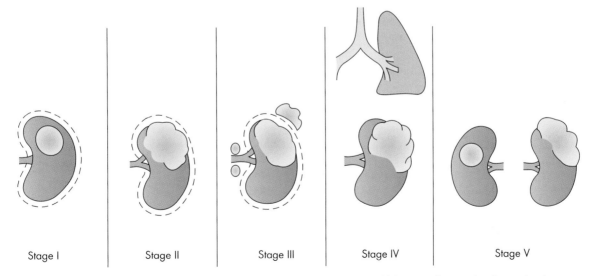

Stage I | Stage II | Stage III | Stage IV | Stage V

Figure 22.3 Staging of Wilms' tumour. Stage I: Tumour confined to the kidney and completely excised macro and microscopically. Stage II: Tumour extending beyond the kidney but completely excised macro- and microscopically. Tumour rupture and spill confined to flank. Stage III: Tumour (a) invading adjacent tissues and incompletely excised; (b) incompletely resected because of local invasion; (c) positive lymph nodes; (d) tumour spill not confined to the flank. Stage IV: Metastatic disease (usually pulmonary). Stage V: Bilateral Wilms' tumours.

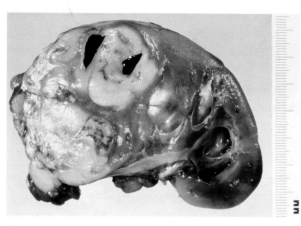

Figure 22.4 Nephrectomy specimen stage II Wilms' tumour. Localised penetration of renal capsule with some tumour extension. Full macroscopic and histological clearance achieved.

chemotherapy and, sometimes, radiotherapy. In unilateral disease, which accounts for 90% of cases, surgery is designed to remove the tumour and kidney intact, to inspect the contralateral kidney and to sample lymph nodes. The procedure is performed via a large transverse abdominal incision so as to expose both kidneys and to allow easy access to the inferior vena cava. After ensuring that no tumour is present in the contralateral kidney, the sequence of surgical steps comprises mobilisation of the colon, identification of the major vessels (i.e. aorta, inferior vena cava, renal artery and vein), ligation of the renal vessels after checking for tumour in the renal vein or inferior vena cava, and removal of the kidney and tumour without rupture (Figure 22.5). Depending on histopathology and surgical staging, a course of chemotherapy is instituted (Table 22.5), the drugs employed including vincristine, actinomycin D and doxorubicin. From 2002, all Wilms' tumours will be managed with pre-operative chemotherapy in the UK. Radiotherapy is used to treat gross abdominal disease and lung secondaries which have not fully responded to chemotherapy.

Complex simultaneous cardiac surgery is occasionally required for cases where inferior vena cava tumour extension has not responded to chemotherapy.

Bilateral Wilms' tumour

- Biopsy
- Chemotherapy
- Radiotherapy.

Bilateral disease is managed initially by biopsies (open or 'Trucut') of both kidneys, followed by chemotherapy intended to minimise the extent of subsequent surgery. Fundamental to the latter is preservation of functioning renal tissue while at the same time excising all tumour, if necessary employing 'workbench' technique. In predisposition syndromes (e.g. Denys–Drash syndrome), where both kidneys inevitably become involved, bilateral nephrectomy is followed by haemo- or peritoneal dialysis. Renal transplantation may follow in the event of 2-year disease-free survival.

These management strategies for unilateral and bilateral disease derive from UK trials. Other regimens employed elsewhere incorporate the same basic principles but have subtly different balances in the burdens of chemotherapy and radiotherapy. The International Society for Paediatric Oncology's regimen, for example, achieves similar results using less radiotherapy but more chemotherapy. Vincristine and adriamycin are administered preoperatively so as to reduce the risk of tumour rupture and the need for subsequent radiotherapy, and whole lung radiation is not routine for stage IV disease. Renal bed irradiation is omitted in cases where local lymph nodes are disease free, and although the local relapse rate is higher this is not at the expense of survival rates, possibly because tumour histology is downgraded by the preoperative chemotherapy.

Survival rates are good for patients with favourable histology (Table 22.6) but less so otherwise (Table 22.7),

Table 22.5 Wilms' tumour: chemotherapy regimens

Stage	Drug	Period
I	V	10 weeks
II	V+A	6 months
III	V+A+D	1 year
IV	V+A+D	1 year

V = vincristine; A = actinomycin D; D = doxorubicin.

Table 22.6 Wilms' tumour (favourable histology) – 5-year survival rates

Stage	5-yr survival (%)
I/II	90
III	80–85
IV	60–80
V (bilateral)	70–80

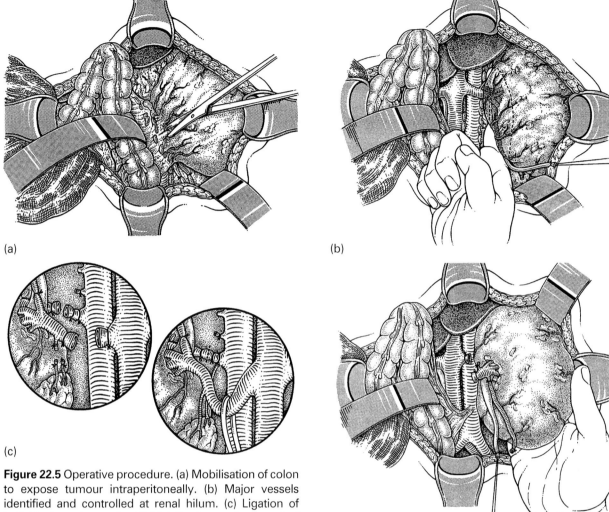

(a)

(b)

(c)

(b)

Figure 22.5 Operative procedure. (a) Mobilisation of colon to expose tumour intraperitoneally. (b) Major vessels identified and controlled at renal hilum. (c) Ligation of individual renal vessels. (d) Mobilisation and removal of kidney. Reproduced from *Rob and Smith's Operative Surgery. Paediatric Surgery*, 5th edition published by Chapman & Hall medical (permission applied for).

in that although improved outcomes have been achieved in patients with clear cell sarcoma, rhabdoid tumours still carry a poor prognosis.

In the event of relapse approximately 50% of patients are still curable, principally those with subdiaphragmatic relapse and who, although treated by

Table 22.7 Wilms' tumour (unfavourable histology) – 5-year survival rates

Tumour type	Survival (%)
Anaplastic	60
Clear cell sarcoma	70–80
Rhabdoid	20

chemotherapy, have received no previous abdominal radiotherapy.

Although Wilms' tumour currently carries an excellent prognosis, the challenge for the future is to maintain such outcomes while at the same time reducing the morbidity inherent in adjuvant chemotherapy and radiotherapy.

Rhabdomyosarcoma

Introduction

Rhabdomyosarcoma, which occurs principally during childhood, arises from undifferentiated mesenchyme. As this is the origin of skeletal muscle, differentiation to tissue resembling mature muscle is a common histological characteristic. Accounting for 10–15% of solid malignant tumours of childhood, rhabdomyosarcoma is rare, affecting 1 in 2 000 000 people annually, with a male preponderance and an increased incidence among Afro-Caribbeans. Although it occurs throughout the body, one-third of tumours arise in the genitourinary tract, in the bladder, particularly the base, or in the prostate, vagina, uterus, or paratesticularly.

Pathology

- Embryonal
- Alveolar
- Pleomorphic.

The aetiology of rhabdomyosarcoma is unknown, although an abnormal gene on chromosome 2q37 may play a role in its development. The conventional histological classification recognises three varieties: embryonal, alveolar and pleomorphic.

An unfavourable prognosis is associated with anaplastic, alveolar and monomorphous round cell histology.

Genitourinary tumours are almost exclusively embryonal, typically with a botryoid configuration (Figure 22.6) and, in girls, classically as a grape-like mass protruding from the vagina. The characteristic feature of differentiated tumours is cross-striations in what appears to be mature skeletal muscle with typical rhabdomyoblasts. Various immunohistochemical markers, improving diagnostic accuracy, are used to demonstrate the presence of myoglobin and desmin. The tumour disseminates principally by local invasion, and less often by lymphatic spread (18%) or by distant metastases (10%).

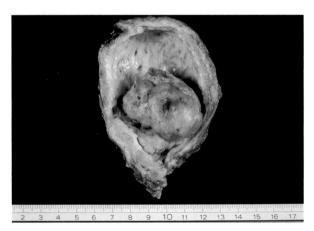

Figure 22.6 Macroscopic appearances of bladder rhabdomyosarcoma in cystectomy specimen.

Clinical presentation

This includes:

- Urinary symptoms, e.g. urgency/frequency
- Abdominal pain and/or mass
- Protruding botryoid vaginal mass.

Rhabdomyosarcoma may occur at any time during childhood, although the uterine form is confined almost exclusively to adolescence, whereas paratesticular tumours arise both in pre- and postpubertal boys.

Tumours at the most common sites (the bladder base and prostate) give rise to urinary frequency, urgency or retention, and similarly tumours of genital origin if forming a pelvic mass. Lesions obstructing the urinary tract may lead to hypertension or to symptoms of renal failure (Figure 22.7).

Haematuria is rare. Vaginal neoplasms may cause correspondingly sited pain or may present as a protruding botryoid mass.

Examination typically finds a lower abdominal mass or a distended bladder.

Investigation

Routine initial investigations comprise chest X-ray, pelvic and urinary tract ultrasonography, cross-sectional imaging (computerised tomography, CT;

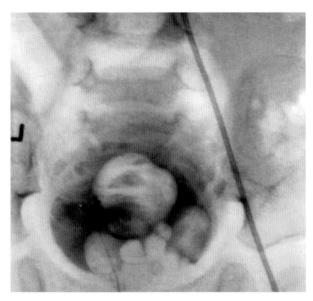

Figure 22.7 Micturating cystourethrogram demonstrating a lobulated filling defect (rhabdomyosarcoma) in the bladder of a 14-month-old child who had presented in renal failure owing to bladder outlet obstruction.

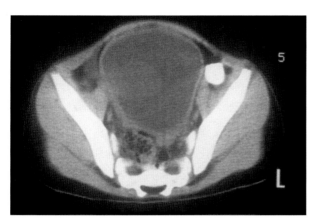

Figure 22.8 CT scan of the pelvis in a child with rhabdomyosarcoma presenting with an abdominal mass (distended bladder).

Figure 22.8) or magnetic resonance imaging (MRI) of the pelvis and chest, radioisotope bone scintigraphy and bone marrow aspiration. Renal function requires assessment in the presence of hydronephrosis.

Although the imaging studies are usually diagnostic, specific histological assessment is essential prior to treatment and the necessary biopsy material may be obtained percutaneously, transurethrally or by open surgery according to circumstances. Endoscopic examination is a further prerequisite in most instances.

Management

- Biopsy
- Chemotherapy and/or radiotherapy
- Organ-sparing surgery.

Management is determined by considerations of histology, anatomy and local or distant spread. Except in rare instances where tumours at a favourable site (e.g. the bladder dome) can be dealt with by excision biopsy, initial treatment comprises chemotherapy, which is followed by surgery preserving, if at all possible, the organ of origin. Chemotherapy regimens involve vincristine, actinomycin D, cyclophosphamide and ifosfamide in various combinations. Radiotherapy, either as an external beam or as a radioactive iridium wire inserted into the urethra or vagina, is employed to treat microscopic disease following surgery or, rarely, as the principal form of treatment in cases where adequate tumour control cannot be achieved without major ablative surgery.

Surgery may take the form of partial cystectomy, submucosal resection of intravesical lesions, or excision of tumour masses adherent to bladder or prostate. Total cystectomy, with or without urethrectomy, represents a salvage procedure to be used only in cases with intravesical, bladder base or prostatic recurrence following chemotherapy, radiotherapy and previous conservative surgery.

Prognosis

The evolution during the last 20 years of multimodal therapies based on collaborative international trials has achieved 70–80% 5-year survival rates. None the less, although such success is achievable while retaining the bladder in some two-thirds of cases, this is not without cost, particularly in respect of persistent urinary frequency and incontinence.

The major challenge for the future lies in improving survival rates while at the same time reducing morbidity, both generally and in relation to local sequelae.

Testicular tumours

This group of rarely metastasising boyhood malignancies, with an incidence of 0.5–2 per 100 000 people, is most conveniently categorised according to the usual age at the presentation. Most come to light as a painless scrotal swelling, sometimes in association with a (usually small) secondary hydrocoele.

Yolk sac tumours

With few exceptions presentation is before 2 years of age, and in most cases treatment amounts to no more than excision of the affected testis after clamping the cord via an inguinal incision. α-Fetoprotein is a sensitive marker of this tumour and, if serum levels do not return to normal following orchidectomy, metastatic spread is likely and may be confirmed by chest X-ray or CT scan. This complication, occurring in 13% of cases, is treatable by chemotherapy.

Teratoma

This, the second most common testicular neoplasm of childhood, also principally affects the very young, 18 months being the mean age at presentation. Orchidectomy is curative, as metastatic disease does not occur in prepubertal boys.

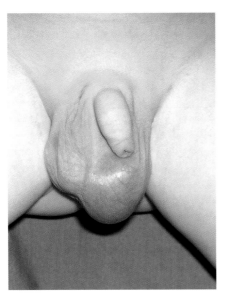

Figure 22.9 Paratesticular rhabdomyosarcoma presenting as a solid testicular swelling.

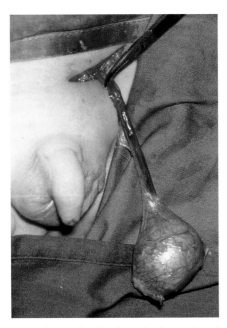

Figure 22.10 Operative findings in the patient in Figure 22.9. As in adults, exploration and orchidectomy should be performed via an inguinal approach and not by a scrotal incision.

Other testicular tumours

Leydig and Sertoli cell tumours usually present between 5 and 10 years of age. Secondary prepubertal testicular tumours are most commonly encountered in patients undergoing treatment for lymphoma or leukaemia: 4% of such patients are so affected.

Germ cell tumours and testicular maldescent

Some 10% of germ cell tumours, which usually arise well beyond childhood, occur in undescended testes, the higher the location of the gonad the greater being the risk. On present evidence, the chance of occurrence is uninfluenced by whether or when orchidopexy has been performed. The contralateral gonad is also at enhanced risk of malignancy.

Paratesticular rhabdomyosarcoma

These account for 10% of solid scrotal mass lesions in childhood. Presentation is with a discrete testicular lump, often in association with a small secondary hydrocoele (Figures 22.9, 22.10). Investigation and treatment run along the lines already described for rhabdomyosarcoma in other locations, and the 3-year survival rate is of the order of 90%.

Key points

- Wilms' tumour now has an excellent prognosis with treatment based on a combination of surgery, chemotherapy and, in some cases, radiotherapy. The challenge for the future is to maintain excellent survival figures while decreasing the morbidity related to intensive treatment regimens.
- Rhabdomyosarcoma is a rare malignancy managed by chemotherapy, radiotherapy and organ-sparing surgery insofar as this is feasible. The difficulty lies in balancing the desirability of localised excision which preserves an intact bladder and urethral sphincter against the risk of local recurrence of an aggressively malignant tumour. Where the tumour is totally excised the long-term prognosis is good.
- Most childhood testicular malignancies can be managed by orchidectomy and close follow-up.

Further reading

Atra A, Ward HC, Aitken K et al. Conservative surgery in multimodal therapy for pelvic rhabdomyosarcoma in children. *Br J Cancer* 1994; 70: 1004–1008

Beckwith JB, Kiviat NB, Bonadiot JF. Nephrogenic rests, nephroblastomatosis and the pathogenesis of Wilm's tumour. *Paediatr Nephrol* 1990; 10: 1–36

Green DM. Wilm's tumour. *Euro J Cancer* 1997; 33: 409–418

Urogenital trauma

23

David FM Thomas

Topics covered
Renal trauma
Ureteric injuries

Bladder injuries
Urethral injuries
Injuries to the external genitalia

Introduction

Although minor injuries to the genitourinary tract are relatively common in childhood major trauma is, fortunately, rare and, with the exception of isolated blunt renal trauma, tends to occur in conjunction with other injuries. Penetrating injuries resulting from gunshot or stab wounds of the type encountered by paediatric urologists in the United States are exceptionally rare in western Europe, where the overwhelming majority of injuries to the urogenital tract in children result from blunt injury. Although the general principles of the management of urological injuries in children follow broadly similar lines to those in adults, the overall management of the injured child demands specialist paediatric expertise and the input of a number of relevant disciplines.

The organisation of trauma services for children is beyond the scope of this book, but it is generally accepted that children with multiple trauma involving the urinary tract should be transferred to a specialist regional centre once their initial condition has been stabilised. Trauma of a minor nature, however, can generally be managed locally, with advice being sought from a specialist paediatric urologist where appropriate.

Although isolated genital injuries often have an innocent explanation, the possibility of sexual abuse, particularly in girls, should never be overlooked, and the involvement of a paediatrician with appropriate expertise should be sought.

Renal trauma

In childhood the kidney is more susceptible to blunt trauma because it lacks the degree of protection afforded to the adult kidney by the bulk of surrounding perirenal fascia and overlying muscle.

Presentation

Isolated renal trauma most commonly results from a sporting or playground injury. In children the extent of the renal injury may not correlate closely with the apparent severity of the trauma, and seemingly insignificant injuries may nevertheless be associated with deceptively severe renal damage. Moreover, children have the capacity to sustain significant blood loss before developing hypotension and other manifestations of hypovolaemia. The presenting clinical features of renal trauma typically include haematuria, loin pain and tenderness, an expanding perirenal mass, and external evidence of injury such as bruising or abrasions.

In children with **multiple injuries** the renal injury may sometimes dominate the clinical picture, but is more commonly overshadowed by coexisting visceral injuries such as splenic or duodenal rupture (Figure 23.1). In these circumstances it is not uncommon for renal contusion or laceration to be identified during the course of abdominal or initial assessment with CT scanning.

Investigations

All children with suspected renal injury should be admitted for observation and monitoring of vital signs. Laboratory tests include **urine microscopy**, **full blood count** and **haematocrit**. Renal trauma is almost invariably accompanied by haematuria, but it should be noted that the severity of the haematuria does not correlate well with the extent of the renal injury.

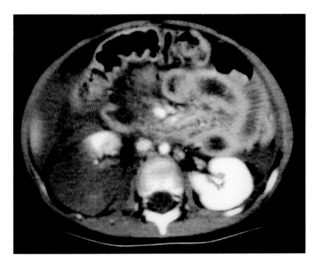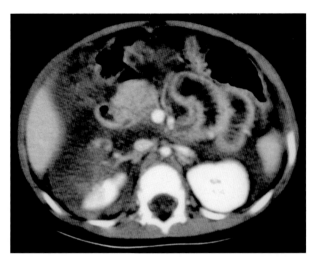

Figure 23.1 CT scan with contrast. Two images demonstrating transection of the upper pole of the right kidney in an 18-month-old child. Seatbelt injury sustained in road traffic accident. An associated duodenal rupture was managed by laparotomy but the renal injury was treated conservatively.

Imaging

In view of the vulnerability of the kidney in children and the potentially deceptive clinical picture in this age group, renal imaging is mandatory in the presence of haematuria or a suspected renal injury. The pattern and extent of imaging, however, may be determined by the overall clinical condition and the availability of imaging modalities. Children with clinical or radiological evidence of a significant renal injury, haemodynamic instability, or evidence of coexisting injuries should be transferred to a specialist centre.

Computerised tomography (CT) with contrast is the imaging modality of choice, particularly where there is any suspicion of coexisting abdominal visceral trauma. CT is now available in all major paediatric centres and most larger district general hospitals. It permits grading of the renal injury and an assessment of renal perfusion (Figure 23.2). Further CT scans may be required to monitor the course of the injury and to guide any decision on possible surgical intervention.

Ultrasound is a reasonable first-line investigation in a child who is clinically stable and who is thought to have sustained only minor renal trauma. However, appearances in the initial phase following injury can appear misleadingly normal. If ultrasound reveals evidence of renal trauma, a CT scan is always advisable to permit a more detailed functional assessment.

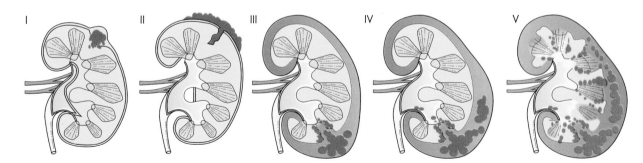

Figure 23.2 Grading of renal trauma. Grade I, renal contusion. Grade II, parenchymal laceration not extending into collecting system. Grade III, parenchymal laceration involving collecting system, perirenal haematoma and extravasation. Grade IV, extensive laceration/parenchymal avulsion injury. Grade V, shattered kidney and/or avulsion of vascular pedicle.

Although the **intravenous urogram (IVU)** has been largely superseded by CT, it remains a useful investigation where CT is not readily available. Unlike CT, however, the IVU provides no additional information on possible injury to other abdominal viscera. **Arteriography** has likewise been largely replaced by CT scanning, and in any event is of little practical value as the prospects of salvaging renal function by revascularisation in avulsion injuries are remote. The interval between devascularisation and even the most prompt surgical intervention invariably exceeds the warm ischaemic time of devitalised renal parenchyma.

Management

The broader aspects of trauma management in children are beyond the scope of this chapter. However, the guiding principles can be defined as follows:

- All children with a suspected or proven diagnosis of renal trauma (even if seemingly trivial) should be admitted for observation, monitoring of vital signs and imaging.
- **Blunt renal trauma should generally be managed conservatively**, but in cases of major renal trauma the possible indications for surgical intervention should be actively reviewed at regular intervals. **Conservative management** of moderate to major renal trauma comprises active monitoring of vital signs, correction of hypovolaemia (with blood if necessary), and reimaging with ultrasound and further CT or other modalities where indicated. Minor injuries require inpatient observation until frank haematuria has resolved.

Indications for surgical intervention are relative rather than absolute and include:

- **Haemorrhage** resulting in haemodynamic instability, particularly if accompanied by an expanding retroperitoneal haematoma or haemoperitoneum;
- **Urinary extravasation** A minor or moderate degree of urinary extravasation is not uncommon and does not, in itself, amount to an indication for surgical exploration. Localised collections can be aspirated or drained percutaneously. Surgical exploration, however, may be warranted if the renal parenchyma is largely intact and there is evidence of a pelvic tear or avulsion of the ureter;

- **'Shattered kidney' (grade V injury)** Even if haemodynamic stability can be achieved, removal of a non-functioning 'shattered' kidney may be justified to hasten recovery and reduce the risk of complications. If there are no other intra-abdominal injuries, exploration can be deferred for a few days rather than undertaken acutely. In the presence of other intra-abdominal injuries, however, a 'shattered' kidney should be removed at the time of laparotomy.
- **Vascular injuries** The prospects of successful revascularisation are minimal in view of the relatively short warm ischaemic time of the kidney. Nevertheless, an attempt at revascularisation might be justifiable in the rare event of devascularisation of a solitary kidney or bilateral injury.

Technical considerations

The kidney should be explored transperitoneally via a midline or upper transverse incision, depending on the age of the child. Laparotomy provides an opportunity to examine the other intra-abdominal viscera for injury and provides better access for vascular control. Prior to exposure of the kidney, the renal artery and vein(s) are identified by their respective points of origin on the aorta and inferior vena cava, and vascular control is achieved by passing vascular slings around the vessels to permit temporary occlusion if required.

The nature and extent of the surgical procedure is determined by the operative findings and may include, for example, repair of a parenchymal laceration with closure of any associated collecting system defect, repair of a pelvic tear, or reanastomosis of an avulsed ureter, or debridement and partial nephrectomy. When renal salvage is not feasible or is not justified by the amount of residual functioning renal tissue, nephrectomy is undertaken. However, **it is crucially important to have previously obtained positive confirmation that a normal functioning contralateral kidney is present before proceeding with nephrectomy.**

Outcome

Early complications include urinoma, infection and abscess formation. Secondary haematuria is not uncommon within the first few weeks of the injury, but is rarely of sufficient severity to require active intervention. Follow-up imaging comprises ultrasound and

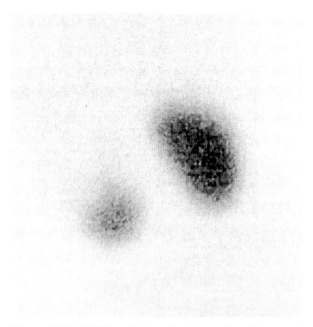

Figure 23.3 DMSA scintigraphy 4 months after renal injury (CT demonstrating right upper pole transection in the patient illustrated in Figure 23.1). DMSA shows complete loss of function in the devascularised lower pole. Differential function right kidney 21%, left kidney 79%.

DMSA – which is best deferred for 2–3 months after the injury (Figure 23.3). **Hypertension** is the principal long-term complication, although the true incidence is difficult to assess because of the lack of reliable long-term data. The overall risk of renal-related hypertension following childhood renal trauma is thought to be low – probably around 2–3% – but the relative risk is likely to be greater when a significant bulk of devascularised tissue has been left in situ. An annual lifelong check of blood pressure is advisable for individuals who have sustained significant parenchymal injuries.

Ureteric injuries

Injuries to the ureter are very rare in children and are more likely to be iatrogenic than traumatic in aetiology. Management is individualised according to the nature and level of the injury. Options include spatulation and end-to-end anastomosis over an indwelling JJ stent; mobilisation of the kidney; nephropexy; and pyeloureterostomy for proximal ureteric injuries. Psoas hitch and ureteric reimplantation may be feasible for injuries to the distal ureter.

Bladder injuries

Penetrating injuries of the bladder are exceedingly rare in children and when they do occur are usually iatrogenic in origin, for example inadvertent damage to the bladder wall during herniotomy. Blunt injuries are similarly rare in this age group and, when they occur, are almost invariably the result of motor vehicle accidents. Spontaneous rupture of the bladder is a recognised and potentially lethal complication of enterocystoplasty, and has also occurred following impaction of a calculus at the bladder neck.

Bladder injuries are traditionally classified according to whether urinary extravasation is confined to the perivesical space (extraperitoneal rupture) or whether there is free leakage of urine into the peritoneum (intraperitoneal bladder rupture).

The presentation of bladder injuries depends on the circumstances in which they have been sustained – for example, iatrogenic bladder perforation during cystoscopy is either recognised during the course of the procedure or becomes apparent as a suprapubic swelling arising out of the pelvis in cases where a catheter has not been left in the bladder postoperatively. Iatrogenic damage to the bladder during herniotomy may be apparent as urinary leakage from the skin incision. Seatbelt injuries present with pain, and major injuries associated with pelvic fractures should be identified during the course of initial evaluation for major trauma. Whenever circumstances permit, the diagnosis should be confirmed by urethral catheterisation and contrast cystography.

Management

Endoscopic extraperitoneal perforation can usually be managed by a period of continuous catheter drainage, but it is advisable to undertake formal repair of any other iatrogenic bladder perforation incurred for example during herniotomy or appendicectomy. Intraperitoneal bladder rupture demands prompt surgical exploration, closure of the bladder defect and, where possible, closure of the overlying peritoneum. Following repair of any bladder injury, continuous postoperative bladder drainage via a urethral or suprapubic catheter should be maintained for a number of days.

The possible diagnosis of bladder perforation or spontaneous rupture should always be actively considered in any patient with a history of bladder augmentation, who subsequently presents with abdominal pain, distension or unexplained systemic ill health and metabolic disturbance.

Urethral injuries

These are generally confined to the male urethra. Three broad mechanisms of injury can be identified:

- Perineal blunt trauma, typically 'stride' or 'straddle' injuries to the bulbar urethra.
- Injuries to the posterior and membranous urethra associated with pelvic fractures (usually road traffic accidents in children).
- Urethral damage resulting from instrumentation or prolonged urethral catheterisation.

Presentation

Blunt trauma – 'straddle injuries'

Children generally present with a history of a traumatic episode and evidence of perineal bruising. Depending on the severity of the injury, the clinical picture may also include urethral bleeding, haematuria or painful urinary retention with bladder distension. Imaging is not usually contributory in the acute phase, although it is advisable to perform an ultrasound scan (and plain X-ray if bony injury is suspected). Ascending contrast urethrography or attempted catheterisation and cystography are not usually tolerated in younger children, but an ascending urethrogram may be feasible in an older boy or adolescent.

Management

Children with suspected or proven urethral injuries should be admitted for observation until the initial discomfort has settled and voiding has been re-established. Where there is evidence of a more severe injury, particularly associated with retention or anuria, the initial management is aimed at establishing bladder drainage and evaluating the severity of the urethral injury.

If the child does not pass urine despite analgesia, the safest course of action is percutaneous insertion of a suprapubic catheter under general anaesthesia. Urethral catheterisation or urethroscopy may be

considered, provided these manoeuvres are undertaken cautiously by an experienced paediatric urologist. However, injudicious attempts at catheterisation or traumatic urethroscopy should be avoided, as this may compound the urethral damage.

After a period of drainage of several days' duration, the urethra is then visualised by contrast descending cystography (and, ideally, an ascending urethrogram). If there is no evidence of extravasation or disruption, the suprapubic catheter can be clamped and normal urethral voiding re-established. More severe injuries of the bulbar urethra are best managed by a sustained period of suprapubic diversion, followed by urethroplasty (see below).

Pelvic fractures

The possibility of injury or disruption of the posterior and/or membranous urethra should be actively considered in any child with a pelvic fracture. As in adults, management of these injuries is controversial, the options comprising:

- Prolonged suprapubic drainage followed by elective urethroplasty or
- Open exploration, debridement and attempted re-alignment approximation of the urethra over a catheter once the initial effects of the injury have subsided, e.g. after 7–14 days.

Post-traumatic urethral stricture

The treatment options are summarised in Figure 23.4 and comprise:

- **Optical urethrotomy** (Figure 23.4a) This is best suited to short, diaphragm-like strictures. Using a 'cold knife' blade mounted on a paediatric or neonatal resectoscope with a 0° or 5° end-viewing lens, the stricture is visualised, and if necessary a ureteric catheter passed through the central lumen to enable the blade to be positioned accurately. The stricture is then incised under vision with radial cuts. A silicone catheter is left in situ for 48–72 hours postoperatively.

  Although optical urethrotomy can be repeated it is unlikely to prove curative if the stricture recurs despite two or three episodes of treatment.
- **Urethroplasty** The length and severity of the stricture is delineated preoperatively by a combination of cystography and urethrography, and by

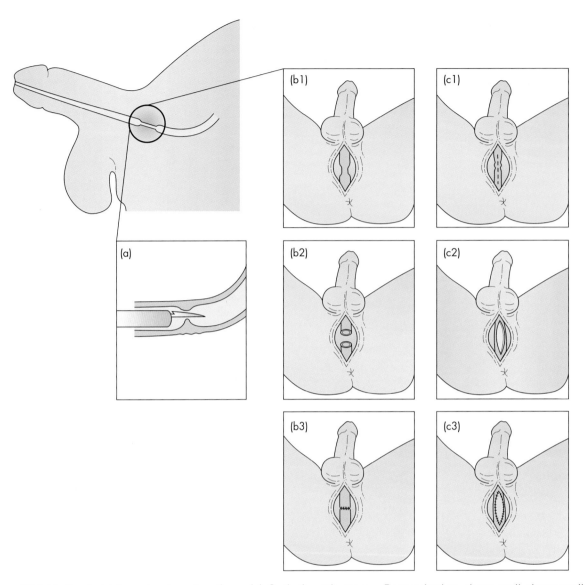

Figure 23.4 Urethral stricture: treatment options. (a) Optical urethrotomy. Best suited to short, well circumscribed strictures. Stricture incised with radial cuts using a cold knife blade mounted on a paediatric resectoscope. (b) 1 Perineal exposure of the bulbar urethra; 2 excision of the strictured segment, mobilisation of healthy urethra; 3 end-to-end primary anastomotic urethroplasty over a silicone catheter. (c) 1 Perineal exposure of the strictured bulbar urethra; 2 incision to lay open strictured segment ('stricturotomy') extended into adjacent healthy urethra; 3 onlay graft of buccal mucosa sutured into the defect.

instrumentation at the time of surgery. A perineal approach usually gives adequate exposure, but an abdominoperineal or transpubic approach may be required for strictures resulting from pelvic fracture injuries. The techniques of choice in children comprise:
– excision of the strictured urethral segment, mobilisation of the urethra and end-to-end anastomosis (Figure 23.4b);

– incision ('laying open') of the stricture and onlay grafting, ideally with a free graft of buccal 'mucosa', or alternatively with a pedicled or free skin graft (Figure 23.4c).

The surgical management of urethral strictures should only be undertaken by paediatric or reconstructive urologists with extensive experience of urethral reconstructive surgery.

Genital injuries

These are uncommon but typically result from playground injuries or animal bites. Scrotal lacerations and severe blunt scrotal trauma should be explored under general anaesthesia to permit debridement and inspection of the testis. When a testicular injury is identified, devitalised tissue is excised, the tunica albuginea repaired, and the scrotum then closed in layers, with attention to haemostasis. Intravenous broad-spectrum antibiotics should be administered for 48 hours postoperatively.

Penile injuries should be managed according to their site and severity. The possibility of sexual abuse should not be overlooked.

Injuries to the female external genitalia, such as stride or straddle injuries, may result in bruising and superficial laceration of the perineum and external genitalia. A short period of suprapubic or urethral catheter drainage may be required in severe cases until the initial early oedema and bruising have resolved. Long-term complications such as strictures are not encountered in girls, as the female urethra is less anatomically vulnerable than in the male. Sexual abuse (rape or attempted rape) is an important cause of genital injury in girls, and for this reason the circumstances of the injury should always be actively investigated in any girl presenting with unexplained genital trauma.

Key points

- Potentially serious renal trauma can occur after seemingly insignificant injury. All children with suspected renal trauma should be admitted for observation, imaging and evaluation.
- Most renal injuries can be managed conservatively, but in cases of severe renal trauma the indications for possible surgical intervention should be actively reviewed at regular intervals.
- The surgical management of post-traumatic urethral strictures should only be undertaken by an experienced paediatric or reconstructive urologist.
- The possibility of sexual abuse should always be considered in any child presenting with an injury to the external genitalia.

Further reading

Brown SL, Elder JS, Spirnak JP. Are pediatric patients more susceptible to major renal injury from blunt trauma? *J Urol* 1998; 160: 138–140

Connor JP, Hensle TW. Trauma to the urinary tract. In: O'Donnell B, Koff SA (eds) *Pediatric urology*, 3rd edn. Oxford: Butterworth–Heinemann, 1997; 696–708

Kardar AH, Sundin T, Ahmed S. Delayed management of posterior urethral disruption in children. *Br J Urol* 1995; 75: 543–547

McAninch JW, Safir MH. Genitourinary trauma. In: Weiss RM, George NJR, O'Reilly PH (eds) *Comprehensive urology*. London: Mosby, 2001; 637–650

Adolescent urology

24

Christopher RJ Woodhouse

Topics covered
Vesicoureteric reflux
Bladder exstrophy
Hypospadias
Female genital reconstruction

Posterior urethral valves
Prune-belly syndrome
Enterocystoplasty
Spina bifida

The major anomalies of the genitourinary tract are now largely amenable to reconstruction in infancy or childhood, and from a paediatric point of view the results are generally good. However, there may be a legacy of potential problems in adolescence and adult life, and although it is neither feasible nor necessary for all paediatric urological patients to be followed indefinitely, it is important to recognise those at particular risk of late complications or lifelong disability. Wherever possible, paediatric urologists should work with their adult urological colleagues and general practitioners to ensure that these patients benefit from continuity of follow-up and specialist care.

Vesicoureteric reflux

The implications of vesicoureteric reflux during adult life are best considered in relation to the following categories of patients:

- Adults whose vesicoureteric reflux has either resolved spontaneously or been surgically corrected in childhood. If there is no renal damage these patients do not require follow-up.
- Adults whose vesicoureteric reflux has either ceased spontaneously or has been corrected in childhood, but in whom reflux nephropathy is present. For these patients lifelong follow-up of blood pressure is needed. By 18 years of age hypertension exists in 11% of patients with unilateral scarring, and 18% of those with bilateral scars. By 27 years this figure has risen to 23%. If the severity of renal damage is

sufficiently severe to reduce the glomerular filtration rate (GFR) to below 40 ml/min/1.73 m^2, late renal failure may be inevitable owing to hyperperfusion of the surviving nephrons. In general, pregnancy does not affect the incidence of either hypertension or renal failure. However, girls already on the brink of renal failure may suffer acute and irreversible deterioration in pregnancy.

- Individuals whose vesicoureteric reflux persists after puberty. There is no consensus on management and the evidence of the few long-term studies is somewhat contradictory. The author favours surgical reimplantation in females to minimise the risk of acquiring reflux nephropathy in pregnancy. Paradoxically, however, it has recently been reported that women who have previously undergone reimplantation are at greater risk of urinary infection in pregnancy than any other group. Whether this is because their urinary tracts were the most damaged originally, or whether it is genuinely related to some aspect of reimplantation, is unknown. In asymptomatic males there seems to be no indication for surgery in the absence of bladder outflow obstruction.
- Adults presenting for the first time with vesicoureteric reflux. Because most are symptomatic, surgical treatment is indicated.

Bladder exstrophy

Most children with exstrophy have an isolated anomaly and generally grow up very well, being both intelligent and well motivated. Despite the excellent results of bladder reconstruction reported from major centres, there remains a lingering suspicion that early diversion is also an acceptable form of management and one with a lower complication rate. Certainly, reconstruction should only be undertaken by surgeons with very wide experience. For this reason, and because of the declining number of new cases, the surgical management of bladder exstrophy now is formally provided on a supraregional basis in England and Wales.

The reconstructed bladder may not be durable into adulthood. Historically, only 23% of children with exstrophy who underwent bladder reconstruction in childhood progressed into adult life without the need for urinary diversion. Of those whose bladder reconstruction did survive beyond childhood, 60% required further reconstruction in adolescence.

Genital reconstruction in exstrophy

Males

The penis in exstrophy is short but of normal calibre. An intrinsic component of the deformity is tight dorsal chordee which, if uncorrected during infancy, will prevent penetrative sexual intercourse. In adults the deformity is investigated by artificial erection, infusing both corpora with saline. Minor defects may be corrected by a ventral Nesbit's procedure, whereas severe penile deformity requires more extensive correction by a Cantwell–Ransley operation.

Females

The vagina is short and lies in a more horizontal plane than normal. The labia are located on the anterior abdominal wall, the introitus is narrowed and the clitoris bifid. Although the labia cannot be repositioned, the overall abnormality can be disguised and patients can have normal sexual function. Fertility is unaffected, but uterine prolapse (procidentia) can be particularly troublesome for up to 50% of women. When one parent has bladder exstrophy the risk of exstrophy or epispadias in their offspring is approximately 1:70.

Hypospadias

The impact of hypospadias surgery on subsequent sexual development is poorly documented, not least because today's adults were reconstructed by techniques that have since been superseded. Surgeons tend to view their own results in an overoptimistic light, sometimes with glowing reports of a straight erection and normal urine stream in 100% of cases. When viewed more objectively, the late results are less impressive and up to 50% of men experience a poor functional or cosmetic outcome.

Where there is a gross persisting abnormality, notably chordee, intercourse may prove to be impossible. By contrast, when the impairment is essentially cosmetic in nature sexual debut and intercourse may be nearly normal. Impairment of semen quality has been reported in up to 50% of men, although there does not appear to be a corresponding increase in the incidence of infertility.

Following repair of penoscrotal or perineal hypospadias (often presenting initially as ambiguous genitalia) intercourse is possible but ejaculation is poor and infertility common.

In one controlled study, boys with a history of hypospadias were found to be 'underachievers'. These findings, however, have not been confirmed by other authors and are unlikely to be representative of the current outcome for boys treated by newer forms of single-stage reconstruction.

Female genital reconstruction of ambiguous genitalia

The timing and nature of female genital reconstruction for conditions such as congenital adrenal hyperplasia is a source of growing controversy. Historically, very few studies have attempted to document the long-term functional and psychological outcome of feminising genitoplasty and vaginoplasty performed in childhood. However, evidence is accumulating from recent follow-up studies which challenges some of the assumptions underpinning the current approach to female genital reconstruction, particularly the belief that one-stage surgery in childhood will suffice. It is increasingly clear that the majority of young women will require further vaginal surgery, ranging from simple introital revision to complex vaginoplasty, to permit normal comfortable intercourse (Figure 24.1). Furthermore, impaired clitoral sensation is not uncommon. Continuity of follow-up from childhood into early adulthood is essential with further care being undertaken in a centre specialising in adolescent

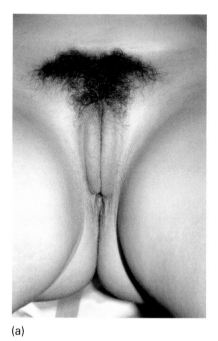 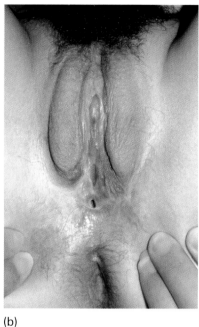

(a)　　　　　　　　　　　　　　(b)

Figure 24.1 Postpubertal outcome of feminising genitoplasty for the correction of virilisation associated with congenital adrenal hyperplasia. Single-stage feminising genitoplasty previously undertaken in the first year of life. (a) External cosmetic outcome satisfactory, with no visible phallic hypertrophy and normal appearance of labia created from 'scrotalised' skin. (b) Retraction of the labia reveals introital scarring, requiring introitoplasty to permit normal, comfortable intercourse.

gynaecology to ensure access to relevant specialist expertise and appropriate psychological support.

Posterior urethral valves

Bladder function

The long-term consequences of posterior urethral valves (PUV) are largely attributable to the damage inflicted on the bladder by obstructed voiding in utero, and in the neonatal period before valve resection. Bladder dysfunction in these patients is characterised by loss of compliance, detrusor instability and reduced functional capacity. Many adolescents later develop chronic retention. The impact of PUV varies in severity. Although some boys experience normal or near-normal bladder function the potential for bladder damage should not be overlooked, as it may not be manifest until adolescence or early adult life. The symptoms of the 'valves' bladder are familiar to all urologists, notably frequency, urgency and incontinence. What may not be recognised, however, are the relentless effects upon the kidney.

Renal function

The progressive nature of renal failure in boys with a history of posterior urethral valves has been recognised for many years, the incidence of impaired renal function being approximately 6% at 5 years of age,

25% at 10 years and 50% at 15 years. It should be noted that a normal plasma creatinine at the onset of puberty is not a guarantee that it will remain normal at the end. In addition to congenital renal dysplasia and renal damage caused by the unrelieved obstruction before valve resection, the kidneys, as described above, may be subjected to ongoing damage from the poorly compliant bladder.

Obstructive uropathy of the pattern seen in boys with PUV is associated with damage to the medulla, resulting in renal tubular concentration defects and polyuria. A vicious cycle can ensue, with the bladder accommodating large volumes of dilute urine by remaining full for longer periods throughout the day. In turn, this leads to prolonged high storage pressures, further worsening the renal damage. Predictors of poor prognosis include clinical presentation before the age of 1 year (including prenatal diagnosis), daytime incontinence after 5 years of age, and persistent bilateral reflux and polyuria. Recent studies provide some support for the hypothesis that the risk of renal failure may be significantly reduced by aggressive management of bladder dysfunction, employing anticholinergics, self-catheterisation and clam cystoplasty to achieve this goal.

Ejaculation

As with the bladder, the prostate may be damaged by back pressure occurring before the obstruction is relieved by valve resection. This is subsequently manifest in reduced semen quality and poor ejaculation, which occur in up to 50% of men with a history of PUV. The seminal abnormality is characterised by lack of liquefaction, low sperm count, poor motility and high pH (up to 9.5). The effect on fertility is unknown, but up to a third of patients experience some difficulty in achieving paternity. Dilatation of the posterior urethra prevents adequate pressure being generated at the beginning of orgasm, so that ejaculation is less forceful than normal or even absent.

Transplantation

When the function of a 'valve' bladder is sufficiently abnormal to destroy two native kidneys, with resultant end-stage renal failure, a transplanted kidney is also more likely than usual to suffer a similar fate. Previous renal transplant data indicated that 5-year graft survival was approximately 50% less in PUV patients than in other transplant recipients. Currently, 5-year graft survival rates are comparable, although PUV patients do experience more infections and have higher levels of plasma creatinine than other recipients, especially from 7 years post transplant.

It is essential that any underlying bladder abnormality is corrected before proceeding to renal transplantation.

Prune-belly syndrome

This distinctive disorder is obvious at birth from the appearances of the abdominal wall (Figure 24.2). Whereas in the past infants with this condition were regularly referred to paediatric urologists, the last decade has seen a dramatic decline in new cases which is thought to reflect the introduction of routine ultrasound fetal anomaly screening and termination of the affected pregnancy.

There are three components to the syndrome:

● Bilateral undescended testes
● Absence of the muscle of the anterior abdominal wall
● Functional and anatomical anomalies of the urinary tract.

Although each carries potential implications for long-term development, most prune-belly patients

nevertheless grow well and tend to be tall. A range of associated anomalies, notably skeletal, have been described in association with the syndrome, although these are seldom of great clinical significance.

Undescended testes

During the 1950s and 1960s it was believed that the testes in prune-belly syndrome were so intrinsically abnormal that the prospect of fertility did not merit serious consideration. Similarly, it was (misguidedly) believed that these testes were too dysplastic to carry an appreciable risk of malignant transformation. Orchidopexy was therefore delayed, either until some major reconstruction was performed or until late childhood. This approach was supported by the observation that men with prune-belly syndrome were invariably sterile and that their testicular biopsies showed Sertoli cells only.

However, it is now appreciated that some germ cells are present and hence the outlook for paternity may not be wholly bleak. The presence of sperm in the semen has been documented, and there has been at least one pregnancy using intracytoplasmic sperm injection, resulting in twins (one was normal but the other had multiple non-urological anomalies).

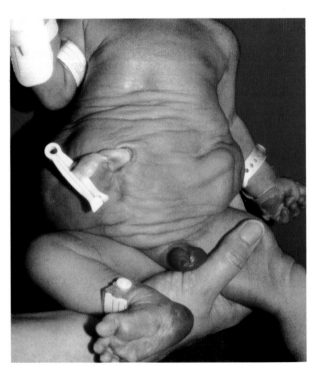

Figure 24.2 Characteristic appearance of the abdominal wall in a newborn infant with prune-belly syndrome.

A number of cases of testicular germ cell neoplasia have now been documented in men with prune-belly syndrome, and so nowadays similar considerations apply to the timing of orchidopexy in prune-belly syndrome as to other forms of undescended testes.

The abdominal wall

The literature concerning the value of abdominal wall reconstruction during childhood is contradictory. Although it is possible to produce some improvement in the cosmetic appearance of the wrinkled skin, it is doubtful whether there is any long-term benefit. Tightening of the skin alone is a pointless exercise without underlying muscular or fascial support. Operations have been devised involving more extensive abdominal wall reconstruction, but again the benefits are arguable.

In adolescents and adults the abdomen is protuberant, resembling a premature 'pot belly' (Figure 24.3). However, this does not give rise to functional problems other than an inability to sit up directly from the lying position. The author's prune-belly syndrome patients are capable of a full range of physical activities and include a long-distance cyclist and a mountaineer.

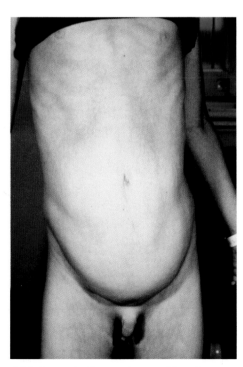

Figure 24.3 Prune-belly syndrome. The appearance of the abdominal wall in later childhood and adolescence improves spontaneously, although some surgeons favour surgical correction (abdominoplasty).

The kidneys

Long-term renal function is largely dependent on the severity of any underlying renal dysplasia and whether surgical intervention is required in childhood. Among the adult patients in the author's practice who had minimal surgery as children, 17 of 21 have normal renal function with a mean GFR of 85 ml/min/1.73 m^2 when assessed at an average age of 24 years. Four patients are in end-stage renal failure and another four are hypertensive. Early aggressive reconstruction had been confined to those boys with significant renal impairment from birth. Of these patients, eight are now adults, of whom five are in end-stage renal failure.

Bladder function is generally maintained satisfactorily, although cystitis may occur, in which event investigation is indicated with the principal aim of determining whether there is residual urine in the bladder after voiding. If this problem is found it is most important to identify and treat any possible outflow obstruction, either in the urethra or at the level of the bladder neck. Despite marked dilatation of both ureters and pelvicaliceal systems, upper tract obstruction is very uncommon.

Enterocystoplasty

All urinary reservoirs constructed of intestine carry the same variety of long-term complications, which can be attributed mainly to the fact that intestinal epithelium is poorly adapted to long-term contact with urine. Hyperchloraemic acidosis occurs in up to 14% of patients, although a higher percentage have a metabolic acidosis with respiratory compensation. Anaemia occurs in 8% of patients following enterocystoplasty, and vitamin B$_{12}$ deficiency becomes a potential risk after 5 years, especially if terminal ileum has been used.

Calculi develop in 12–15% of reconstructed bladders. Contributory factors include infection, self-catheterisation and retained urinary mucus.

Abnormalities of calcium metabolism and bone development are of particular concern in children. Delayed growth in height (but not in weight) has been documented in 20% of children after enterocystoplasty but almost all patients will have regained their expected height by the end of puberty. It is unclear whether this phenomenon is independently related to the enterocystoplasty rather than the underlying condition, which in the case of spinal dysraphism often has a profound impact on skeletal growth. Ureterosigmoidostomy in rats has been reported to be associated with impaired development of the femora, which can be averted by the continuous administration of antibiotics. In contrast, enterocystoplasty results in significant loss of bone mineral density and expansion of the marrow cavity regardless of antibiotic administration. Further research is needed to establish the full extent of the impact on bone metabolism of enterocystoplasty and modified forms of ureterosigmoidostomy.

Although rare, perforation of a reconstructed bladder is a serious complication which may prove lethal if recognition is delayed or treatment inadequate. The diagnosis can be made on clinical grounds, aided by diagnostic aspiration of any abdominal fluid collection identified on ultrasound. Unless there is improvement within a few hours on a regimen of antibiotics, intravenous fluids and continuous bladder drainage, laparotomy is essential.

The incidence of malignancy in patients with ureterosigmoidostomies is 22% after a mean interval of 20 years. The interaction of urine and faecal bacteria in the sigmoid has been shown to result in the presence of nitrosamine and other known carcinogens. Although low concentrations of such urinary carcinogens have also been identified in bladders following enterocystoplasty, the overall risk of malignancy is likely to be lower. At present the experimental evidence remains inconclusive, but in the clinical setting it is clear that children who have undergone enterocystoplasty require careful long-term follow-up into adult life.

Spina bifida

Patients with spina bifida have a spectrum of disabilities, ranging from virtual normality to wheelchair dependence and poor intelligence. During childhood a heavy burden falls upon the parents, but independent self-care should always be the long-term objective. Achieving this goal depends on:

- Adaptation of daily living to permit self-sufficiency in tasks such as dressing, washing and performing routine household chores;
- Bowel and bladder management;
- Sexual education;
- General education.

The urologist should play a role in all four aspects of general development.

Daily living

Parents tend to be overprotective. Only 15% of spina bifida patients undertake the types of household chores undertaken by their normal siblings and 16% do not even acquire a basic level of self-sufficiency. Twenty-eight per cent of females are not taught hygenic management of menstruation. Up to 46% of individuals with spina bifida develop pressure sores at some time.

Bowel management

Even the mildest neurological deficit leads to incompetence of the anal sphincter. Faecal continence is usually dependent on acquiring a pattern of 'controlled constipation'. The concept of the antegrade contenence enema (ACE) has been an important advance in the management of the neuropathic bowel.

Bladder control

Only a small percentage of individuals are continent without resort to clean intermittent catheterisation, which in many cases is in addition to reconstructive procedures. It is most important that any intervention needed to impart continence be completed before puberty, as the natural tendency is for continence to deteriorate rather than to improve (Figure 24.4). Very few adults with spina bifida, especially females, can

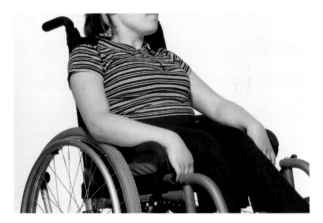

Figure 24.4 A wheelchair-bound spina bifida patient who had previously undergone bladder augmentation in childhood but became unable to access her urethra to perform self-catheterisation. Continence achieved following Mitrofanoff procedure. Where possible, definitive continent reconstruction should be completed before or shortly after the onset of puberty.

acquire the skills needed for urethral self-catheterisation if not taught in childhood. Moreover, about 10% of wheelchair-bound patients become unfit for radical surgery in adulthood because of inadequate respiratory reserve.

Sexual development – females

The impact of spina bifida on sexual function is closely related to the level of the spinal cord lesion and the severity of the associated neuropathic bladder. Most females whose neurological impairment is below L2 are normal, as are most of those who are continent of urine. In contrast, only about 20% of women with higher levels of cord damage or with urinary incontinence experience normal sexual function. None the less, two-thirds form steady sexual relationships, regardless of the degree of handicap or continence. Pregnancies are difficult, with high rates of urinary infection and deterioration in bladder function. Although the overall risk of neural tube defect among offspring is 1:23 (1:50 for sons and 1:13 for daughters) this can be significantly reduced by dietary folic acid supplements for 3 months prior to conception. Few spina bifida patients will accept antenatal screening and termination of affected pregnancies.

Sexual development – males

All males with intact sacral reflexes and urinary continence are potent. Of those with absent sacral reflexes, 64% of those whose primary neurological level is below D10 are potent, but the figure falls to 14% in men with higher neurological levels. The nature of arousal and erection in these patients remains to be fully explored. Early reports suggest that sildenafil (Viagra) may have a potential role in treating erectile dysfunction in some cases. Semen can be obtained from impotent men by electroejaculation, but semen analysis in these circumstances invariably reveals azoospermia. Despite these drawbacks 60% of adult males with spina bifida have a regular sexual partner regardless of their degree of mobility or continence.

General education and social adaptation

The main adverse factors in these areas are:

- Mental handicap
- Poor manual dexterity
- Inappropriate schooling
- Overprotective parents.

The two latter can be overcome if they are recognised and if appropriate support is provided. The presence of neuropathic bladder and bowel and the overall level of neurological deficit (excluding intellectual impairment) have little direct bearing on educational potential and social integration.

Key points

- Individuals with evidence of renal scarring (reflux nephropathy) should undergo lifetime measurement of blood pressure. Closer monitoring is required for those with severe scarring who are at risk of renal impairment.
- Approximately one-third of boys with posterior urethral valves are destined for renal failure by the time of adolescence or adult life.
- Young women who have undergone feminising genital reconstruction in childhood should be followed up and their subsequent care transferred to a specialist adolescent gynaecology unit.
- The incidence of new cases of prune-belly syndrome has fallen dramatically following the introduction of antenatal screening.
- Enterocystoplasty may be associated with stones and metabolic disturbances. The true risk of malignancy in reconstructed bladders may not be apparent for some decades.
- The measures needed to restore urinary continence in patients with spina bifida should be commenced during childhood and completed before adulthood.

Further reading

Creighton SM, Minto CL, Steele SJ. Objective cosmetic and anatomical outcomes at adolescence of feminising surgery for ambiguous genitalia done in childhood. *Lancet* 2001; 138: 124–127

Diseth H, Bjordal R, Schultz A, Stange M, Emblem R. Somatic function, mental health and psychological functioning in 22 adolescents with bladder exstrophy and epispadias. *J Urol* 1998; 159: 1684–1690

Dorner S. Sexual interest and activity in adolescents with spina bifida. *J Child Psychol Psychiatr* 1997; 18: 229–237

Mansfield JT, Snow BW, Cartwright PC, Wadsworth K. Complications of pregnancy in women after reimplantation for vesicoureteric reflux. *J Urol* 1995; 154: 787–790

Mureau MA, Slijper FME, van der Meulen JC, Verhulst FC, Slob AK. Psychosexual adjustment of men who underwent hypospadias repair: a norm-related study. *J Urol* 1995; 154: 1351–1355

Parkhouse HF, Barrett TM, Dillon MJ et al. Long-term outcome of boys with posterior urethral valves. *Br J Urol* 1988; 62: 59–62

Woodhouse CRJ. *Long-term paediatric urology*. Oxford: Blackwell Scientific, 1991

Woodhouse CRJ. The sexual and reproductive consequences of congenital genitourinary anomalies. *J Urol* 1994; 152: 645–651

Woodhouse CRJ, Hinsch R. The anatomy and reconstruction of the adult female genitalia in classical bladder exstrophy. *Br J Urol* 1997; 79: 618–622

Index